Granulomatous disease
Otorhinolaryngology, Head and Neck

Sanjana Vijay Nemade
Kiran Jaywant Shinde

Granulomatous diseases in Otorhinolaryngology, Head and Neck

Springer

Sanjana Vijay Nemade
Department of ENT
Smt. Kashibai Navale Medical College
and General Hospital
Pune, India

Kiran Jaywant Shinde
Department of ENT
Smt. Kashibai Navale Medical College
and General Hospital
Pune, India

ISBN 978-981-16-4049-0 ISBN 978-981-16-4047-6 (eBook)
https://doi.org/10.1007/978-981-16-4047-6

This Springer imprint is published by the registered company Springer Nature Singapore Pte Ltd.
The registered company address is: 152 Beach Road, #21-01/04 Gateway East, Singapore 189721, Singapore

It is my genuine gratefulness and warmest regard that I dedicate this work to the institution "Smt Kashibai Navale Medical College and General Hospital" that nurtured a teacher, clinician, and surgeon in me.

Preface

Granulomatous diseases are rare inflammatory diseases in the head and neck region. They often have systemic manifestations that affect organs throughout the body. Granulomatous diseases have a varied aetiology that includes autoimmune, infectious, idiopathic, reactive, neoplastic, and hereditary causes. They present primarily as nodules, mass, or an ulcerative lesion, with symptoms secondary to the lesion, such as pressure symptoms. The characteristic feature is the presence of a "granuloma" that is created by a chronic immunologic process resulting clinically in localized nodular inflammation. Until the advent of immunohistochemistry, flow cytometry, and advanced molecular techniques, this group of diseases was collectively lumped into a "catch-all" category of destructive diseases. Advances in endoscopic technology and laboratory evaluation have led to a better understanding and more appropriate disease-specific care. Many of these conditions can be very aggressive, and timely diagnosis is facilitated by a high index of suspicion, endoscopy with biopsy, serology, and molecular assays.

This manual includes the description of the granulomatous diseases of the head and neck, with their characteristic features, necessary investigations, and management. It includes a wide variety of infective, idiopathic, neoplastic, hereditary, reactive, and various other types of chronic granulomatous reaction in the head and neck region. Further, the description is supported with all illustrations including clinical photographs, radiological pictures, and histopathological and microbiological images showing characteristic and differentiating features. This book also elaborates the important medical and surgical management of the granulomatous diseases. Every chapter ends with the "Essential features" of that particular granulomatous disease. It will certainly help the postgraduate medical students to remember the salient differentiating features of the diseases. It will assist the clinicians as well, for the early diagnosis and management of the patients with chronic granulomatous diseases.

Pune, India — Sanjana Vijay Nemade
Pune, India — Kiran Jayawant Shinde

Acknowledgement

Conflicts of Interest and Source of Funding: No

Introduction

Granulomatous inflammation is a unique form of chronic inflammation. Any process that results in granuloma formation in the body may be termed *granulomatous*. By definition, a granuloma is a nodular inflammatory lesion. Histologically, granulomas are aggregates of mononuclear inflammatory cells or modified macrophages, which are usually surrounded by a rim of lymphocytes, fibroblasts, and multinucleated giant cells. Granulomas typically form to protect the host from persistent inflammatory stimuli, which if ongoing may produce locally inflammatory and destructive effects. Granuloma formation may be the primary result of a disease or a secondary disease association.

Robert Koch developed a method of staining and identified bacteria; thus, he was able to differentiate between infectious and non-infectious granulomatous diseases. The advent of modern pathology with improved microscopic staining techniques and communication between researches spawned this new category of "granulomatous diseases" in the early twentieth century. Granulomatous diseases have a varied aetiology that includes autoimmune, infectious, idiopathic, hereditary, and neoplastic causes. Sometimes, it may develop as a reaction to endogenous elements such as cholesterol or exogenous chemicals, foreign body, trauma, or other environmental triggers. Many rheumatic and connective tissue disorders are associated with secondary granulomatous manifestations. The clinical findings associated with granulomatous inflammation are usually variable and often indistinct. In the head and neck, granulomatous diseases may affect the orbits, sinonasal cavities, salivary glands, aerodigestive tract, temporal bone, cerebrum, cranial nerves, or skull base.

Granulomatous diseases of the head and neck are classified as follows:

Class	Subclass	Disease	Causative organism
Autoimmune	–	GPA (Wegener's granulomatosis)	–
		Churg-Strauss syndrome	
		Behcet's disease	
Infectious	Bacteria	Tuberculosis	*Mycobacterium*
		Syphilis	*Treponema pallidum*
		Leprosy	*Mycobacterium leprae*
		Actinomycosis	*Actinomyces Israelii*
		Rhinoscleroma	*Klebsiella rhinoscleromatis*
		Cat-scratch disease	*Bartonella henselae*
		Lyme disease	*Borrelia burgdorferi*
		Tularemia	*Francisella tularensis*
	Fungus	Aspergillosis	*Aspergillus Fumigatus* and *Aspergillus Flavus*. Other species such as *A. niger*, *A. terreus*, and *A. nidulans*
		Mucormycosis	Mucor, Rhizopus, Absidia, and Cunninghamella
		Rhinosporidiosis	*Rhinosporidium seeberi*
		Candidiasis	*Candida albicans* (most common)
		Blastomycosis	*Blastomyces dermatitidis*
		Histoplasmosis	*Histoplasma capsulatum*
		Cryptococcosis	Cryptococcus neoformans
		Coccidioidomycosis	Coccidioides immitis and Coccidioides posadasii
		Paracoccidioidomycosis	*Paracoccidioides brasiliensis*
	Protozoa	Leishmaniasis	Leishmania

Class	Subclass	Disease	Causative organism
Idiopathic		Sarcoidosis	
		Crohn's disease	
		Orofacial granulomatosis	
Hereditary		CGD—Chronic granulomatous disease	
Neoplastic		NK/T-cell lymphoma (midline lethal granuloma)	
Reactive		Reparative giant cell granuloma	
		Cholesterol granuloma	
		Chemical granuloma (cocaine, talc, beryllium, tattoo)	
		Foreign body granuloma	
		Pyogenic granuloma	
Other		Relapsing polychondritis	
		Langerhans cell histiocytosis (LCH)	
		Systemic lupus erythematosus (SLE)	
		Rheumatoid arthritis	

Clinical Features of Granulomatous Diseases

Granulomatous diseases cause a great range of symptoms not only in head and neck but also throughout the body. Because ear, nose, and throat manifestations predominate, patient usually presents to an otorhinolaryngologist in the first visit. Although similar histologically, these diseases require a thorough approach because of a wide variety of disease processes.

Ear—Diffuse inflammatory process due to vasculitis may present with acute or chronic otitis media, sudden or gradual hearing impairment. Conductive hearing loss is attributed to the expansion of the inflammatory procedure to the middle ear and eustachian tube. It may result from granulomatous nasopharyngeal involvement, secondary eustachian tube dysfunction, and serous otitis media. Sensorineural hearing loss occurs due to vasculitis of the auricular artery or its cochlear branch. Mixed hearing loss is often seen because of the toxic action of inflammatory products from the middle ear or direct granulomatous involvement of the inner ear. Tympanomastoid involvement may extend to petrous apex or to middle and posterior cranial fossa in case of destructive lesions. Facial nerve palsy has been shown to complicate the course of many connective tissue disorders. Melkersson-Rosenthal syndrome and rheumatologic diseases such as sarcoidosis have been most commonly associated with facial nerve palsy, which accompanies other manifestations of active disease in the majority of cases. Auricular chondritis is often associated with inflammatory reaction.

Aerodigestive tract involvement—Manifestations in the nose and paranasal sinuses may vary from allergic rhinitis, sinonasal polyposis, diffuse mucosal thickening, and mucocutaneous ulcers to granulomatous mass with or without bony destruction of the septum, turbinates, and palate. Remodelling and destruction of sinus walls may also be seen. Symptoms include nasal obstruction, rhinorrhea, crusting, epistaxis, anosmia/hyposmia, and oroantral fistula. Deep mucosal ulcers of the tongue, cheeks, and palate, gingivitis, and "strawberry gingival hyperplasia" are common in many granulomatous diseases. It may present as granulomatous mass sessile or pedunculated, necrotizing lesions with bony destruction. These lesions may extend to involve the oropharynx, hypopharynx, or larynx causing airway obstruction. Pulmonary involvement is very common in most of the granulomatous diseases. The cricoarytenoid joint can be potentially affected during the course of various inflammatory arthropathies. Symptoms of aerodigestive tract involvement include dysphagia, odynophagia, burning sensation in throat, recurrent deep mucosal ulcers, hoarseness of voice, dyspnoea, haemoptysis, cough, and neck abscess either due to primary lesion or suppurative lymphadenitis.

Salivary gland enlargement is other common manifestation of granulomatous disease. Parotid and/or submandibular glands are unilaterally or more often bilaterally affected. Glands are firm, non-tender, and usually diffusely enlarged on physical examination (lymphoepithelial sialadenitis).

The temporomandibular joint can be affected during the course of inflammatory arthropathies such as RA. Common ocular manifestations vary from episcleritis, scleritis, and conjunctivitis to granulomatous lesions and nodules. Symptoms as a result of intracranial granulomatous mass include seizures, confusion, disorientation, memory loss, cranial nerve paralysis, and visual and speech disturbances. Meningitis and raised intracranial tension are the common manifestations. Disseminated disease and multisystem involvement may lead to gastrointestinal, hepatobiliary, genitourinary, and cardiac manifestations.

Diagnosis of Granulomatous Diseases

A detailed history, including family history and a thorough physical examination, is necessary for primary clinical diagnosis.

The diagnosis is aided by:

- Culture and/or biopsy of the tissue for causative organism and histopathological evaluation is the gold standard diagnostic modality. Microscopy and culture is particularly helpful in infective granulomatous diseases, where the characteristic appearance of infective agent is delineated. On histopathology, granuloma is a compact collection of mononuclear inflammatory cells or modified macrophages, which are usually surrounded by a rim of lymphocytes and often contain giant cells. It can be caseating or non-caseating granuloma. Caseating granulomas are usually seen in tuberculosis, syphilis, cat-scratch disease, actinomycosis, blastomycosis, cryptococcosis, and coccidioidomycosis. Non-caseating granulomas are encountered in leprosy, sarcoidosis, Crohn's disease, reactive granulomas, and foreign body granulomas.
- Imaging—Radiographs, computerized tomography (CT scan), MR imaging, and PET scan show characteristic features. Imaging findings include

sinonasal opacification, ocular and other soft-tissue masses, osseous erosion, airway narrowing, lymphadenopathy, salivary gland infiltration, and intracranial involvement. Vascular involvement may also be evident, with displacement, narrowing, or occlusion of arteries and veins. Some radiologic findings of granulomatous processes have a considerable overlap with findings of malignancy, and a radiologic differential diagnosis inclusive of both is critical to avoid incorrect clinical treatment.
- Haematocrits, serum antibody detection/serum markers, and molecular assays such as polymerase chain reaction help in prompt and accurate diagnosis.
- Other tests may be required as per the clinical presentation of the disease, such as pulmonary function tests, endoscopic evaluation, audiological tests, and ophthalmologic evaluation.

Treatment of Granulomatous Diseases

Treatment varies according to the disease. Infective disease needs antimicrobial therapy.

Systemic or intralesional corticosteroids help to regress the inflammation. It may also be sufficient for localized or limited mucocutaneous involvement. Steroid-sparing medications may be used, especially in patients who present with refractory or chronic disease.

Immunomodulators such as anti-TNF-α therapy may be beneficial for short-term therapy, but long-term benefits remain unclear.

Surgical excision of the granulomas is required in many cases. Laser excision is the preferred treatment for mucosal oral granulomas.

Bibliography

1. Gotmare S, Tamgadge A, Bhalerao S, Pareira T, Tamgadge S. Granulomatous diseases of the oral tissues. Sci J. 2007;1.
2. Alawi F. Granulomatous diseases of the oral tissues: differential diagnosis and update. Dent Clin North Am. 2005;49:203–21.
3. Saccucci M, Di Carlo G, Bossu M, Giovarruscio F, Salucci A, Polimeni A. Autoimmune diseases and their manifestations on oral cavity: diagnosis and clinical management. J Immunol Res. 2018:6061825.
4. Kenechi Nwawla O, Nadgir R, Fujita A, Sakai O. Granulomatous disease in the Head and Neck: developing a differential diagnosis. Radiographics. 2014;34(5). https://doi.org/10.1148/rg.45130068.
5. Lee KJ. Essential otolaryngology. Chapter 12. Granulomatous diseases of Head and Neck.
6. Emmanuelli JL. Infectious granulomatous diseases of the Head and Neck. Am J Otolaryngol. 1993;14(3):155–67.
7. Razek AAKA, Castillo M. Imaging appearance of granulomatous lesions of Head and Neck. Eur J Radiol. 2010;76(1):52–60.

Contents

About the Authors

Sanjana Vijay Nemade, MBBS, MS(ENT), FCPS(ENT)

Designations: Professor and Head, Department of ENT—SKNMC&GH; Head, Criteria II (Teaching-Learning and Evaluation-NAAC), SKNMC&GH; Core member of Learning Management System, SKNMC&GH; Core member of Medical Education Unit, SKNMC&GH.

Dr. Sanjana Nemade completed her undergraduate education from B.J. Medical College, Pune and postgraduate education from Topiwala National Medical College, and BYL Nair hospital, Mumbai. She has achieved the "Mumbai University award" for being topper in the postgraduate examination. At present, she is working as professor and Head, ENT at SKN Medical College and general hospital, Pune. With 18 years of teaching experience, she is an outstanding talent in all ENT and Head Neck surgeries with special interest in endoscopic and bronchoscopic surgeries. Performing intense qualitative work in research, she has been qualified with "Advanced diploma in clinical research". She has published more than 15 peer- reviewed articles in international Pubmed indexed journals, more than 25 articles in national Pubmed indexed journals and has authored 2 books.

Authored books:

1. "Syndromes and eponymous signs in ENT." Dr. Sanjana Nemade, Dr. Kiran Shinde
2. "Emergencies in ENT and Head Neck." Dr. Sanjana Nemade, Dr. Kiran Shinde.

Kiran Jayawant Shinde, MBBS, MS(ENT)

Designations: Former Professor & Head, Department of ENT-SKNMC&GH.

Dr. Kiran Shinde completed his undergraduate and postgraduate education from B.J. Medical College, Pune. He has 38 years of teaching experience in the field of otorhinolaryngology. He has trained many undergraduate and postgraduate students in his career. Along with ENT and head neck surgeries, he is an expert in bronchoscopic foreign body removal. He has published more than 20 articles in national and international journals and has authored 2 books. His achievements have been recognized by various awards.

Part I

Autoimmune Granulomatous Diseases

1 Granulomatosis with Polyangiitis-GPA (Wegener's Granulomatosis)

Abstract

Granulomatosis with polyangiitis (GPA, formerly Wegener's granulomatosis) is a rare necrotizing vasculitis. It is a multisystem disorder often affecting the upper and lower respiratory tract and the kidneys, with a mortality of over 90% if untreated. The etiology of GPA remains unclear, and current hypotheses are based on the notion of environmental triggers, frequently infectious, in genetically susceptible individuals. According to the EULAR criteria, upper airway involvement can be assessed in the presence of chronic or bloody nasal discharge, recurrent epistaxis/crusts/granulomata, septal perforation or sinus inflammation. The sinonasal disease is a common presenting feature of GPA. Longstanding disease can lead to septal perforation and saddle nose deformity. Other manifestations of ear, nose, and throat involvement include otitis, mastoiditis, oral ulcers or granulomata, mucocele, hearing loss and subglottic stenosis. Diagnosis is based on characteristic clinical and pathological findings, usually in association with anti-neutrophil cytoplasm antibody (ANCA) directed against neutrophil and monocyte proteinase 3 (PR3) or myeloperoxidase (MPO). Treatment aims to induce remission with immunosuppressants such as Rituximab or Cyclophosphamide in combination with high-dose corticosteroids for several months to years. Surgical interventions should be reserved for the treatment of complications in the acute stages of the disease.

Synonyms
Midline granulomatosis; Necrotizing respiratory granulomatosis; Pathergic granulomatosis; Wegener's disease (former); Wegener's granulomatosis (former).

1.1 Background

Granulomatosis with polyangiitis (GPA), previously known as Wegener's granulomatosis (WG) [1], is a systemic autoimmune disease of unknown etiology characterized by necrotizing granulomatous inflammation and vasculitis affecting mainly small blood vessels. Scottish otolaryngologist "Peter McBride" (1854–1946) first described the condition in 1897. The full clinical picture was first presented by "Friedrich Wegener" (1907–1990), a German pathologist [2].

The clinical manifestations of GPA can be very heterogeneous, often affecting the upper respiratory tract, lungs, and kidneys. Otorhinolaryngology manifestations are seen in more than 70% of patients. Upper respiratory

S. V. Nemade, K. J. Shinde, *Granulomatous diseases in Otorhinolaryngology, Head and Neck*,
https://doi.org/10.1007/978-981-16-4047-6_1

tract involvement generally precedes pulmonary or renal involvement [2, 3].

The classic triad of full-blown Wegener's granulomatosis (WG) consists of the following:

- Necrotizing granulomatous inflammation of the upper and lower respiratory tracts
- Systemic vasculitis of small arteries and veins
- Focal glomerulonephritis [4]

1.2 Epidemiology

The incidence is 10–20 cases per million per year. It is exceedingly rare in Japan and in African Americans [5]. The most common ages of presentation of GPA are the sixth and seventh decades of life, but it can appear at any age, with similar frequency between genders in adult age [2].

1.3 Etiopathogenesis

The cause of GPA is unknown, although microbes, such as bacteria and viruses, as well as genetics have been implicated in its pathogenesis [6].

It causes inflammation of blood vessels associated with poorly formed granulomas, necrosis, and giant cells. Bacterial colonization with *Staphylococcus aureus* has been believed as an initiating factor of autoimmunity. Mutations in the genes PTPN22, CTLA4, and human leukocyte antigen may influence the risk of developing GPA. It has been widely accepted as anti-neutrophil cytoplasmic antibodies (ANCAs) are responsible for the inflammation in GPA. In vitro studies have found that ANCAs can activate neutrophils, increase their adherence to endothelium, and induce their degranulation that can damage endothelial cells. This anti-neutrophilic process can cause extensive damage to the vessel wall, particularly arterioles [2, 7].

1.4 Clinical Features

Otorhinolaryngological presentation in patients with GPA ranges between 72.3% and 99% of cases [8].

1.4.1 Sinonasal Features

The nose and paranasal sinuses are involved in up to 80% of Wegener's granulomatosis (WG) cases. Severity varies from mild nasal obstruction to nasal collapse [1, 8].

Nasal signs and symptoms include mucosal edema with nasal obstruction, rhinorrhea, septal ulcers, crusting, and epistaxis (due to vasculitis of Kiesselbach's plexus.). Chronic sinusitis affects 40–50% of patients with sinonasal disease. Secondary bacterial or fungal sinusitis is common. The examination may reveal nasal mucosal irregularity ("cobblestone" or "granular"appearance), ulcers, thick crusts, or friable mucosa (Fig. 1.1).

Osseocartilaginous destruction may be revealed by the following:

- Saddle nose deformity (Fig. 1.1)
- Septal perforation, septal necrosis and destruction (Fig. 1.1)
- Pain at the nasal dorsum, which suggests chondritis [2–5]

1.4.2 Oropharyngeal Features

Oral or pharyngeal involvement occurs in up to 6% of patients. Mucosal ulcerations are the most common oral lesions. Buccal ulcers are common, but they may occur on the tongue, palate, or pharynx. Ulcers are persistent, not recurrent (Fig. 1.2) [11].

Gingivae are striking red, with variably described white, yellow, or blue areas. Characteristic strawberry gingival hyperplasia has been suggested as an early manifestation of the disease. There is delayed healing of oral

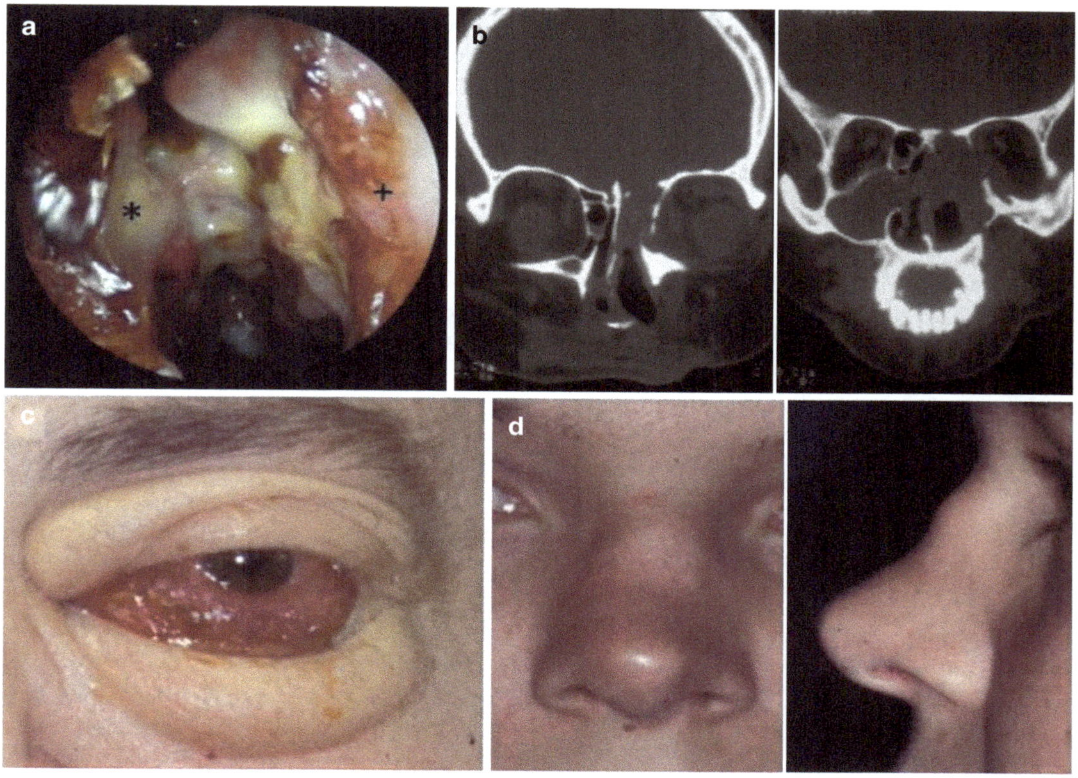

Fig. 1.1 (**a**) Nasal cavity in GPA with granulations, destruction, bacterial infection, left nasal cavity. (nasal septum*, lateral nasal wall+), (**b**) CT scan of the same patient, destruction of the orbital wall and frontal skull base, (**c**) The same patient with orbital cellulitis, (**d**) Saddle nose deformity in GPA [22]

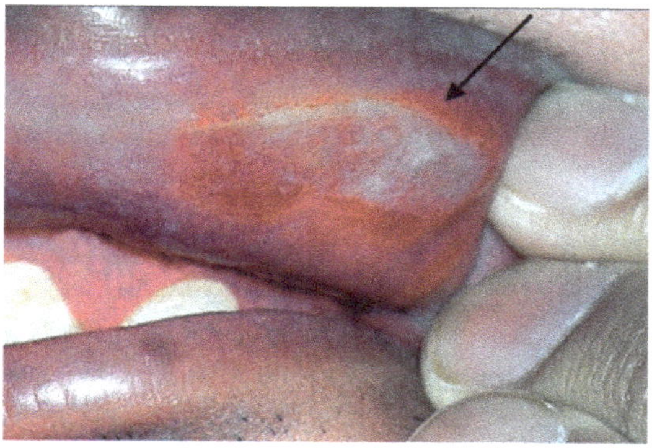

Fig. 1.2 Ulcers with erythematous margins is typical early manifestation of Wegener's granulomatosis

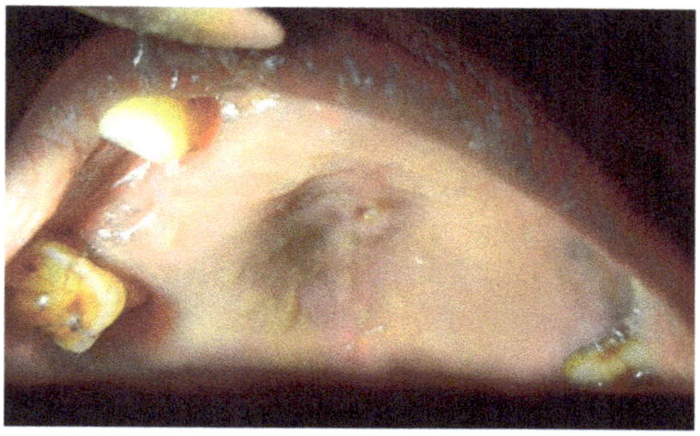

Fig. 1.3 Oronasal fistula secondary to midline destruction

wounds. In time, the underlying bone can be involved, leading to lose teeth. Rarely, oronasal fistula (Fig. 1.3), oroantral fistula, osteonecrosis of the palate, and labial mucosal nodules may occur [10].

1.4.3 Laryngotracheal Involvement

It varies in severity, from hoarseness of voice to stridor and life-threatening obstruction. Subglottic stenosis is the most characteristic and serious laryngeal lesion. It occurs in 16–20% of all patients with WG and up to 50% of pediatric patients with WG, and can be the only presenting manifestation of WG. Subglottic region is prone to develop granulomas due to limited blood supply and turbulent airflow. All patients with subglottic granuloma and stenosis should be evaluated for the presence of cytoplasmic anti-neutrophil cytoplasmic antibodies (c-ANCA) and perinuclear ANCA (p-ANCA) as part of the routine laboratory workup [12].

1.4.4 Otological Features

Otologic involvement occurs in 25–40% of patients during the course of Wegener's granulomatosis (WG). Otitis media is the most common otologic manifestation.

- Serous otitis media is the most prevalent type and is usually secondary to associated nasal disease and subsequent Eustachian tube dysfunction. Up to 30% of patients with WG require tympanostomy during the course of their disease. Suppurative otitis media or mastoiditis may supervene, with symptoms that manifest as chronic otorrhea, hearing loss and postauricular pain.
- Primary middle ear disease may result from necrotizing granuloma and vasculitis of the middle ear resulting in middle ear granulation tissue, tympanic perforation, and chronic otorrhea. It can lead to extensive tympanic scarring or granulomatous occlusion that results in persistent conductive hearing loss. It is sometimes mistaken for otologic tuberculosis. The condition improves only with the use of glucocorticoid or cytotoxic agents.
- Edema or erythema of the auricle may resemble relapsing polychondritis [9].

1.4.4.1 Hearing Loss

Conductive hearing loss is secondary to otitis media. Sensorineural hearing loss is less common. The suggested mechanisms include cochlear nerve compression by adjacent granuloma, cochlear immune-complex deposition, and local vasculitis that involves cochlear vessels. Sensorineural hearing loss is usually bilateral and profound, however, it is reversible with glucocorticoids or cytotoxic agents [10, 11].

1.4.4.2 Vertigo or Disequilibrium

Vertigo or disequilibrium is rarely reported in WG. Possible causes include the following:

1. Vasculitis of the vestibular inner ear
2. Granulomatous neuritis of the vestibular portion of cranial nerve VIII (CN VIII)
3. Vestibular deposition of immune complexes
4. Central cerebral or cerebellar involvement by WG [11]

1.4.4.3 Facial Paralysis

Facial paralysis is mostly associated with primary Wegener granulomatosis (WG) of the middle ear or mastoid. It is caused by necrotizing vasculitis of the vasa nervorum or neuritis due to granulomatous involvement of the middle ear and mastoid (Figs. 1.4 and 1.5). Facial neuropathy in the absence of middle ear disease is suggested to be due to neuritis or vasculitis.

Multiple cranial neuropathies involving VI, VII, IX, and XII cranial nerves have been reported in patients with large cranial base lesions and destruction of the petrous portion of the temporal bone [11].

1.4.5 Salivary Gland Involvement

Involvement of the salivary glands is rare in Wegener's granulomatosis (WG). It typically occurs early in the course of the disease.

Extensive involvement of the salivary glands may produce sufficient destruction to simulate Sjogren syndrome. When involved, submandibular or parotid glands enlargement is evident [13].

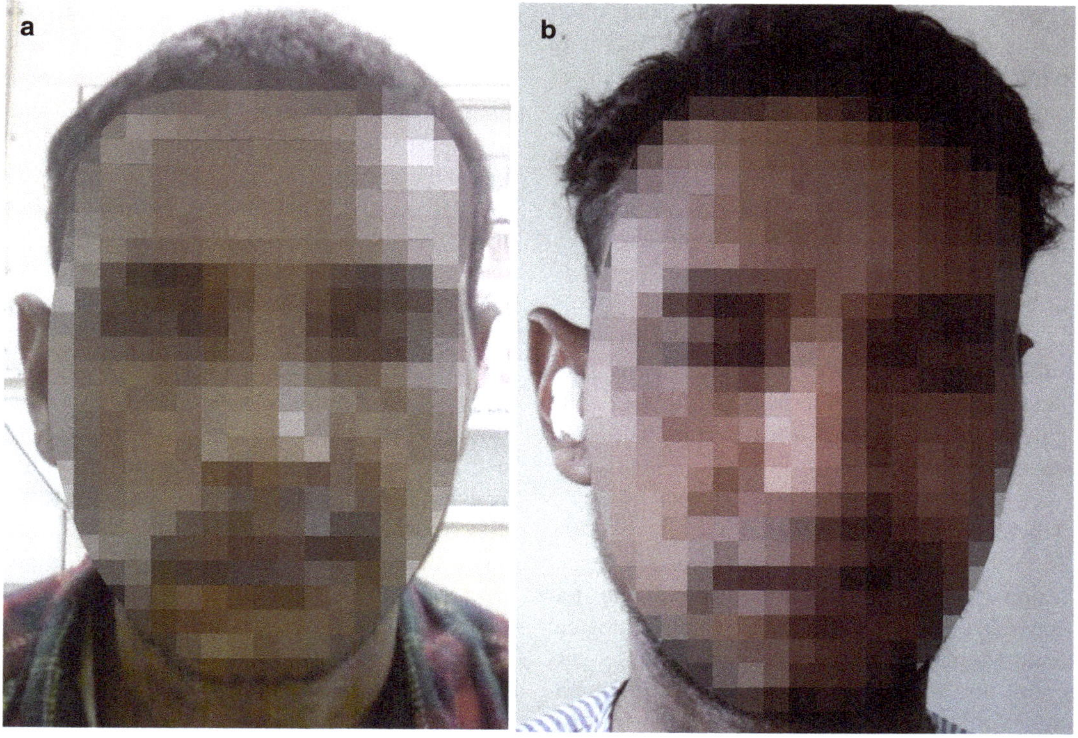

Fig. 1.4 (**a**) Facial paralysis due to right ear involvement with GPA. (**b**) Improvement in facial nerve function 1 week after tympanomastoidectomy

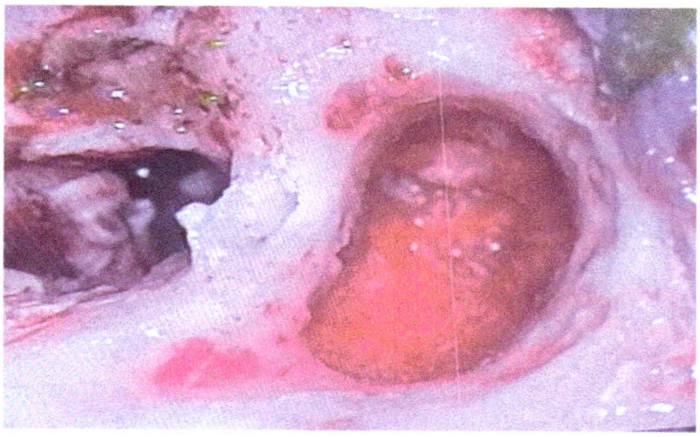

Fig. 1.5 Intraoperative photograph showing mastoid cavity full of reddish granulations

1.4.6 Other System Involvement

- Kidney: Rapidly progressive glomerulonephritis (75%), leading to chronic kidney disease.
- Lungs: Pulmonary nodules (referred to as "coin lesions"), infiltrates (often interpreted as pneumonia), cavitary lesions, haemopysis, and rarely bronchial stenosis.
- Arthritis: Pain or swelling (60%), often initially diagnosed as rheumatoid arthritis.
- Skin: Subcutaneous nodules (granulomas) on the elbow, purpura, various others (see cutaneous vasculitis).
- Nervous system: Occasionally sensory neuropathy (10%) and rarely mononeuritis multiplex.
- Heart, gastrointestinal tract, brain, and other organs are rarely affected.
- Up to 8% of patients may develop a retro orbital tumor, sometimes by extension of sinus lesions or else by the appearance of primary granulation tissue in that area [14].

1.5 Diagnosis

1.5.1 Classification Criteria for GPA

The American College of Rheumatology Classification Criteria for GPA are useful criteria that have been used since inception to classify GPA as a separate disease from other forms of systemic vasculitis and to facilitate clinical research with a standardized group of patients (Table 1.1). The criteria have limitations because they may not distinguish GPA from microscopic polyangiitis (MPA) and vasculitis mimics [15, 16].

The presence of two or more of these four criteria yields a sensitivity of 88% and specificity of 92% [15].

The diagnosis of GPA is performed based on suggestive clinical symptoms (head and neck manifestations, characteristics associated with pulmonary and/or renal involvement). The diagnosis is confirmed by:

1.5.1.1 Histopathology

Biopsy of sinonasal lesions, oral ulcers, laryngeal lesions/granulomas, middle ear granulations tissue is helpful to reveal typical histopathological features such as the presence of small vessel vasculitis and necrotizing granulomatous inflammation with giant multinucleated cells. These may occur together or in isolation (Fig.1.6) [18].

1.5.1.2 Serology

ANCA are antibodies whose targets are the two main components of neutrophil granulocytes: monocyte proteinase 3 (PR3) serine and myeloperoxidase (MPO). Anti-PR3 antibodies (c-ANCA) are virtually pathognomonic for WG, while anti-myeloperoxidase (MPO) antibodies (p-ANCA) are more suggestive of other necrotizing primary vasculitis, mainly in microscopic polyangiitis.

There are two types of tests to detect ANCA—immunofluorescence or ELISA (enzyme-linked immunosorbent assay). Immunofluorescence distinguishes between anti-PR3 and anti-myeloperoxidase based on staining pattern (the first are associated with c-ANCA and the second with p-ANCA). Detection through ELISA (presence of anti-PR3 or else anti-myeloperoxidase) provides greater specificity. However, when both methods are combined, the sensitivity and specificity for the diagnosis of GPA increase up to 90% and 98%, respectively. The severity of AAV (ANCA-associated vasculitis) can be assessed using a disease activity instrument such as the Birmingham Vasculitis Activity Score (BVAS), which can categorize GPA as mild, moderate, severe, or life-threatening depending on the extent of the organ involvement [15, 17].

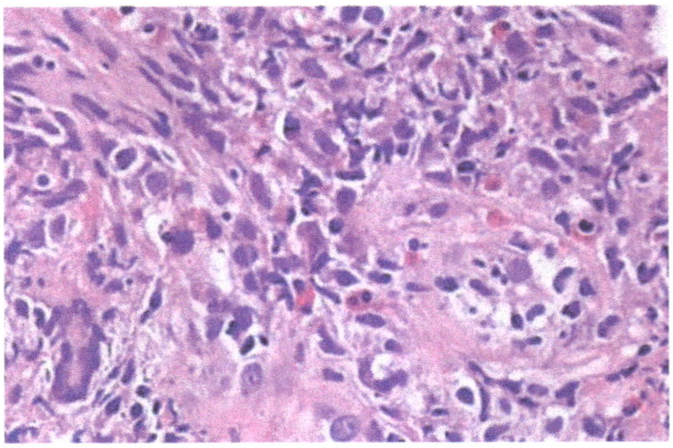

Fig. 1.6 Histopathology reveals the presence of granulomatous inflammation with scattered giant cells and vasculitis

Table 1.1 ACR classification criteria for granulomatosis with polyangiitis (formerly, Wegener's Granulomatosis)

	Classification criteria	
1	Nasal or oral Inflammation	Painful or painless oral ulcers or purulent or bloody nasal discharge.
2	Abnormal chest Radiograph	Pulmonary nodules, fixed pulmonary infiltrates or pulmonary cavities
3	Abnormal urinary sediment	Microscopic haematuria with or without red cell casts
4	Granulomatous inflammation	Biopsy reveals vasculitis and perivascular granulomatous inflammation

1.5.1.3 Endoscopy

Diagnostic nasal endoscopy helps in the early detection of granulomatous inflammation and the extent of the destruction. It also aids in taking a biopsy of the nasal mass. Direct laryngoscopy may show edematous mucosa or bland scar. Biopsy specimens generally demonstrate only fibrosis and inflammation, without evidence of vasculitis. Subglottic specimens have been reported as showing evidence of WG in 5–15% of biopsies [18]. Bronchoscopy is helpful in the evaluation of alveolar hemorrhage, infection, endotracheal and endobronchial granulomas, tracheal stenosis.

- Audiological evaluation for detection of the type and severity of hearing loss

1.5.1.4 Imaging:

CT scan—In the initial inflammatory stage, the sinonasal mucosal changes are non-specific, similar to chronic inflammatory changes. Later in the granulomatous stage, granuloma depicts as soft tissue mass on CT scan. In the chronic phase, the sinus walls often become thick, and a double cortical line with central marrow can be seen. The walls of the residual paranasal sinuses (especially maxillary) become markedly thick while the sinus volume is gradually reduced, the nasal septum is perforated, and the turbinates appear truncated and shortened. Also, there are destructive lesions in the hard palate, alveolus with sinonasal-oral fistulas, or complete nasal septum destruction (Fig. 1.8). This is attributed to granulomatous lesions within the wall of the small blood vessels that lead to the obliteration of the lumen and to avascular necrosis with subsequent bone destruction, often involving midline structures. CT neck may reveal a circumferential narrowing of the subglottis. The stenotic segment can be limited to the subglottis or extend 3–4 cm inferiorly into the trachea. HRCT temporal bone helps to delineate the granulomatous destruction of the mastoid and petrous apex (Fig. 1.7).

MRI scan—MRI scan of paranasal sinuses may show soft tissue mass with hypointensity on both T2- and T1-weighted images with variable degrees of contrast enhancement [17]. MRI brain

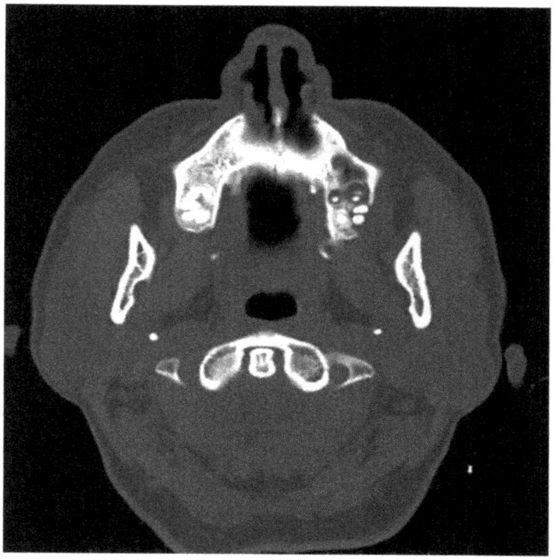

Fig. 1.8 CT scan (axial view) showing destructive lesion in the left alveolus

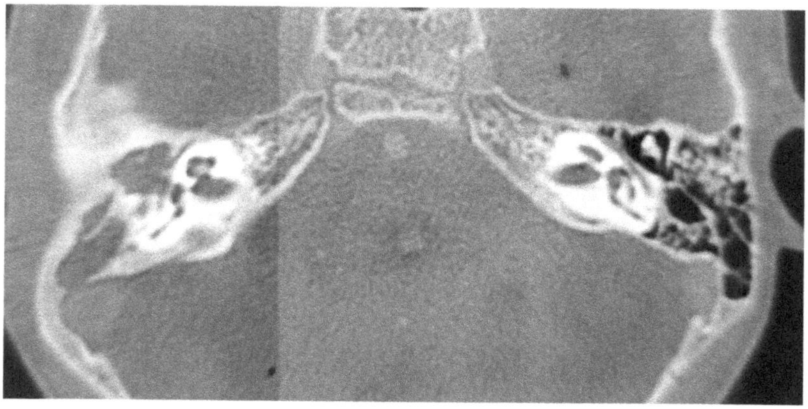

Fig. 1.7 HRCT temporal bone of GPA patient showing opacified right tympanomastoid air cells with the destruction of tympanic portion of facial canal and sinus plate

is the preferred imaging modality for cranial nerve palsy (most commonly facial nerve) with or without meningitis.

1.5.1.5 Pulmonary Function Tests:

Spirometry, Plethysmography, and diffusing capacity should be performed.

1.6 Treatment

Treatment depends on severity and system involvement.

Induction of remission in GPA is approached as follows:

- Immunosuppressants such as Rituximab or cyclophosphamide in combination with high-dose corticosteroids [19]. Both pulsed cyclophosphamide (15 mg/kg IV every 2–3 weeks) and daily cyclophosphamide (2 mg/kg/day) produce similar remission rates; however pulsed cyclophosphamide administration has been considered as a less toxic alternative to daily cyclophosphamide. Rituximab (375 mg/m^2) once a week is alternative to cyclophophamide. Methylprednisolone is given as 1000 mg IV, followed by oral prednisolone 1 mg/kg/day tapered to 5 mg/day by 6 months.
- Methotrexate (20–25 mg weekly oral or subcutaneous) with high-dose corticosteroids, in non-organ threatening or non-life-threatening GPA.
- Plasmapheresis is sometimes recommended for very severe manifestations of GPA, such as diffuse alveolar hemorrhage and rapidly progressive glomerulonephritis (as seen in pulmonary-renal syndrome). The use of plasmapheresis in those with GPA and acute kidney failure (renal vasculitis) might reduce progression to end-stage kidney disease at 3 months [17, 18].

Therapy for remission is usually indicated for 3–6 months.

1.6.1 Maintainance of Remission

- Azathioprine (2 mg/kg/day) is safer than and as effective as, cyclophosphamide in maintaining remission.
- Methotrexate (20–25 mg weekly, oral, or subcutaneous) is used for maintenance of remission if the serum creatinine level is less than 1.5 mg/dL.
- Leflunomide (20–30 mg/day) is as effective as methotrexate, but is associated with more adverse effects [17, 18].

The treatment duration of maintenance therapy varies between individuals. In most instances, it is given for a minimum of 2 years and then tapered towards discontinuation.

- Supportive treatment depending upon the system involved:
- Sinonasal disease—Nasal irrigation, nasal corticosteroid spray, and antibiotics if infection occurs. If perforation of the nasal septum occurs (or saddle nose deformity), then surgical repair is recommended [18, 20].
- Surgical interventions are reserved for the treatment of complications in the acute stages of the disease. On remission (at least 6 months), reconstructive surgery is performed in cases of destruction (e.g., saddle nose, naso-facial, naso-orbital, and naso-oral fistulas).
- Tympanostomy for serous otitis media and Tympanomastoidectomy for middle ear and mastoid involvement are necessary.
- Subglottic stenosis and laryngeal granulomas require intralesional corticosteroids, tracheostomy, or surgical reconstruction. Methylprednisolone acetate injection combined with the serial passage of blunt dilators has been shown to be another effective means of managing subglottic stenosis that is refractory to medical treatment [16, 20].
- Early detection of sensorineural hearing loss may be treated with corticosteroids such as

Prednisolone (0.8–1 mg/kg/day) and is tapered slowly over a period of 2–3 weeks [21].

- Treatment of other system involvement may require coordinated efforts of a team of specialists such as pulmonologists, immunologists, rheumatologists, nephrologists, dermatologists, neurologists, and cardiologists [20].

1.7 Essential Features

- Granulomatosis with polyangiitis (GPA), previously known as Wegener's granulomatosis (WG) [1] is a systemic autoimmune disease of unknown etiology characterized by necrotizing granulomatous inflammation and vasculitis affecting mainly small blood vessels. anti-neutrophil cytoplasmic antibodies (ANCAs) are responsible for the inflammation in GPA.
- The disease can affect all organs of the body; however upper and lower respiratory tracts and kidneys are affected primarily. Otorhinolaryngology manifestations are seen in more than 70% of patients.
- The nasal manifestations range from nasal obstruction, rhinorrhea, septal ulcers, crusting, and epistaxis, sinusitis to osseocartilaginous destruction leading to septal perforation and saddle nose deformity. Mucosal ulcerations are the most common oral lesions, followed by strawberry gingival hyperplasia. Laryngeal manifestations vary in severity, from hoarseness of voice to stridor secondary to subglottic stenosis. Otological features range from serous otitis media, the most frequent manifestation to chronic otitis media, sensorineural hearing loss, vertigo, and facial paralysis.
- Disease progression, further systemic manifestations, and serological investigations in an interdisciplinary framework aid the correct diagnosis.
- The gold standard for diagnosis is the histopathology of the lesions showing the presence of small vessel vasculitis and necrotizing granulomatous inflammation. Detection of ANCA by immunofluorescence or ELISA supports the diagnosis.
- Treatment aims to induce remission with immunosuppressants such as Rituximab or Cyclophosphamide in combination with high-dose corticosteroids for several months to years.
- Surgical interventions should be reserved for the treatment of complications in acute stages of the disease, such as tympanostomy, mastoidectomy, tracheostomy, or sinus surgery. Upon remission (at least 6 months), reconstructive surgery should be performed in cases of destruction (e.g., saddle nose, naso-facial, and naso-oral fistulas).

References

1. Falk RJ, et al. Granulomatosis with polyangiitis: an alternative name for Wegener's granulomatosis. Arthritis Rheum. 2011;63:863–4.
2. González-Gay MA, García-Porrúa C. Epidemiology of the vasculitides. Rheum Dis Clin N Am. 2001;27:729–49.
3. Tsuzuki K, et al. Difficulty of diagnosing Wegener's granulomatosis in the head and neck region. Auris Nasus Larynx. 2009;36:64–70.
4. García-Porrua C, et al. Unilateral submandibular swelling as unique presentation of Wegener's granulomatosis. Rheumatology (Oxford). 2001;40:953–4.
5. Jennette JC, et al. Nomenclature of systemic vasculitis: proposal of an international consensus conference. Arthritis Rheum. 1994;37:187–92.
6. Seo P, Stone JH. The antineutrophil cytoplasmic antibody-associated vasculitis. Am J Med. 2004;117:39–50.
7. Watts RA, et al. Prevalence and incidence of Wegener's granulomatosis in the UK general practice research database. Arthritis Rheum. 2009;61:1412–26.
8. McDonald TJ, DeRemee RA Head and neck involvement in Wegener's granulomatosis. ANCA-associated systemic vasculitis: immunological and clinical aspects, pp. 309–313.
9. Tsuzuki K, et al. Difficulty of diagnosing Wegener's granulomatosis in the head and neck region. Auris Nasus Larynx. 2009;36:64–70.
10. Gubbels SP, et al. Head and neck manifestations of Wegener's granulomatosis. Otolaryngol Clin N Am. 2003 Aug.;36(4):685–705.
11. Cadoni G, et al. Wegener's granulomatosis: a challenging disease for otorhinolaryngologists. Acta Otolaryngol. 2005 October;125(10):1105–10.

12. Gluth MB, et al. Subglottic stenosis associated with Wegener's granulomatosis. Laryngoscope. 2003 August;113(8):1304–7.
13. Cummings CW, et al. Otolaryngology – Head and neck surgery. 4th ed. St. Louis, MO: Mosby; 2005. pp. 934–936; 1493–1508
14. Kuan EC, Suh JD. Systemic and odontogenic etiologies in chronic rhinosinusitis. Otolaryngol Clin North Am (Review). 2017;50(1):95–111.
15. Lutalo PMK, Dçruz DK. Diagnosis and clasiification of granulomatosis with polyangitis (aka Wegener's granulomatosis). J Autoimmunity. 2014;48–49:94–8.
16. Takagi D, et al. Otologic manifestations of Wegener's granulomatosis. Laryngoscope. 2002;112:1684–90.
17. Marzano AV, et al. Granulomatous vasculitis. Giornale Italiano di Dermatologia e Venereologia (Review). 2015, April;150(2):193–202.
18. Schonermarck U, et al. treatment of ANCA-associated vasculitis. Nature Rev Nephrol (Review). 2014, January;10(1):25–36.
19. Metzler C, et al. Elevated relapse rate under oral methotrexate versus leflunomide for maintainance of remission in wegener's granulomatosis. Rheumatology. July 2007;46(7):1087–91.
20. Holle JU, et al. Rituximab for refractory granulomatosis with polyangiitis (Wegener's granulomatosis): comparison of efficacy in granulomatosis versus vasculitic manifestations. Ann Rheum Dis. 2012;71:327–33.
21. Hoffman GS, et al. Wegener granulomatosis: an analysis of 158 patients. Ann Intern Med. 1992;116:488–98.
22. Laudien, M. Orphan diseases of the nose and paranasal sinuses: Pathogenesis – clinic – therapy. GMS Curr Top Otorhinolaryngol Head Neck Surg. 2015; 14: Doc04. Published online 2015 Dec 22. https://doi.org/10.3205/cto000119

2 Churg-Strauss Syndrome

Abstract

Eosinophilic granulomatosis with polyangiitis (Churg-Strauss, EGPA) is a systemic small-to-medium-sized vasculitis associated with asthma and eosinophilia. Histologically EGPA presents tissue eosinophilia, necrotizing vasculitis, and granulomatous inflammation with eosinophil tissue infiltration. EGPA commonly involves the upper airway and lung parenchyma, peripheral neuropathy, cardiac disorders, and skin lesions. The pathogenesis of EGPA is multifactorial. The disease can be triggered by exposure to a variety of allergens and drugs, but a genetic background has also been described, particularly an association with HLA-DRB4. The disease progresses in 3 phases. The prodromal (or allergic) phase lasting for months to many years is characterized by various allergic reactions, asthma, allergic rhinitis and sinusitis. The eosinophilic phase is characterized by multisystem involvement—especially the lungs, gastrointestinal tract, and skin. The vasculitis phase is characterized by widespread inflammation of various blood vessels (vasculitis) and presents with renal, neurological, and cardiovascular system involvement. Six Diagnostic criteria are established by the American College of Rheumatology. The anti-neutrophil cytoplasmic antibodies (ANCA) are positive in 40% of cases, especially in those patients with clinical signs of vasculitis. EGPA has a good response to glucocorticoids, although the combination of glucocorticoids and immunosuppressants (e.g., cyclophosphamide, azathioprine) is needed in most cases.

Synonyms

Eosinophilic granulomatosis with polyangitis (EGPA); CSS; Allergic granulomatous and angiitis; Allergic angiitis and granulomatosis [1, 2].

2.1 Background

Churg-Strauss syndrome (CSS) is a rare necrotizing vasculitis of unknown etiology that affects small to medium-sized blood vessels. This syndrome is characterized by bronchial asthma, hypereosinophilia and extravascular eosinophilic granulomas [3]. It was first described by "Churg" and "Strauss" in 1951 as an allergic angiitis and granulomatosis [4].

Churg-Strauss syndrome is a disorder marked by blood vessel inflammation. This inflammation can restrict blood flow to vital organs and tissues, sometimes permanently damaging them. The exact cause of Churg-Strauss syndrome is unknown. It is likely that overactive immune system response is triggered by a combination of genes and environmental factors, such as allergens or certain medications. Instead of simply

S. V. Nemade, K. J. Shinde, *Granulomatous diseases in Otorhinolaryngology, Head and Neck*,
https://doi.org/10.1007/978-981-16-4047-6_2

protecting against invading organisms such as bacteria and viruses, the immune system overreacts and targets healthy tissue, causing widespread inflammation. Asthma is the most common sign of Churg-Strauss syndrome. ENT manifestations are in the form of allergic rhinitis, nasal polyposis, otitis media, recurrent laryngitis and progressive sensorineural hearing loss. The disorder can also cause a variety of other problems, such as hay fever, rash, gastrointestinal bleeding, and pain and numbness in the hands and feet. Churg-Strauss syndrome is rare and has no cure, but steroids and immunosuppressant drugs can definitely restrict the progress of disease [3–5].

2.2 Epidemiology

It is estimated as 1.3 per 100,000 population with no gender predilection [2, 6].

CSS usually occurs between 14 and 75 years of age, with the peak incidence occurring in middle-aged individuals, although children can be affected as well [7]. The annual incidence in the general population is estimated to be between 2.4 and 4.0 per million people [5, 6].

Although pediatric cases have also been described, no family clustering or ethnic predisposition has been clearly found [8].

2.3 Etiopathogenesis

It is an autoimmune disorder and is grouped under ANCA-associated vasculitis. The frequency of HLA-DRB4 allele is a genetic risk factor for the development of CSS [5, 6]. Myeloperoxidase (MPO) specific perinuclear (P) ANCA can be detected in a subset of patients, but the titer insufficiently represents the course of the disease. Interleukin 5 secreted by T-cells under B-cell influence appears to play an important role, especially for the survival of eosinophils in EGPA [5]. Daives et al. suggested that arboviral infection-related superantigens might stimulate the production of ANCA that attacks host tissues because of molecular mimicry or some other abnormality of immune tolerance [6]. It is characterized by eosinophilic infiltration, necrotizing vasculitis of small and medium-sized vessels, and extravascular granuloma formation [5, 6].

2.4 Clinical Features

It varies from mild symptoms to life-threatening complications. Churg-Strauss syndrome has three stages:

- The prodromal (or allergic) phase is characterized by various allergic reactions. Affected people may develop asthma, allergic rhinitis and/or repeated episodes of sinusitis. Otitis media and laryngitis can be associated. This phase can last from months to many years.
- The eosinophilic phase is characterized by the accumulation of eosinophils in various tissues of the body—especially the lungs, gastrointestinal tract and skin.
- The vasculitis phase is characterized by widespread inflammation of various blood vessels (vasculitis). Chronic vasculitis can cause narrowing of blood vessels, which can reduce blood flow to organs. Inflamed blood vessels can also become thin and fragile (potentially rupturing) or develop a bulge (aneurysm) [2, 5]. In this stage, sudden sensorineural hearing loss, facial paralysis, labyrinthitis, or vestibular neuronitis may be the ontological manifestations secondary to vasculitis [9].
- Nonspecific symptoms: Many people may have nonspecific symptoms such as fatigue, fever, weight loss, night sweats, abdominal pain, and/or joint and muscle pain.
- Upper respiratory system: Severe asthma, pansinusitis, sinonasal polyposis (Fig. 2.1, 2.2), transient patchy lung lesions. Allergic rhinitis, rhinosinusitis, and nasal polyposis have long been associated with CSS [10–13].
- Neurological symptoms: Neurological symptoms such as pain, tingling or numbness. Progressive sensorineural hearing loss.
- Skin lesions: Purplish skin lesions, a rash with hives, and/or small bumps (especially on the elbows) due to accumulation of eosinophils in the dermis.
- Gastrointestinal symptoms: Abdominal pain, diarrhea, bleeding, and acalculous cholecysti-

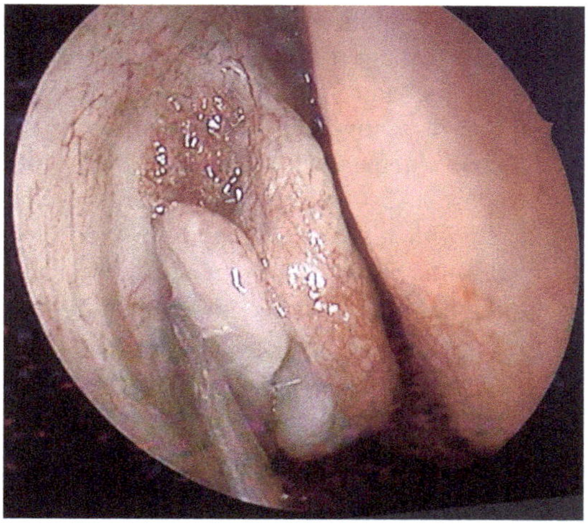

Fig. 2.1 Nasal endoscopic picture of ethmoidal polyps

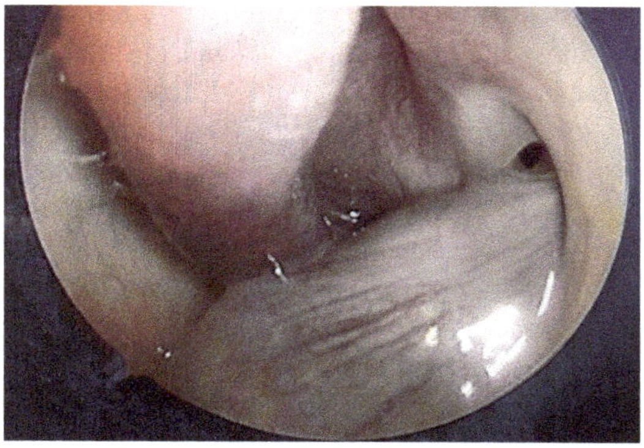

Fig. 2.2 Nasal endoscopic picture of maxillary polyp coming out of the maxillary ostium

tis due to eosinophilic gastroenteritis or mesenteric ischemia due to vasculitis.

- Cardiovascular system: Myocarditis, endomyocardial fibrosis and in severe cases, cardiac failure.
- Musculoskeletal: Joint pain (arthralgia), muscular pain (myalgia), or even arthritis can occur, usually during the vasculitic phase.
- Renal: Renal involvement is rare but may cause glomerulonephritis [2, 5, 14].

2.5 Diagnosis

Diagnosis is on the basis of criteria established in 1990 by the American College of Rheumatology for identifying Churg-Strauss syndrome.

2.5.1 The Six Criteria

The syndrome is considered to be present if a person has four of the six criteria.

- Asthma.
- Eosinophilia. A count higher than 10% is considered abnormally high.
- Mononeuropathy or polyneuropathy causes numbness or pain in the hands and feet. Migratory spots or lesions on a chest X-ray (pulmonary infiltrates). These lesions typically move from one place to another or come and go. On chest X-rays, the lesions mimic pneumonia.
- Acute or chronic sinusitis.
- Extravascular eosinophils: Tissue biopsy of either skin or a removed nasal polyp may show the presence of eosinophils outside the blood vessels.

The nasal mucosa is thus early and regularly involved in the disease process.

2.5.2 Endoscopy

Nasal endoscopy may reveal polyps (Figs. 2.1 and 2.2), nasal secretions, hyperplasia of the inferior turbinates, synechia, and crust formation. Changes in the nasal mucous membranes like edematous swelling of vulnerable or nonspecific mucosal irritation are commonly seen [5].

Bronchoscopy with bronchoalveolar lavage may show the presence of eosinophilic inflammation, obviating the need for lung biopsy [15].

2.5.3 The Birmingham Vasculitis Activity Score (BVAS)

It is a validated tool for the assessment of disease activity in patients with many different forms of vasculitis. The BVAS includes scored items grouped into nine organ systems which capture a broad spectrum of clinical manifestations from vasculitis. Only features attributed to active vasculitis are considered. The BVAS is part of the OMERACT core outcome measures for use in clinical trials of anti-neutrophil cytoplasmic antibody (ANCA)- associated vasculitis [16, 17].

2.5.4 Blood Cells and Biomarkers

- Eosinophilia—The active phase is characterized by marked peripheral blood eosinophilia (>1500 cells/μL or >10%). Eosinophilia correlates with disease activity and relapses [13, 18].
- C-reactive protein (CRP) and erythrocyte sedimentation rate (ESR) are also higher in the active phase [18].
- Serum total IgE levels are elevated in most patients, but they lack specificity for common allergens. Recent data have shown that serum IgG4 levels were high in 75% of patients with active EGPA, better correlating with its activity than IgE [12, 13, 18].
- ANCA may appear several years before the onset of vasculitis. The perinuclear immunofluorescence (p-ANCA) pattern is usually found in 74–90% of EGPA ANCA- positive cases, especially anti-MPO antibodies. The remaining cases are anti-cytoplasmic ANCA (c-ANCA) corresponding to anti-proteinase-3 or mixed patterns antibodies (p- ANCA + c-ANCA) [18].
- Emerging biomarkers—Plasma levels of eotaxin3 (at cut-off level of 80 pg/ml) has the sensitivity and specificity of 87.5% and 98.6%, respectively, for the diagnosis. It is a reliable biomarker to assess therapeutic response. As CSS involves several mechanisms with high heterogeneity and different therapeutic responses, biomarkers, and endotyping help to determine the optimal primary therapeutic modality, select a good responder to a specific treatment, and predict treatment outcomes [19, 20].

2.5.5 Imaging

X-ray chest, computerized tomography (CT) thorax help to delineate pulmonary pathology. Various patterns commonly found in the thorax are lobar or segmental opacity, diffuse interstitial or miliary patterns, migratory infiltrates of the lower lobe or subpleural, hilar, or mediastinal lymphadenopathy, pleural effusion, and pulmonary hemorrhage, ground-glass opacity and hyperinflation [21].

CT and MRI Paranasal sinuses help to look for sinonasal polyposis (Figs. 2.3a, b and 2.4) HRCT temporal bone and MRI is warranted in case of otological manifestations.

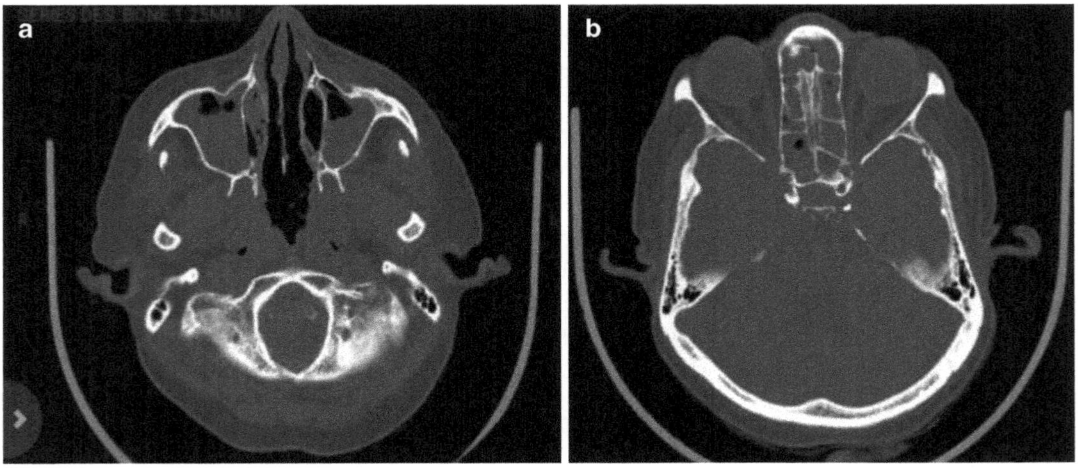

Fig. 2.3 (**a**) CT PNS axial view showing polypoidal mucosal thickening in bilateral maxillary sinuses. (**b**) CT PNS axial view showing hyperdense opacities in bilateral anterior and posterior ethmoidal sinuses suggesting polyposis

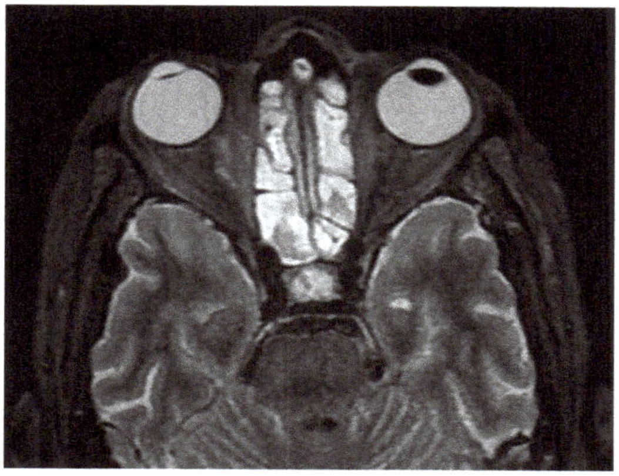

Fig. 2.4 MRI PNS axial view showing hyperintense opacities in bilateral anterior and posterior ethmoidal sinuses suggesting polyposis

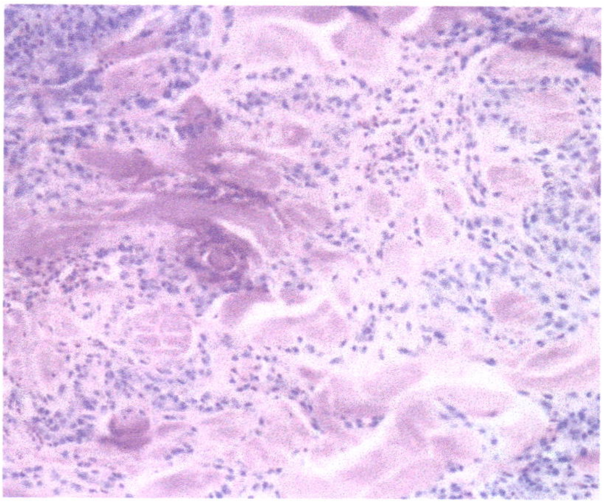

Fig. 2.5 Histopathology revealing tissue eosinophilia and extravascular granulomas

2.5.6 Histopathology

Histopathological examination of biopsy taken from nasal mass, lungs, skin or muscle, to confirm or rule out the presence of vasculitis [3, 6]. Three major histological features are suggestive of CSS: necrotizing vasculitis, extravascular necrotizing granulomas, and tissue eosinophilia (Fig. 2.5) [22].

2.5.7 Other Tests

- In case of hearing loss, audiometric evaluation is necessary.
- Pulmonary function tests: An obstructive or restrictive pattern predominates depending on whether the airway or parenchyma is involved. Airflow measurements are performed according to the treatment of asthma. A reduction of diffusion capacity should lead to the consideration of thromboembolic complications [23].

2.6 Treatment

Churg-Strauss syndrome is not completely curable disease, but certain medications may reduce the severity of symptoms.

"Five Factors Score" (FFS) is used as prognostic index for CSS, although it has not been validated internationally [24].

- Cardiomyopathy
- Gastrointestinal involvement
- Central nervous system involvement
- Proteinuria (>1 g/24 h)
- Serum creatinine (>150 mmol/L)

2.6.1 Oral Corticosteroids and Immunosuppressants

The presence of one or more risk factors (FFS ≥ 1) indicates a worse prognosis and those patients are usually treated with glucocorticoids and immunosuppressants. Cyclophosphamide (6-12 pulses) has been successfully used for induction of remission in patients based on the FFS. Azathioprine or methotrexate can also be used in place of cyclophosphamide.

The patients with FFS = 0 are usually treated with oral corticosteroids such as prednisolone alone.

Immune globulin—Given as a monthly infusion, immune globulin is generally given to people who do not respond to other treatments. High doses of intravenous immunoglobulin are usually used in combination with plasma exchange [18].

Biological Therapies (Monoclonal Antibodies)—B-cell depletion with drugs such as Rituximab, a chimeric anti-CD20 monoclonal antibody, effectively induces remission that alter the immune system's response seem to improve symptoms and decrease the number of eosinophils. It has been studied in small trials, and its long-term safety and efficacy are still unknown [18].

Surgical Management—Functional endoscopic sinus surgery (FESS) for pansinusitis and sinonasal polyposis is indicated [1, 5, 18].

2.6.2 Supportive Therapy

Antihistaminics with Montelukast—For the treatment of allergic rhinitis, asthma, and nasal polyposis

Steroid Nasal Spray: Local treatment to alleviate the symptoms and to prevent the progress of the nasal disease.

2.7 Essential Features

- Rare, systemic, small to medium vessel granulomatous vasculitis.
- Clinically presents with asthma, blood eosinophilia exceeding 1500/mm^3, evidence of vasculitis involving two or more organs and sinonasal polyposis or pansinusitis.
- The disease progresses in three phases. The prodromal phase, eosinophilic phase, and vasculitis phase.
- The prodromal (or allergic) phase lasting for months to many years is characterized by various allergic reactions, asthma, allergic rhinitis and sinusitis.
- The eosinophilic phase is characterized by multisystem involvement—especially the lungs, gastrointestinal tract, and skin.
- The vasculitis phase is characterized by widespread inflammation of various blood vessels (vasculitis) and presents with renal, neurological and cardiovascular system involvement.
- American College of Rheumatology has provided six diagnostic criteria for Churg-Strauss syndrome. The presence of four of six criteria makes the diagnosis.
- Renal manifestations occur in 45% of those with the diagnosis. May cause multisystem involvement.
- Birmingham Vasculitis Activity Index (BVAS) includes an assessment of the head and neck region and the severity of disease progression.
- Microscopic features include fibrinoid necrosis, necrotizing vasculitis and extravascular eosinophil-rich granulomatous inflammation.
- Associated with HLA-DRB4 and anti-neutrophil cytoplasmic antibodies (ANCA).
- Antihistaminics with montelukast and steroid nasal spray give symptomatic improvement.
- In severe manifestations with risk factors, immunosuppressants (e.g., cyclophosphamide, glucocorticoids, azathioprine), B-cell depleting agent Rituximab, anti-IL5 antibody Mepolizumab is recommended.
- Surgical management is with FESS for pansinusitis and sinonasal polyposis.

References

1. Reid AJ, et al. Churg Strauss syndrome in a district hospital. Q J Med. 1998;91:219–29.
2. Guillevin L, et al. Prognostic factors in polyarteritis nodosa and Churg-Strauss syndrome: a prospective study in 342 patients. Medicine. 1996;75:17–28.
3. Bacciu A, et al. Ear, nose and throat manifestations of Churg-Strauss syndrome. Acta Otolaryngol. 2006 May;126(5):503–9.
4. Lanham JG, et al. Systemic vasculitis with asthma and eosinophilia: a clinical approach to the Churg-Strauss syndrome. Medicine. 1984;63:65–81.
5. Laudien M Orphan diseases of the nose and paranasal sinuses: Pathogenesis-clinic-therapy. GMS Curr Top Otorhinolaryngol Head Neck Surg. 2015; 14: Doc04. Published online 2015 Dec 22. https://doi.org/10.3205/cto000119
6. Davies DJ, Moran JE. Segmental necrotizing glomerulonephritis with antineutrophil antibody: possible arbovirus eitiology? BMJ. 1982;285:606.
7. Maeda Y, et al. Churg-Strauss syndrome associated with necrotizing crescentic glomerulonephritis in a diabetic patient. Intern Med. 1997;36:68–72.
8. Zwerina J, et al. Churg-Strauss syndrome in childhood: a systematic literature review and clinical comparison with adult patients. Semin Arthritis Rheum. 2009;39:108–15.

9. Abril A, et al. The Churg Strauss syndrome (allergic granulomatous angiitis): review update. Semin Arthritis Rheum. 2003;33:106–14.
10. Weller PF, et al. The relationship of asthma therapy and Churg-Strauss syndrome: NIH workshop summary report. J Allergy Clin Immunol. 2001;108:175–83.
11. Churg J, Strauss L. Allergic granulomatosis, allergic angiitis and periarteritis nodosa. Am J Pathol. 1951;27:277–301.
12. Lanham JG, et al. Systemic vasculitis with asthma and eosinophilia: a clinical approach to the Churg-Strauss syndrome. Medicine (Baltimore). 1984;63:65–81.
13. Chumbley LC, et al. Allergic granulomatosis and angiitis (Churg-Strauss syndrome): report and analysis of 30 cases. Mayo Clin Proc. 1977;52:477–84.
14. Guillevin L, et al. Churg Strauss syndrome: Clinical study and long term follow-up of 96 patients. Medicine. 1999;78:26–37.
15. Szczeklik W, et al. Lung involvement in Churg-Strauss. syndrome as related to the activity of the disease. Allergy. 2010;65:1484–5.
16. Suppiah R, et al. A cross-sectional study of the Birmingham Vasculitis activity score version 3 in systemic vasculitis. Rheumatology (Oxford). 2011;50:899–905.
17. Merkel PA, et al. The OMERACT core set of outcome measures for use in clinical trials of ANCA-associated vasculitis. J Rheumatol. 2011;38:1480–6.
18. Izquierdo-Domínguez A, et al. Churg-strauss syndrome or eosinophilic granulomatosis with Polyangiitis. Sinusitis. 2016;1(1):24–43. https://doi.org/10.3390/sinusitis1010024.
19. Ninomiya T, et al. Periostin as a novel biomarker for postoperative recurrence of chronic rhinosinitis with nasal polyps. Sci Rep. 2018;8:11450. https://doi.org/10.1038/s41598-018-29612-2.
20. Kato Y, et al. The expression and functional analysis of CST1 in intractable nasal polyps. Am J Respir Cell Mol Biol. 2018;59:448–57. https://doi.org/10.1165/rcmb.2017-0325OC.
21. Jeong YJ, et al. Eosinophilic lung disease: a clinical, radiological and pathological view. Radiographic. 2007;27:617–37.
22. Guillevin L, et al. Clinical findings and prognosis of polyarteritis nodosa and Churg -Strauss angiitis: a study in 165 patients. Br J Rheumatol. 1988;27:258–64.
23. Bottero P, et al. The common allergens in the Churg-Strauss syndrome. Allergy. 2007;62:1288–94.
24. Guillevin L, et al. The five-factor score revisited: assessment of prognoses of systemic necrotizing vasculitides based on the French Vasculitis study group (FVSG) cohort. Medicine. 2011;90:19–27.

3 Behcet's Disease

Abstract

Behcet's disease is a rare, chronic inflammatory disorder characterized by varied manifestations including oral ulcers, genital ulcers, ocular inflammation, pathergy test, skin disease including papulopustular lesions and erythema nodosum. In addition to its principal clinical symptoms, Behcet's disease can clinically manifest in many other major organ systems, such as the vascular, gastrointestinal, and musculoskeletal systems. Behcet's disease is unique among vasculitides in that it has the ability to affect small, medium, and large vessels. The disease appears to involve an autoimmune response triggered by exposure to an infectious agent. Demographic characteristics, clinical features, and famillialfamilial occurrence of the disease differ due to environmental and/genetic factors. Diagnosis is based on clinical criteria established by the International Study Group for Behcet's Disease (ICBD) The treatment approach depends on the individual patient, severity of disease, and major organ involvement. Corticosteroid therapy with or without cytostatic drugs are is commonly used depending on the severity and morbidity of the disease.

Synonyms

Behcet's syndrome; malignant aphthosis; Behcet's triple symptom complex [1].

3.1 Overview

Behcet's disease (BD) is a multisystemic, relapsing inflammatory disorder with vasculitis as the main feature. It is usually considered to be a condition affecting the oral cavity, eyes, and genitals "Hulusi Behcet," the Turkish dermatologist and scientist first described this disease in 1937. He first recognized the three main symptoms of the disease in one of his patients [1, 2]. Behcet's disease may present with features other than the classic triad of symptoms. Increased awareness of the clinical features within the head and neck region enables early diagnosis and treatment of this potentially serious condition [1].

3.2 Epidemiology

It is a rare disease with an estimated global incidence to be about 0.1 to 3 cases for every 100,000 people. Globally, males are affected more frequently than females. The prevalence of this disease increases from North to South. It follows a more severe course in patients with an early age of onset, particularly in patients with eye and gastrointestinal involvement [2, 3].

S. V. Nemade, K. J. Shinde, *Granulomatous diseases in Otorhinolaryngology, Head and Neck*,
https://doi.org/10.1007/978-981-16-4047-6_3

3.3 Etiopathogenesis

The primary mechanism of the damage is autoimmune vasculitis, which by definition is an overactive immune system that targets the patient's own blood vessels. Vasculitis resulting in occlusion of the vessels leads to organ damage. The involvement of a subset of T cells (Th17) seems to be important. The primary cause is not well known. The genetic association with the GIMAP (GTPase of the immunity-associated protein) family of genes on the long arm of chromosome 7 (7q36.1) has been reported. The genes implicated are GIMAP1, GIMAP2, GIMAP4 [3].

3.4 Clinical Features

Aphthous oral ulcers- This is the most common presentation of disease (95% of patients). The ulcer has sharp borders surrounded by an erythematous rim and a base covered with yellow-white colored pseudomembrane (Fig. 3.1).

Ulcers are classified into three groups according to ulcer diameter, but these three morphological forms are recognized as parts of the same spectrum. Minor aphthae are shallow mucosal ulcers with a diameter of <10 mm, which may be found in groups, usually on the nonkeratinized section of oral mucosa (lateral sides and ventral surface of the tongue, mouth floor.

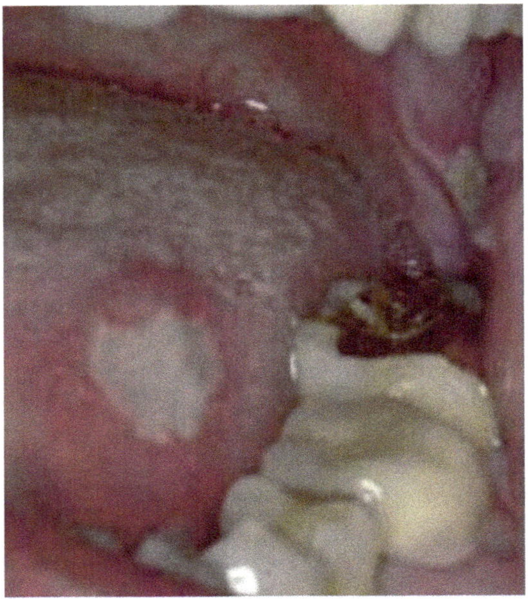

Fig. 3.1 Tongue ulcer covered with a yellowish white membrane and with erythematous margins

Major aphthous ulcers have similar morphologies, but they have a larger diameter (×10 mm), are deeper than the minor variants, and tend to heal with scarring [2, 4]. Herpetiform aphthae are pinpoint shaped, very small, and shallow mucosal ulcers and tend to occur in crops. Sometimes they may converge and form large ulcers with irregular borders [5].

Genital ulcers- Genital ulcers are present in 90 % of patients with Behcet's disease. Usually larger than oral aphthae, genital ulcers of BD have similar clinical features. These ulcers may persist for weeks and can be very painful. The most common places for genital ulcerations are the scrotum and the shaft of the penis in men and the major and minor labia in women. Genital ulcers have irregular borders, are deeper than oral aphthae, and heal with scarring and occasionally causing fistulae extending to the urethra or bladder [6–8].

Eye involvement- Ocular involvement is seen in 50% of patients. Posterior uveitis, anterior uveitis, or retinal vasculitis are common manifestations. Anterior uveitis presents with painful eyes, conjunctival redness, hypopyon, and decreased visual acuity, while posterior uveitis presents with painless decreased visual acuity and visual field floaters [9].

Optic nerve involvement in Behcet's disease is rare, typically presenting as progressive optic atrophy and visual loss. Papilledema as a result of dural sinus thrombosis [10] and atrophy resulting from retinal disease, have been characterized as secondary causes of optic nerve atrophy in Behcet's disease [9].

Signs and symptoms of acute optic neuropathy include painless loss of vision which may affect either one or both eyes, reduced visual acuity, reduced color vision, relative afferent pupillary defect, central scotoma, swollen optic disc, macular edema, or retrobulbar pain [9].

Sensorineural hearing loss- It is very rare and maybe the manifestation of VIII cranial nerve involvement secondary to vasculitis [11].

Cutaneous involvement- Papulopustular lesions (PPLs) are the most common cutaneous manifestation of Behcet's disease PPLs are observed on the trunk, face, and extremities. PPLs are "pseudofolliculitis or papulopustular lesions; or acneiform nodules observed in post-adolescent patients not receiving corticosteroid treatment" [12, 13].

Nodular lesions located on the lower extremities resembling erythema nodosum are frequently seen in Behcet's disease patients; Erythema nodosum-like lesions (ENLs) are rather common. ENLs manifest mostly in females. Other than lower extremities, ENLs are reported on the face and neck. ENLs do not ulcerate and heal in 2–3 weeks. The main difference between erythema nodosum and ENL is the existence of vasculitis and necrobiosis in the latter [12, 13].

The term "pathergy" is used to define the cutaneous hyper-reactivity to minimal trauma. A positive pathergy reaction is characterized by an erythematous, indurated papule at the site of trauma, which usually evolves into a sterile pustule. Pathergy is one of the diagnostic criteria for Behcet's disease and is accepted as a sign for the active disease [8, 14].

Behcet's disease may also affect major vessels. The most common arterial lesions are occlusions or stenosis and aneurysms or pseudoaneurysms. Subcutaneous thrombophlebitis is another common cutaneous manifestation of BD.

3.4.1 Other System Involvement

- CNS involvement shows aseptic meningitis due to vascular thromboses such as dural sinus thrombosis and organic brain syndrome manifesting with confusion, seizures, and memory loss. Sudden hearing loss (Sensorineural) is often associated with it [15]. Dural venous sinus thrombosis may subsequently lead to secondary optic atrophy [13].
- Lung involvement is typically in the form of hemoptysis, pleuritis, cough, or fever, and in severe cases can be life-threatening if the outlet pulmonary artery develops an aneurysm which ruptures causing severe vascular collapse and death from bleeding in the lungs [15].
- GI manifestations include abdominal pain, nausea, and diarrhea with or without blood, and they often involve the ileocecal valve [15].
- Arthritis is seen in up to half of people with BD.

3.5 Diagnosis

Clinical diagnosis of Behcet's disease is based on clinical findings including oral and genital ulcers, skin lesions such as erythema nodosum, acne, or folliculitis, ocular inflammatory findings, and a pathergy reaction.

According to the International criteria for Behçet's disease (ICBD) - point score system: scoring ≥ 4 indicates Behcet's disease [8, 10].

- Oral aphthosis: 2 points (oral aphthous ulcers of any shape, size, or number at least 3 times in any 12 months period)
- Ocular lesions: 2 points (eye inflammation such as iritis, uveitis, retinal vasculitis)
- Genital aphthosis: 2 points (including anal ulcers and spots in the genital region and swollen testicles or epididymitis in men)
- Skin lesions: 1 point (papulo-pustules, folliculitis, erythema nodosum, acne in post-adolescents not on corticosteroids).
- Positive pathergy test: 1 point. (Papule >2 mm dia. 24–48 h or more after needle-prick). The pathergy test has a specificity of 95–100%, but the results are often negative in American and European patients

- Neurological manifestations: 1 point.
- Vascular manifestations: 1 point.

3.5.1 Histopathology

Biopsy of oral/genital ulcers usually has similar histopathological features of all variants of aphthous oral ulcers, hence has a limited value in the differential diagnosis. Lymphocytes, macrophages, and neutrophils are observed at the base of an ulcer (Fig. 3.2). At the periphery of the ulcer base, the infiltrate may penetrate into the epidermis. Some recently published direct immunofluorescence (DIF) studies report IgM and C3 deposits in the perivascular region with or without granular C3 deposits at the dermo-epidermal junction in the perilesional skin of aphthous ulcer in Behcet's disease patients [8, 17]

3.5.2 Other Tests

- Inflammatory markers such as ESR and CRP may be elevated.
- A complete ophthalmic examination may include a slit lamp examination, optical coherence tomography to detect nerve loss, visual field examinations, fundoscopic examination to assess optic disc atrophy and retinal disease, fundoscopic angiography, and visual evoked potentials, which may demonstrate increased latency.
- Optic nerve enhancement may be identified on Magnetic Resonance Imaging (MRI) in some patients with acute optic neuropathy. However, a normal study does not rule out optic neuropathy.
- Cerebrospinal fluid examination for elevated protein level with or without pleocytosis. Imaging including angiography may be indicated to identify dural venous sinus thrombosis as a cause of intracranial hypertension and optic atrophy [4, 10].

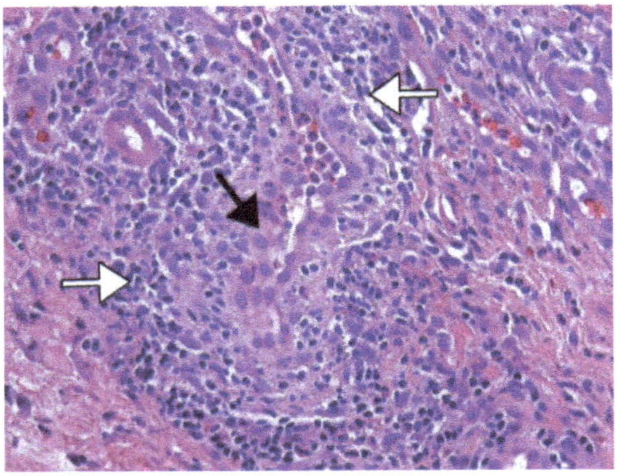

Fig. 3.2 Endothelial cell swelling (black arrow) and perivascular inflammatory cell infiltrate (white arrows) [16]

3.6 Treatment

Treatment aims at reducing inflammation and controlling the immune system.

3.6.1 Pharmacotherapy

- High-dose corticosteroid therapy is often used for severe disease manifestations. The most commonly used dose is 5 mg/kg every 6–8 weeks and repeated infusions are required to maintain long-term remission.
- Anti-TNF therapy such as Infliximab, Etanercept, may be useful in people with mainly skin and mucosal symptoms.
- Interferon-alpha-2a: This immunosuppressive therapy is alternative to steroids, particularly for genital and oral ulcers as well as ocular lesions. Azathioprine, when used in combination with interferon alpha-2b also shows promise. Colchicine can be useful for treating some genital ulcers, erythema nodosum, and arthritis. Benzathine-penicillin may also reduce new arthritic attacks.
- Thalidomide has also been used due to its immune-modifying effect. Dapsone and

Rebamipide have been found to carry beneficial results for mucocutaneous lesions [15, 18].
- IV Immunoglobulins could be a treatment for severe or complicated cases [18].

3.6.2 Surgery

Surgical treatment of arterial manifestations of BD bears many pitfalls, since the obliterative endarteritis may lead to the formation of pseudoaneurysms at the site of puncture in case of angiography or endovascular treatment. Invasive treatment should not be performed in the acute and active phases of the disease when inflammation is at its peak. The disease activity is monitored by relapsing symptoms, ESR (erythrocyte sedimentation rate), and serum levels of CRP (C-reactive protein) [19].

3.7 Essential Features

- Behcet's disease (BD) also known as Behcet's syndrome is a multisystemic, relapsing inflammatory disorder mainly affecting the oral cavity, genitalia, and eyes.
- Oral ulcerations (95% of cases) on lips, gingival, buccal mucosa, and tongue.
- Genital ulcers (90% of cases), Erythema nodosum-like lesions, healing with hyperpigmentation.
- Acne-like papulopustular lesions on the face, upper trunk, and extremities.
- Recurrent asymmetric mono or oligoarthritis, arthralgia, usually involving lower extremities, resolves with no deformity or erosion.
- Ocular involvement (50% of cases), mainly posterior or panuveitis and retinal vasculitis.
- Superficial and deep venous thrombosis.
- Variable gastrointestinal, neurologic involvement in 5% of patients.
- According to the International criteria for Behcet disease (ICBD) point score system [Oral aphthosis (2), genital aphtosis (2), ocular lesions (2), pathergy reaction (1), neurological involvement (1), skin involvement (1) and vascular manifestations (1)], scoring ≥ 4 indicates Behcet's disease.
- Treatment is tailored to each patient's clinical manifestations.
- Corticosteroids are useful in controlling acute manifestations.
- Cytotoxic medications are indicated in patients with ocular, central nervous system, and vascular disease.

References

1. Behcet H. Uber rezidivierende, aphthöse, durch ein virus verursachte Geschwüre am Mund, am uge und an den Genitalien. Dermatol Wochenschr. 1937;105:1152–7.
2. Gül A, et al. Familial aggregation of Behcet's disease in Turkey. Ann Rheum Dis. 2000;59(8):622–5.
3. Kapsimali VD, et al. Etiopathogenesis of Behçet's disease with emphasis on the role of immunological abberations. Clin Rheumatol. 2010;29:1211–6.
4. Alpsoy E, et al. Mucocutaneous lesions of Behçet's disease. Yonsei Med J. 2007;48(4):573–85.
5. Oh SH, et al. Comparison of the clinical features of recurrent aphthous stomatitis and Behçet's disease. Clin Exp Dermatol. 2009;34(6):e208–12.
6. Melikoglu M, et al. The uniquatures of vasculitis in Behçet's syndrome. Clin Rev Allergy Immunol. 2008;35(1–2):40–6.
7. Escudier M, et al. Number VII Behçet's disease (Adamantiades syndrome). Oral Dis. 2006;12(2):78–84.
8. Alpsoy E, et al. Review of the chronology of clinical manifestations in 60 patients with Behçet's disease. Dermatology. 2003;207(4):354–6.
9. Kansu T, et al. Optic neuropathy in Behçet's disease. J Clin Neuroophthalmol. 1989;9(4):277–80.
10. International Study Group for Behçet's Disease. Criteria for diagnosis of Behçet's disease. Lancet. 1990;335(8697):1078–80.
11. Jorizzo JL, et al. Mucocutaneous criteria for the diagnosis of Behcet's disease: an analysis of clinicopathologic data from multiple international centers. J Am Acad Dermatol. 1995;32(6):968–76.
12. Hatemi G, et al. Behçet's syndrome: a critical digest of the 2012–2013 literature. Clin Exp Rheumatol. 2013;31(3 Suppl 77):108–17.
13. Fujikado T, Imagawa K. Dural sinus thrombosis in Behçet's disease--a case report. Jpn J Ophthalmol. 1994;38(4):411–6.
14. Varol A, et al. The skin pathergy test: innately useful? Arch Dermatol Res. 2010;302(3):155–68.
15. Beales IL. Gastrointestinal involvement in Behçet's syndrome. Am. J. Gastroenterol. 1998;93(12):2633.

16. McDonald DR, et al. Behçet's disease. CMAJ. 2007 Apr 24;176(9):1273–4. https://doi.org/10.1503/cmaj.061136.
17. Kose. Direct immunofluorescence in Behçet's disease: a controlled study with 108 cases. Yonsei Med J. 2009;50(4):505–11.
18. Matsuda T, et al. Efficacy of rebamipide as adjunctive therapy in the treatment of recurrent oral aphthous ulcers in patients with Behcet's disease: a randomised, double-blind, placebo-controlled study. Drugs in R&D. 2003;4(1):19–28.
19. Genadiev GG, et al. Surgical treatment of Angio-Behçet H Behcet's disease. InTech. 2017; https://doi.org/10.5772/intechopen.68664. isbn: 978-953-51-3225-7

Part II

Infective Granulomatous Diseases

Tuberculosis

4

Abstract

Tuberculosis (TB) is a chronic granulomatous, infectious, and communicable disease caused by *Mycobacterium tuberculosis*. India is the highest TB burden country in the world, with an estimated more than 2 million cases annually. Two major disease patterns are primary tuberculosis and secondary tuberculosis. Primary TB is characterized by the Ghon complex. Secondary TB causes florid and widespread granulomatous inflammation. Extra-pulmonary manifestations can occur in primary or secondary TB evolving from pulmonary focus or by haematogenic dissemination. Out of the extra pulmonary manifestations of tuberculosis, otorhinolaryngology, head and neck manifestations are mainly in the form of cervical lymphadenopathy being the commonest, otitis media, granulomatous lesions of hypopharynx and larynx, oral cavity ulcers and granulomas, oropharyngeal lesions and nasal gra nulomas. The diagnostic gold standard for active tuberculosis (TB) is the detection of *Mycobacterium tuberculosis* by sputum/secretions smear microscopy, culture, or molecular methods. HRCT help in early diagnosis by delineating nodular infiltrates, abscess, and granulomatous lesions. Interferon-γ (IFN-γ) release assays (IGR s) can reliably detect active disease and latent TB infection. Ribosomal RNA probes and DNA PCR assays allow identification within 24 h. WHO recommended standardized regimens for anti-TB treatment include five essential medicines isoniazid (H), rifampicin (R), pyrazinamide (Z), ethambutol (E), and streptomycin (S).

Synonyms
Koch's infection, Phthisis, Phthisis pulmonalis [1, 2].

4.1 Background

Tuberculosis is classified as one of the granulomatous inflammatory diseases. It is an infectious and contagious disease caused by a bacterium, *Mycobacterium tuberculosis*, also called Koch's Bacillus (KB). "Robert Koch" identified and described the bacillus causing tuberculosis, M. tuberculosis, on March 24, 1882 [1]. He received the Nobel Prize in 1905 for this discovery [1]. World Tuberculosis Day is marked on March 24 each year, the anniversary of Koch's original scientific announcement. Tuberculosis is a widespread public concern and is particularly the disease affecting the urban poor. It generally affects the lungs, but extrapulmonary manifestations are also common. Most of the infections do not have symptoms, in which case it is known as latent tuberculosis. The classic symptoms of active TB are a chronic cough with hemoptysis, night

S. V. Nemade, K. J. Shinde, *Granulomatous diseases in Otorhinolaryngology, Head and Neck*,
https://doi.org/10.1007/978-981-16-4047-6_4

sweats, and weight loss. Infection of other organs can cause a wide range of symptoms [1, 2].

4.2 Epidemiology

Tuberculosis (TB) continues to remain one of the most pressing health problems in India. India is the highest TB burden country in the world, accounting for one-fifth of the global incidence with an estimated more than 2 million cases annually [3]. Undiagnosed and mismanaged TB is partly responsible for this. Globally, it is very prevalent; approximately 1.7 billion people are infected with 9 million new cases a year with an estimated 1.6 million deaths [3]. TB is more common in men than in women, affecting in particular adults in economically productive age groups [4].

4.3 Etiopathogenesis

Tuberculosis is spread through the air when patients with active infection coughs, speaks, spits, or sneezes. People with the latent disease do not spread disease. The most important risk factor globally is HIV; 13% of all people with TB are infected by the virus. Tuberculosis is closely linked to both overcrowding and malnutrition, making it one of the principal diseases of poverty. Chronic lung disease, alcoholism, and diabetes mellitus (threefold increase) are another significant risk factors. Silicosis increases the risk about 30-fold. Those who smoke cigarettes have nearly twice the risk of TB compared to nonsmokers. Certain medications, such as corticosteroids and chemotherapeutic agents, are other important risk factors, especially in the developed world. Genetic susceptibility also exists [3, 4].

The causative organism, *Mycobacterium tuberculosis* (MTB), is a small, aerobic, nonmotile bacillus. The high lipid content of this pathogen accounts for many of its unique clinical characteristics. The M. tuberculosis complex (MTBC) includes four other TB- causing mycobacteria: *M. bovis, M. africanum*, M. canetti, and M. microti [5]. In the developing world, *M. bovis* causes oropharyngeal and intestinal TB.

TB infection begins when the mycobacteria reach the alveolar air sacs of the lungs, where they invade and replicate within endosomes of alveolar macrophages. Macrophages identify the bacterium as foreign and attempt to eliminate it by phagocytosis. During this process, the bacterium is enveloped by the macrophage and stored temporarily in a membrane-bound vesicle called a phagosome. The phagosome then combines with a lysosome to create a phagolysosome. In the phagolysosome, the cell attempts to use reactive oxygen species and acid to kill the bacterium. However, M. tuberculosis has a thick, waxy mycolic acid capsule that protects it from these toxic substances. M. tuberculosis is able to reproduce inside the macrophage and will eventually kill the immune cell. It is characterized by the formation of granulomas.

The granuloma may prevent the dissemination of the mycobacteria and provide a local environment for the interaction of cells of the immune system. Another feature of granulomas is the development of abnormal cell death (necrosis) in the center of tubercles. It has the texture of soft, white cheese and is termed caseous necrosis [4–6].

4.3.1 There are Two Major Patterns of Disease with TB

- Primary Tuberculosis: It is seen as an initial infection, usually in children. The initial focus of infection is a small subpleural granuloma accompanied by granulomatous hilar lymph node infection. Together, these make up the Ghon complex. In nearly all cases, these granulomas resolve, and there is no further spread of the infection.
- Secondary Tuberculosis: It is seen mostly in adults as reactivation of previous infection (or reinfection), particularly when health status declines. The granulomatous inflammation is much more florid and widespread. Typically, the upper lung lobes are most affected, and cavitation can occur.

According to the site of involvement, TB is classified into

- Pulmonary TB—the most common presentation.
- Extrapulmonary TB—Extrapulmonary manifestations can occur in primary or secondary TB evolving from pulmonary focus or by haematogenic dissemination. This includes tuberculosis of organs other than the lungs, such as lymph nodes, upper airway, ears, abdomen, genitourinary tract, skin, joints and bones, meninges, etc. [5]

4.4 Clinical Features

Constitutional symptoms include fever, chills, night sweats, loss of appetite, weight loss, and fatigue [7]. ENT involvement is seen in primary TB as a result of primary infection or hematogenous spread from pulmonary TB [6, 8].

4.4.1 Laryngeal TB

It is the most common ENT manifestation. Common sites are the vocal folds, followed by the vestibular folds and may involve the epiglottis, the aryepiglottic fold, the arytenoids, the posterior commissure and the subglottis [7]. Tuberculous lesions are ulcerofungative, ulcerative, nonspecific inflammations, or polypoid masses that can develop into granulomatous lesions causing airway obstruction. These lesions are seen most frequently in the posterior glottis (Fig. 4.1 but have been seen throughout the larynx and may be difficult to distinguish from cancerous lesions [9]. Perichondritis and cartilage destruction of the epiglottis and laryngeal cartilages may lead to turban-shaped epiglottis and mouse nibbled vocal cords. Symptoms of the early phase are dysphonia, cough, hemoptysis. In the late phase, dysphonia and dyspnoea are the primary symptoms [7, 10].

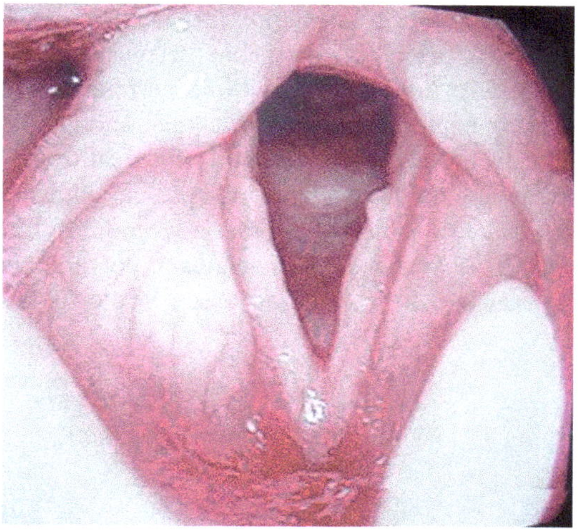

Fig. 4.1 A small nodular lesion in the posterior third of the left vocal fold [9]

4.4.2 TB of Cervical Lymph Nodes

Tuberculous lymphadenitis may result from dissemination via the bloodstream of bacillary pulmonary foci, as well as from the bacilli gaining entrance via the tonsils, dental or pharyngeal foci. It is located most frequently in the cervical, supraclavicular, hilar, mediastinal and retropharyngeal regions. However, any lymph node may be affected. Cervical lymphadenopathy is most common, and the anterior cervical chain is more common amongst cervical lymph nodes. Node is firm rubbery, becoming more firm and matted as disease progresses. Infrequently node presents as a fluctuant mass with draining sinuses (Fig.4.2) [11]. Matted lymph nodes are usually encountered in two-thirds of TB patients and bilateral nodes in one-third of patients.

4.4.3 Aural TB

Tuberculous otitis media is the common presentation. Spread of infection is hematogenous, lymphatic or direct extension from the nasopharynx through the Eustachian tube and externally, by perforation of the tympanic membrane.

The classic triad of presentation is painless otorrhea, which is persistent despite multiple courses of antibiotics, multiple perforations of the tympanic membrane (Fig. 4.3a), and peripheral facial palsy. However, this classical triad is often absent, and patients may present with single large or subtotal perforation (Fig. 4.3b). It is usually associated with abundant polypoid or avascular pale granulation tissue in the middle ear and mastoid. Other symptoms are otalgia and hearing loss. Currently, its presentation has become polymorphic. The complications are peripheral facial paralysis, retro-auricular fistula, labyrinthitis, meningitis, tuberculous osteomyelitis of the petrous pyramid, subperiosteal, cerebral or cerebellar abscess, acute mastoiditis and cellulites [7, 12, 13].

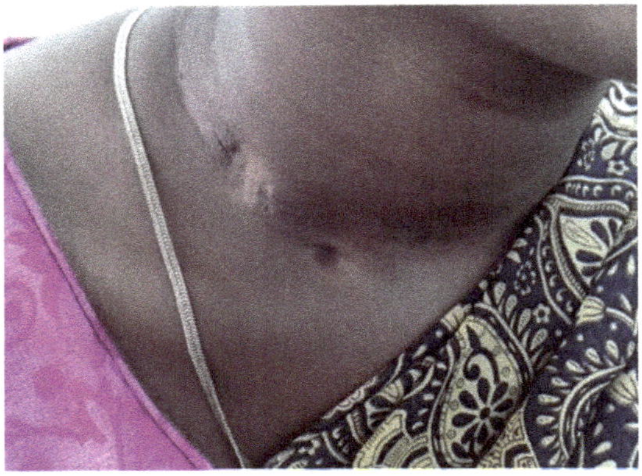

Fig. 4.2 Tuberculous sinuses in the neck [11]

4.4.4 Nasal TB

Nasal TB is an extremely rare form. It presents as three entities—nodular form (lupus vulgaris), ulcerative form, or sinus granuloma. Lupus vulgaris is the most common form. It is caused by direct inoculation, involving the skin and mucosa, with nodules (apple jelly nodules). The ulcerative form presents with ulcers over the cartilaginous part of the nasal septum, presenting with nasal obstruction and may progress to septal perforation (Fig. 4.4). Sinus granuloma presents with a mass in the paranasal sinuses [8, 9].

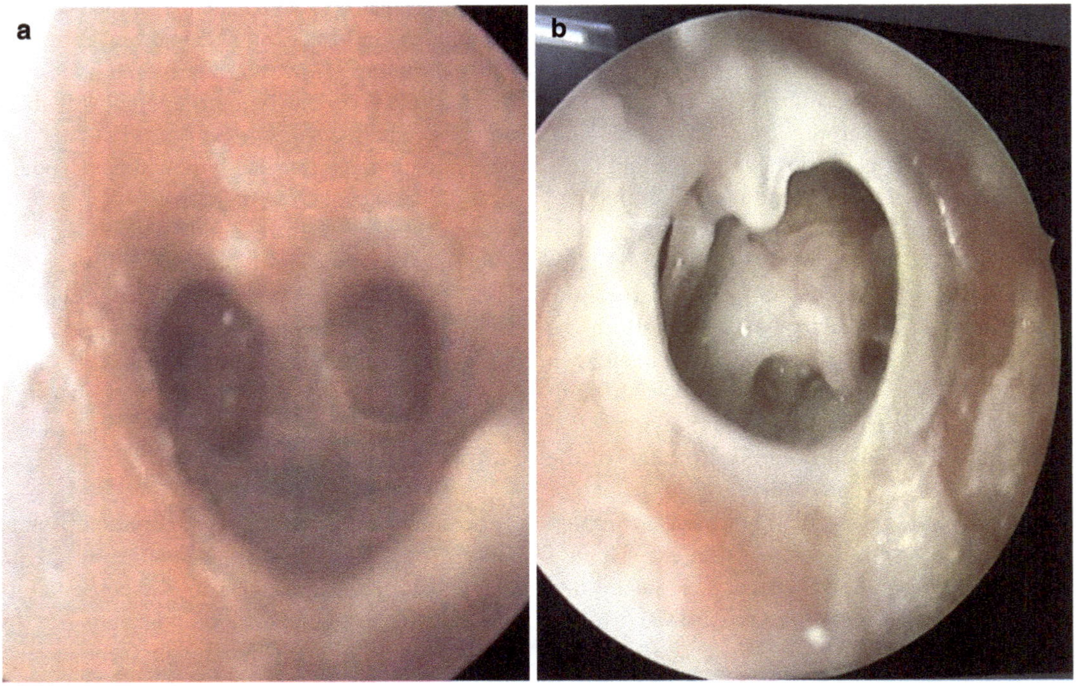

Fig. 4.3 Tuberculous otitis media with (**a**) multiple perforations (**b**) single large perforation

Common symptoms are rhinorrhea and nasal obstruction. Rarely, nasal mass, epistaxis, dryness and crusting, epiphora, recurrent polyps, and nasal skin ulcers (Fig. 4.5) may occur [8, 12].

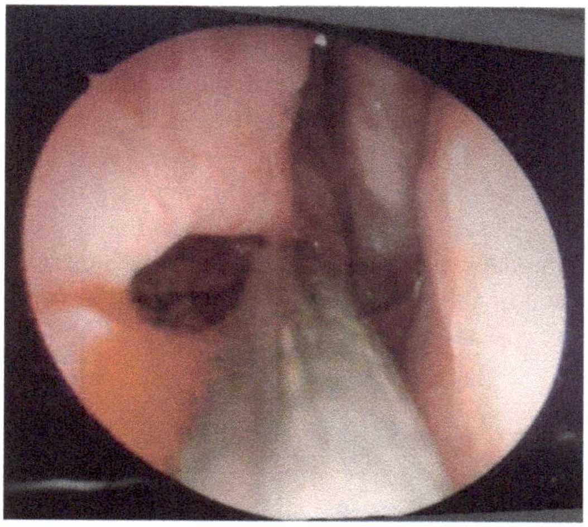

Fig. 4.4 Nasal endoscopic view showing perforation in the cartilaginous part of the septum

4.4.5 TB in the Oral Cavity and Oropharynx

It is rare representing 0.1–5% of total TB infections. In presents as deep nonhealing solitary ulcer with irregular borders, often simulating malignancy (Fig. 4.6).

Tongue is the most common site of involvement, followed by gums, hard and soft palate, lips, maxilla and mandible. The integrity of the oral mucosa, the cleaning action of the saliva, the presence of oral saprophytes and submucosal

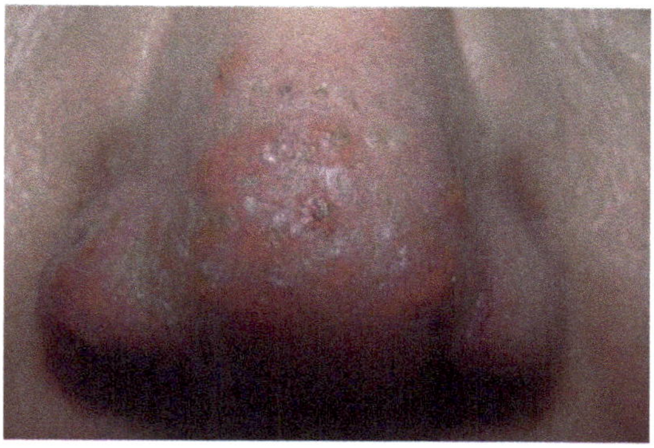

Fig. 4.5 Reddish ulcerative lesion on the nose [9]

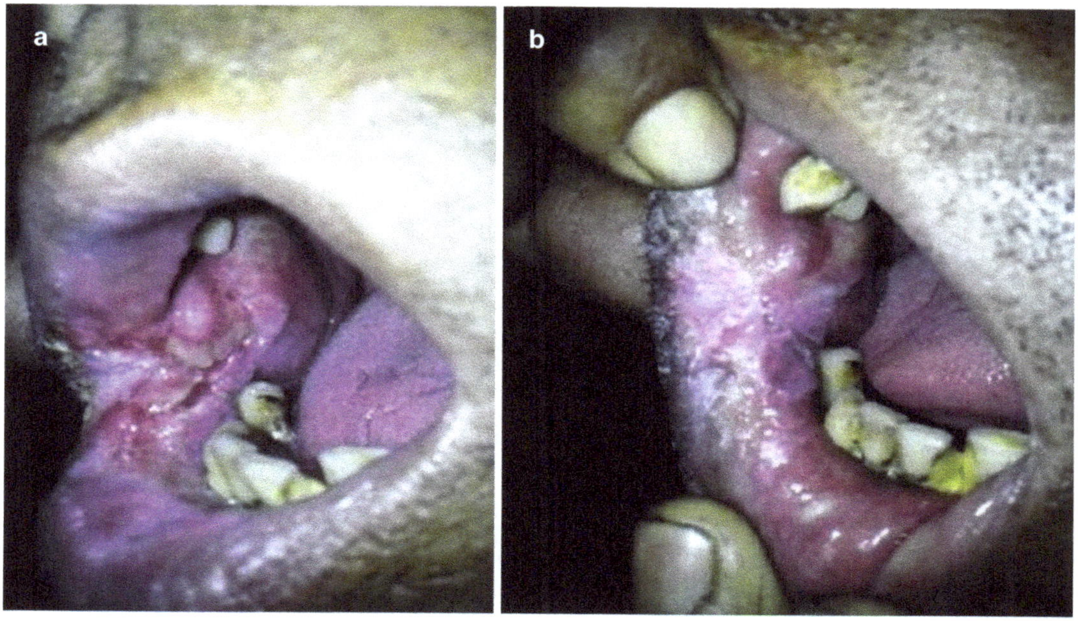

Fig. 4.6 (**a**) before treatment of the tuberculous ulcer; (**b**) after treatment [11]

antibodies represent a natural resistance to the invasion of *Mycobacterium tuberculosis*. Oral trauma, tooth extraction, inflammatory conditions and poor hygiene represent gateways [8, 12].

Tuberculosis of tonsil causing unilateral hypertrophy of tonsil with the ulcerative erythematous surface may occur.TB Involving Salivary Glands:

Primary TB is a relatively common cause of granulomatous disease of the salivary glands. Generally, it affects one side, and the usual target is the parotid gland. The primary form can occur in two ways: acute suppurative sialadenitis or chronic sialoadenitis. Secondary tuberculosis, unlike the primary form, often involves the submandibular and the sublingual glands than the parotid gland [13].

4.5 Diagnosis

The presence of nontender cervical adenopathy should raise the index of suspicion. Accurate diagnosis depends on the results of skin testing, demonstration of acid-fast bacilli on cytology, culture and evidence of granulomatous inflammation on histopathology. Clinical diagnosis is aided by endoscopic examination such as nasopharyngoscopy, direct laryngoscopy and bronchoscopy.

4.5.1 Microscopy and Culture

Fine needle aspiration cytology(FNAC) will be useful on suspected neck swellings such as lymphadenopathy or salivary gland swellings [14]. FNAC is a safe, minimally invasive procedure that does not require hospital admission and can be easily performed by healthcare professionals trained in this technique.

Culture—The acid-fast bacillus is cultured from the body secretions such as sputum, nasal secretions, ear discharge, laryngotracheal secretions, bronchial lavage, pus from the discharging sinuses, lymph node aspirates or the swab collected from nose, throat, and laryngeal ulcers. Since MTB retains certain stains even after being treated with an acidic solution, it is classified as an acid-fast bacillus. The most common acid-fast staining techniques are the Ziehl–Neelsen stain and the Kinyoun stain, which dye acid-fast bacilli a bright red that stands out against a blue background (Fig. 4.7). Auramine-rhodamine stain and Fluorescence microscopy are also used [7, 14].

4.5.2 Histopathology

Biopsy of the ulcerative lesions, apple jelly nodules, or granulations in the middle ear may reveal a typical histopathological picture showing macrophages, T lymphocytes, B lymphocytes, and fibroblasts aggregating to form granulomas, with lymphocytes and multinucleated giant cells surrounding the infected macrophages with or without caseation (Fig. 4.8) [13–15].

4.5.3 Imaging

Chest radiographs may show a patchy or nodular infiltrate. TB may be found in any part of the lung, but upper lobe involvement is most common. The lordotic view may better demonstrate apical abnormalities.The following patterns may be seen on chest radiographs [16]:

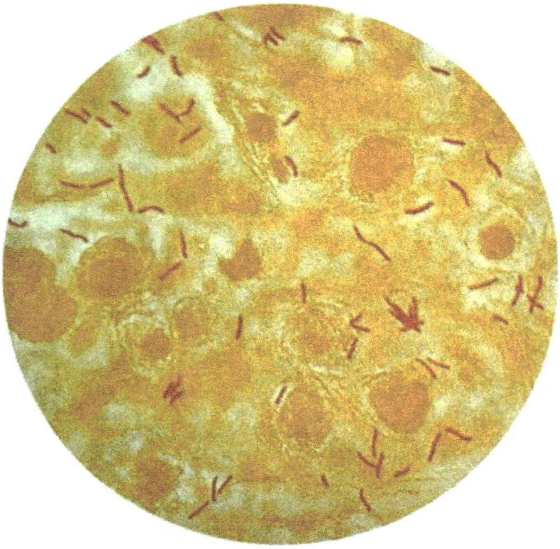

Fig. 4.7 Bright red acid-fast bacillus in sputum

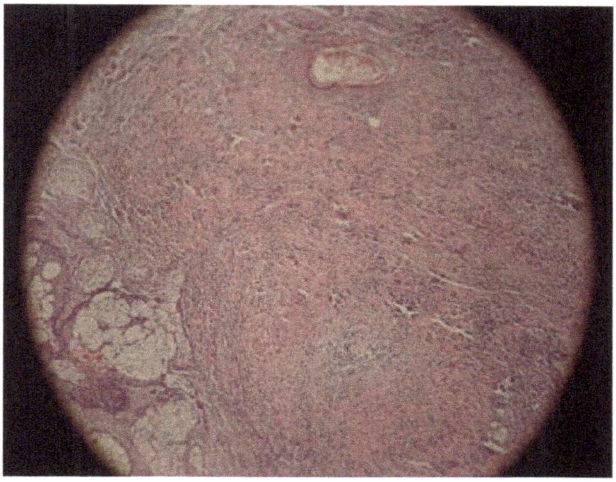

Fig. 4.8 TB histopathology Caseating granulomatous reaction, epithelioid cells, lymphocytes, and a few giant cells [9]

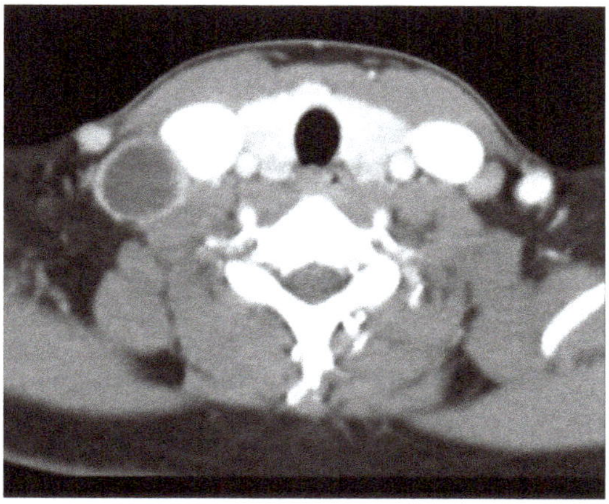

Fig. 4.9 CT neck (Axial view) showing a lymph node mass and liquefication on the right side

- Cavity formation—Indicates advanced infection and is associated with a high bacterial load.
- Noncalcified round infiltrates—May be confused with lung carcinoma.
- Homogeneously calcified nodules (usually 5–20 mm)—Tuberculomas; represent old infection rather than active disease.
- Miliary TB—Characterized by the appearance of numerous small, nodular lesions that resemble millet seeds on chest radiography.

In addition to chest X-rays, radiological examination of the soft tissue neck, chest, cervical spine and mastoids should also be carried out [7, 13].

CT neck may reveal calcified lymph nodes or matted lymphadenopathy with central liquefaction (Figs. 4.9 and 4.10). Soft tissue lesions and abscesses involving the oropharynx, hypopharynx and larynx are also well delineated on CT (Fig. 4.11).

CT paranasal sinuses delineate the sinonasal granulomas and the destruction. High-resolution CT scan of the temporal bone may demonstrate destruction of the ossicular chain, sclerosis of the mastoid cortex, and opacification of the middle ear and mastoid air cells (Fig. 4.12).

Technetium-99m (^{99m} Tc) methoxy isobutyl isonitrile single-photon emission CT (SPECT) scanning for solitary pulmonary nodules yields a high predictive value for distinguishing TB from malignancy. Therefore, it has the potential to serve as a low-cost alternative when positron emission tomography (PET) scanning is not available, especially in endemic areas.

4.5.4 The Mantoux Tuberculin Skin Test

It is often used to screen people at high risk for TB. In the Mantoux test, a standard dose of 5 tuberculin units (TU—0.1 ml) is injected intradermally (between the layers of dermis) on the

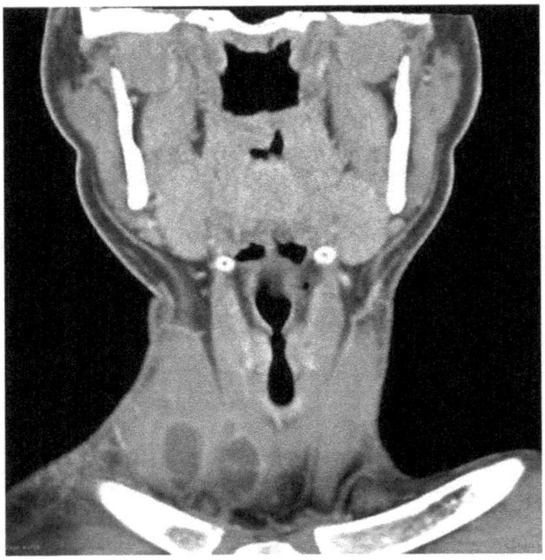

Fig. 4.10 CT neck (Coronal view) showing suppurative (central liquefication) matted lymph nodes in the right supraclavicular region

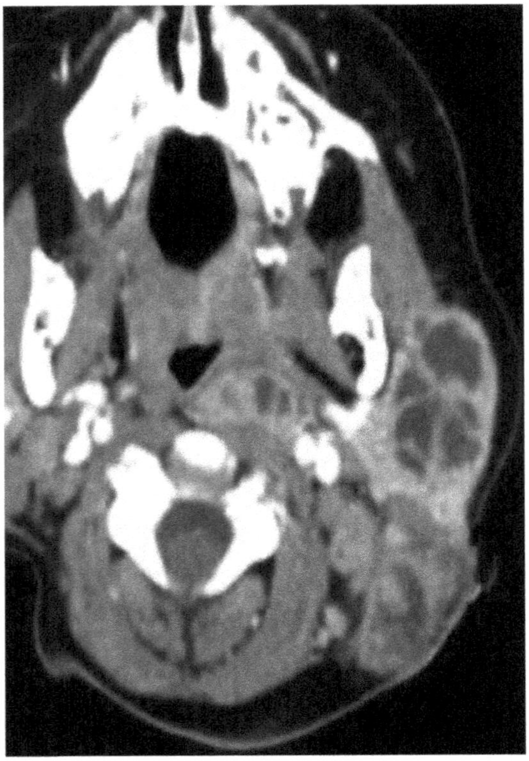

Fig. 4.11 Tuberculous lesion in the oropharynx with parapharyngeal abscess and lymphadenopathy

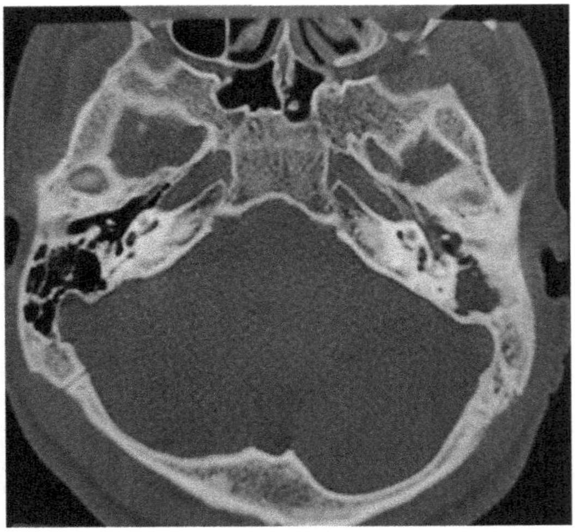

Fig. 4.12 HRCT temporal bone (axial view) showing left tympanomastoid opacification

flexor surface of the left forearm midway between elbow and wrist. When placed correctly, the injection should produce a pale wheal of the skin, 6–10 mm in diameter. The result of the test is read after 48–96 h, but 72 h (3rd day) is the ideal. This intradermal injection is termed the Mantoux technique. A person who has been exposed to the bacteria is expected to mount an immune response in the skin containing the bacterial proteins [17].

Those who have been previously immunized with the Bacille Calmette-Guerin vaccine may have a false-positive test result. The test may be falsely negative in those with sarcoidosis, Hodgkin's lymphoma, malnutrition, and most notably, active tuberculosis [9].

4.5.5 Serology

Detection of serum antibodies (Abs) to MTB antigens (TB serology) offers an alternative method for diagnosing TB. Serology does not require a specimen from the site of disease and can be scaled up into a rapid, robust, inexpensive format requiring limited laboratory infrastructure. Depending on antigens included in the serologic test, as well as study design, subjects, and site, sensitivity estimates range from 10% to 90%, and specificity estimates range from 47% to 100% [18].

Table 4.1 Recommended doses of first-line antituberculosis drugs for adults and children [21]

Drug	Recommended dose			
	Daily		3 times weekly	
	Dose and range (mg/kg body weight)	Maximum (mg)	Dose and range (mg/kg body weight)	Daily maximum (mg)
Isoniazid (H)	5 (4–6)	300	10 (8–12)	–
Rifampicin (R)	10 (8–12)	600	10 (8–12)	600
Pyrazinamide (Z)	25 (20–30)	–	35 (30–40)	–
Ethambutol (E)	Children 20 (15–25) adults 15 (15–20)	–	30 (25–35)	–
Streptomycin	15 (12–18)		15 (12–18)	

Interferon-gamma release assays, on a blood sample, are recommended in those who are positive to the Mantoux test. These are not affected by immunization or most environmental mycobacteria, so they generate fewer false-positive results [9, 18].

Interferon-γ (IFN-γ) release assays (IGR s)—The most current IGRAs are QuantiFERON®-TB Gold In-Tube (QFT; Cellistis, Ltd. Carnegie, Australia) and T-Spot TB (Oxford Immunotec, Marlborough, MA) [19]. QFT is an in vitro, enzyme-linked immunosorbent assay (ELISA), whereas T-Spot TB is an enzyme-linked immunospot assay; both have received regulatory approval in the United States for diagnosis of TB. IGRAs can reliably detect active disease and latent TB infection, but they cannot differentiate between the two. Therefore, a positive test result suggests that there is a high risk for current or future active tuberculosis. Conversely, a negative result suggests that TB infection is unlikely [19, 20].

4.5.6 Molecular Assay

4.5.6.1 Nucleic Acid Amplification Tests

Deoxyribonucleic acid (DNA) probes specific for mycobacterial ribosomal RNA identify species of clinically significant isolates after recovery. In tissue, polymerase chain reaction (PCR) amplification techniques can be used to detect *M tuberculosis*-specific DNA sequences and, thus, small numbers of mycobacteria in clinical specimens [11, 18].

Ribosomal RNA probes and DNA PCR assays allow identification within 24 h. The DNA probes are approved for direct testing on smear-positive or smear-negative sputa. However, smear-positive specimens yield higher sensitivity [18].Treatment

The standardized regimens for anti-TB treatment recommended by WHO include five essential medicines designated as "first line:" isoniazid (H), rifampicin (R), pyrazinamide (Z), ethambutol (E), and streptomycin (Table 4.1).

WHO recommends the use of fixed-dose combinations (FDCs) of drugs for the treatment of all TB patients. Several advantages of FDCs over individual medicines (or single-drug formulations) have been identified:

- Prescription errors are likely to be less frequent.
- Fewer tablets need to be ingested, which may encourage adherence to treatment.
- Patients cannot select which medicines to take (when treatment is not observed).
- Poor bioavailability of rifampicin has been found in some FDCs. The use of drug combinations of assured quality (including proven bioavailability) is essential; these medicines may be obtained through the Global Drug Facility (GDF) [21].

4.5.7 Latent TB

It is treated with either isoniazid alone or a combination of isoniazid with either Rifampicin or Rifapentine. The treatment takes at least three months. People with latent infections are treated to prevent them from progressing to active TB disease later in life [22, 23].

4.5.8 New Cases of Active TB

For treatment of new cases of pulmonary or extrapulmonary TB, WHO recommends a standardized regimen consisting of two phases. The initial (intensive) phase uses four drugs (isoniazid, rifampicin pyrazinamide and ethambutol—HRZE) administered for two months. This is followed by a continuation phase with two drugs (isoniazid and rifampicin—HR) for four months or, exceptionally, with two drugs (isoniazid and ethambutol—HE) for six months when adherence to treatment with rifampicin cannot be ensured. The preferred continuation-phase regimen is four months of rifampicin and isoniazid (4HR) administered daily or three times weekly [21].

In the continuation phase, a self-administered regimen comprising daily treatment with six months of isoniazid and ethambutol (6HE) is an option if adherence to treatment with isoniazid and rifampicin (HR) cannot be ensured; for example, in mobile populations and for patients with very limited access to health care. However, in a comparative international multicentre clinical trial, 6HE was found to be inferior to the 4HR continuation phase regimen. [21, 24]

4.5.9 Previously Treated Cases

Drug resistance is more likely to develop in previously treated patients (i.e., patients who have been treated for longer than one month) who continued to be or who became sputum smear (or culture) positive. Ideally, all previously treated patients should be assessed for drug susceptibility before initiating therapy [21].

4.5.9.1 The Standard Re-treatment Regimen Consists of

- Five drugs in the initial phase (rifampicin, isoniazid, pyrazinamide, ethambutol, and streptomycin). The initial phase is administered for 3 months, with all five drugs administered for the first two months. Streptomycin is discontinued after 2 months, and the four remaining drugs are given in the third month. WHO recommends daily administration of drugs in the initial phase.
- Three drugs in the continuation phase (rifampicin, isoniazid, and ethambutol). The continuation phase is administered for 5 months, daily or intermittently, three times a week [21].

4.5.10 Treatment of Drug-Resistant Tuberculosis

- Symptoms and radiographic findings do not differentiate multidrug-resistant TB (MDR-TB) from fully susceptible TB. MDR-TB should be suspected if the patient has a history of previous treatment for TB, was born in or lived in a country with a high prevalence of MDR-TB, has a known exposure to an MDR-TB case, or is clinically progressing despite standard TB therapy.
- Antibiotic sensitivity testing is mandatory to rule out multiple drug-resistant TB (MDR-TB). If MDR-TB is detected, treatment with at least four effective antibiotics for 18–24 months is recommended. Totally drug-resistant TB is resistant to all currently used drugs. It was first observed in 2003 in Italy but now has been widely reported, especially in Iran and India. Bedaquiline is found to be useful in multiple drug-resistant TB [19, 25].

4.5.10.1 Medication Administration

Directly observed therapy (DOT), i.e., having a health care provider watch the person take their medications, is recommended by the World Health Organization (WHO) in an effort to reduce the number of people not appropriately taking antibiotics [26].

4.5.10.2 Duration of Treatment

The recommended duration of treatment is guided by smear and culture conversion. The minimal recommendation is that treatment lasts for at least 18 months after culture conversion; extension to 24 months may be indicated in chronic cases with extensive pulmonary damage [21, 24].

The principles of anti-TB treatment are the same irrespective of HIV status. Although ethambutol and isoniazid are included in recommendations for the continuation phase, short-course regimens that contain rifampicin throughout have better outcomes, and reduce the risk of TB recurrence. The use of thioacetazone is contraindicated in HIV-infected individuals because of the risk of fatal hypersensitivity reactions and is discouraged by WHO because of the risk of severe toxicity. Ethambutol should replace thioacetazone, especially in areas where HIV is prevalent [21].

4.5.10.3 Surgical Management

It is usually required for complications of tuberculosis and includes excision of upper airway granulomas to maintain airway patency, tracheostomy in case of extensive laryngeal granulomas, drainage of neck abscess and tympanomastoidectomy for tuberculous otitis media.

4.5.10.4 Vaccination

Albert Calmette and Camille Guerin, in 1906, invented an immunization against tuberculosis called Bacille Calmette-Guerin (BCG) [25] Till now, it has been the most widely used vaccine. In children, it decreases the risk of getting the infection by 20% and the risk of infection turning into the active disease by nearly 60% [25].

4.6 Essential Features

- Tuberculosis (TB) is a chronic granulomatous, infectious, and communicable disease caused by *Mycobacterium tuberculosis*. In the developing world, *M. bovis* causes oropharyngeal and intestinal TB.
- Very prevalent, approximately 1.7 billion people are infected with 9 million new cases a year, with an estimated 1.6 million deaths.
- Transmission is from person to person via airborne droplets, and infections may be dormant for years.
- AIDS patients are more susceptible to TB and have more severe disease.
- There is also increased risk with alcoholism, immunosuppression (immunotherapy with
- TNF antagonists, lymphoma, especially Hodgkin lymphoma), chronic renal disease and chronic lung disease.
- Two major disease patterns are primary tuberculosis and secondary tuberculosis.
- Primary TB is characterized by the Ghon complex. Secondary TB causes florid and widespread granulomatous inflammation.
- Extrapulmonary manifestations can occur in primary or secondary TB evolving from pulmonary focus or by haematogenic dissemination.
- Extrapulmonary manifestations include cervical lymphadenopathy being the commonest, otitis media, granulomatous lesions of hypopharynx and larynx, oral cavity ulcers and granulomas, oropharyngeal lesions and nasal granulomas.
- The acid-fast bacillus is cultured from the body secretions such as sputum, nasal secretions, ear discharge, laryngotracheal secretions, bronchial lavage, pus from the discharging sinuses, lymph node aspirates or the swab collected from nose, throat and laryngeal ulcers.
- Typical histopathological picture shows macrophages, T lymphocytes, B lymphocytes, and fibroblasts aggregating to form granulomas, with lymphocytes and multinucleated giant cells surrounding the infected macrophages with or without caseation.
- HRCT help in early diagnosis by delineating nodular infiltrates, abscess, and granulomatous lesions.
- Interferon-γ (IFN-γ) release assays (IGR s) can reliably detect active disease and latent TB infection.
- Ribosomal RNA probes and DNA PCR assays allow identification within 24 h.
- WHO recommended standardized regimens for anti-TB treatment include five essential

medicines isoniazid (H), rifampicin (R), pyrazinamide (Z), ethambutol (E), and streptomycin (S).

- Multidrug-resistant TB and extensive drug-resistant TB have recently emerged as clinical and public health challenges that have come about, at least in part from incomplete compliance with drug treatment regimens.

References

1. McCarthy OR. The key to the sanatoria. J R Soc Med. 2001;94(8):413–7.
2. Ferri FF. Ferri's differential diagnosis : a practical guide to the differential diagnosis of symptoms, signs, and clinical disorders. 2nd ed. Philadelphia, PA: Elsevier/Mosby; 2010. Chapter T. isbn 978-0-323-07699-9
3. Vashishtha VM. Current status of tuberculosis and acute respiratory infections in India: much more needs to be done! Indian Pediatr. 2010;47(1):88–9. https://doi.org/10.1007/s13312-010-0005-6.
4. Hawn TR, et al. Tuberculosis vaccines and prevention of infection. Microbiol Mol Biol Rev. 2014;78(4):650–71.
5. Harris RE. Epidemiology of chronic disease: global perspectives. Jones & Bartlett Learning: Burlington, MA; 2013. p. 682. isbn 978-0-7637-8047-0
6. Organization, World Health. Implementing the WHO stop TB strategy: a handbook for national TB control programmers. Geneva: World Health Organization (WHO); 2008. p. 179. isbn 978-92-4-154667-6
7. Lee KC, Schecter G. Tuberculous infections of head and neck. Ear Nose Throat J. 1995;74(6):395–9.
8. Kumar V, et al. Robbins basic pathology. 8th ed. Philadelphia: Saunders Elsevier; 2007. p. 516–22. isbn 978-1-4160-2973-1
9. Mota LAA, et al. ENT Manifestations in Tuberculosis. Tuberculosis- Expanding knowledge book. Published on July 8th 2015. https://doi.org/10.5772/59664
10. Kommareddi S, et al. Nontuberculous mycobacterial infections: comparison of the fluorescent auramine-O and Ziehl-Neelsen techniques in tissue diagnosis. Hum Pathol. 1984;15(11):1085–9.
11. Sharma S. ENT manifestations in Tuberculosis: an important aspect of ENT practice. Pan African Medical J. 2020 Aug 17;36:295.
12. Golden MP, Vikram HR. Extrapulmonary tuberculosis: an overview. Am Fam Physician. 2005;72(9):1761–8.
13. Harney M, et al. Laryngeal tuberculosis: an important diagnosis. J Laryngol Otol. 2000;114(11):878–80.
14. Sharma SK, Mohan A. Extrapulmonary disease. Indian J Med Res. 2004;120:316–53.
15. Madison BM. Application of stains in clinical microbiology. Biotech Histochem. 2001 May;76(3):119–25.
16. Krishna SB, et al. Laryngeal tuberculosis: a rare case report. J Pharm Biomed Sci. 2014;04(06):497–501.
17. TB Elimination - Tuberculin Skin Testing (PDF). CDC.gov. CDC – National Center for HIV/AIDS, Viral Hepatitis, STD, and TB prevention – division of tuberculosis elimination. October 2011. Retrieved 5 June 2017.
18. Achkar JM, et al. Adjunctive tests for diagnosis of tuberculosis: serology, ELISPOT for site-specific lymphocytes, urinary Lipoarabinomannan, string test, and fine needle aspiration. J Infect Dis. 2011 Nov 15;204(Suppl 4):S1130–41. https://doi.org/10.1093/infdis/jir450.
19. World Health Organization (WHO). Latent tuberculosis infection. Geneva: World Health Organization (WHO); 2018. p. 23. isbn 978-92-4-155023-9
20. Sosa LE, et al. Tuberculosis screening, testing, and treatment of U.S. health care personnel: recommendations from the national tuberculosis controllers association and CDC, 2019. MMWR Morb Mortal Wkly Rep. 2019;68(19):439–43.
21. Implementing the WHO Stop TB strategy: a handbook for national tuberculosis control programmes. Chap. 2.
22. Bento J, et al. Diagnostic tools in tuberculosis. Acta Medica Portuguesa. 2011;24(1):145–54.
23. Diseases, Special Programme for Research & Training in Tropical. Diagnostics for tuberculosis: global demand and market potential. Geneva: World Health Organization (WHO); 2006. p. 36. isbn 978-92-4-156330-7
24. World Health Organization. Guidance for national tuberculosis programmes on the management of tuberculosis in children. Geneva: World Health Organization; 2006. (WHO/HTM/TB/2006.371; WHO/FCH/CAH/2006.7)
25. Jacob JT, et al. Acute forms of tuberculosis in adults. Am J Med. 2009;122(1):12–7.
26. Brennan PJ, Nikaido H. The envelope of mycobacteria. Annu Rev Biochem. 1995;64:29–63.

5 Syphilis

Abstract

Syphilis is a systemic bacterial infection caused by the spirochete Treponema pallidum. Due to its many protean clinical manifestations, it has been named the "great imitator and mimicker." Syphilis is an important synergistic infection for HIV acquisition. Syphilis presents in three stages, denoted as primary, secondary, and tertiary. The primary lesion appears at the site of infection and is characterized by healing ulcers. Since the secondary stage is due to the systemic spread of the spirochetes beyond the primary infection site, early treatment during the primary stage is important. Oral presentation of syphilis, such as ulceration, mucous patches, and maculopapular lesions, is most commonly occurring at the secondary stage and is more seldom a sign of primary disease. Involvement of the central nervous system like cognitive symptoms, ataxia, and paralysis may occur in all stages but is often associated with the tertiary stage. Further typical manifestations of the tertiary stage are gumma and generalized glossitis. A cardiovascular syphilis may also occur in the tertiary stage. Dark field microscopy, serology, in combination with a thorough clinical examination, is commonly used for diagnosis. Benzathine penicillin G still remains the gold standard treatment. Surgical management is in the form of excision of gumma or reconstruction.

5.1 Background

Syphilis is a sexually transmitted disease caused by the bacteria spirochete "*Treponema pallidum*." Although there is some debate about its origin, the symptom complex of syphilis and its sexual transmission was clearly described in the fifteenth century. The disease draws its name from the afflicted shepherd, "Syphilis," whose symptoms were described in the early 1500s by the poet-pathologist "Frascatorius" [1, 2] *Treponema pallidum* was identified as the agent that causes syphilis in 1905 by German scientists, and one year later, the test to diagnose this infection was developed. Its genome was sequenced in 1998 [2].

5.2 Epidemiology

Although the incidence of syphilitic infections has dramatically decreased in the last 40 years, small epidemics of these infections continue to occur [1]. It affects between 700,000 and 1.6 million pregnancies a year, resulting in spontaneous abortions, stillbirths, and congeni-

S. V. Nemade, K. J. Shinde, *Granulomatous diseases in Otorhinolaryngology, Head and Neck*,
https://doi.org/10.1007/978-981-16-4047-6_5

tal syphilis. It is estimated that there are more than 12 million cases per year in the world. The incubation period is usually 21–30 days after contact, although it can vary from 10 to 90 days, depending on the number and virulence of Treponemas and the host response [1, 2]. Syphilis increases the risk of HIV transmission by 2–5 times, and co-infection is common (30–60% in urban centers). Untreated, it has a mortality rate of 8–58%, with a greater death rate in males [3].

5.3 Etiopathogenesis

"*Treponema pallidum*" is a fragile spiral bacterium 6–15 micrometers long by 0.25 micrometers in diameter. It is frequently transmitted when infectious lesions come into contact with abraded skin or mucous membrane. Most commonly, this contact occurs during sexual contact, although materno-fetal transmission in congenital syphilis represents a clear exception. Transmission by blood transfusion or needle sharing is rare. The risk of infection after sexual contact is higher when the infected partner is in the early stages of syphilis; contact with partners with latent disease presents a low risk of transmission [1–3]. In acquired syphilis, *T. Pallidum* rapidly penetrates intact mucous membranes or microscopic dermal abrasions and, within few hours, enters the lymphatics and blood to produce systemic infection. The incubation period from exposure to development of primary lesions, which occur at the primary site of inoculation, averages 3 weeks but can range from 10 to 90 days [1–4].

The clinical sequelae of *T. pallidum* infection are divided into stages. Primary syphilis is defined by the presence of a chancre at the site of treponemal inoculation. Secondary syphilis represents hematogenous spirochete dissemination and is commonly followed by a latent or asymptomatic phase. Following this latent phase, patients may progress to develop symptoms of tertiary syphilis [4, 5].

5.3.1 Primary Syphilis

Primary syphilis is defined by the presence of a lesion referred to as a chancre, at the site of inoculation. These lesions tend to be indurated, ulcerated, and painless. Chancres are seen between 10 and 90 days after inoculation and most commonly occur on the external genitalia but may be noted in the oral, nasal or anal mucosa. The chancre is often accompanied by firm regional lymphadenopathy that is non-tender. Primary lesions heal spontaneously within a few weeks [2–5].

5.3.2 Secondary Syphilis

The clinical manifestations of secondary syphilis result from hematogenous dissemination of the infection and are protean: condyloma lata (papulosquamous eruption), hands and feet lesions, macular rash, diffuse lymphadenopathy, headache, myalgia, arthralgia, pharyngitis, hepatosplenomegaly, alopecia, and malaise. As a result, syphilis has been named the great imitator [2]. Epithelial surfaces are frequently involved, resulting in a wide variety of cutaneous and mucus membrane manifestations.

The condyloma lata is another lesion found in secondary syphilis. These are large, raised, white, or gray lesions found in warm, moist areas. These lesions are found near the site of the original chancre (perineum or anus) and are thought to result from direct rather than hematogenous treponemal spread [5, 6].

5.3.3 Tertiary Syphilis (Gummatous Syphilis)

It is characterized by destructive granulomatous lesions (gummata) that involve epithelial, skeletal, or visceral tissue throughout the body. Cutaneous gummas are indurated, nodular, papulomatous, or ulcerative lesions that form characteristic circles or arcs with peripheral hyperpigmentation [5–7].

5.3.4 Congenital Syphilis

Materno-fetal transmission rates are highly dependent on the stage of maternal syphilis. Children born to parents with primary or secondary syphilis virtually always carry the disease; half are born prematurely or die in the perinatal period, whereas the other half develop congenital syphilis [6–8] Early congenital syphilis occurs within the first 2 years of life. Late congenital syphilis emerges in children older than 2 years. After age 2 years, parents may note problems with the child's hearing and language development and with vision [14–16].

The relationship between HIV and syphilis is more than the concomitant transmission of sexually transmitted diseases [2]. Syphilis produces genital lesions and evokes a systemic inflammatory response; both may lead to increased transmission of HIV [3, 4]. Concomitant infection of HIV is believed to increase the incidence of neurosyphilis and benign tertiary syphilis [5–7]. Patients diagnosed with syphilis should be tested for HIV.

5.4 Clinical Features

5.4.1 Ear Manifestations

The ear is affected in both congenital and acquired syphilis and is a late manifestation of the disease. Characteristic symptoms include unexplained sensorineural hearing loss and Meniere's disease with fluctuating tinnitus and episodic vertigo. Several pathogenic mechanisms have been proposed, such as direct spirochete perilymphatic invasion, temporal bone osteitis, and microvascular inflammation and infarction. Patients with acute meningeal syphilis have a 20% incidence of significant sensorineural hearing loss, which is frequently associated with other cranial neuropathies [9].

The hearing loss of otosyphilis typically begins at high frequency and often progresses to a complete loss of bilateral cochlear and vestibular function.

Middle ear involvement causes fibrosis involving the ossicular chain, especially incudomalleolar joint and stapes footplate. This may lead to conductive hearing loss. Fibrosis between the stapes footplate and membranous labyrinth can result in a false-positive fistula test of Hennebert's sign (a fistula sign without a fistula) [10–12]

5.4.2 The Oral Cavity and Oropharyngeal Manifestations

In primary syphilis, other than the genitalia, the lips are the second most common site of initial spirochete inoculation and chancre formation [12]. Other sites are tongue and tonsil [13]. The mucous patches of secondary syphilis may present throughout the upper aerodigestive tract especially involving lips, tongue, and buccal mucosa (Figs. 5.1 and 5.2). Mucosal lesions may be associated with cutaneous macules on the palms of the hands and brackets (Fig. 5.2a). Secondary syphilis may present as pharyngitis or tonsillitis Hypertrophy of the Waldeyer's ring with associated adenopathy is common.

Tertiary syphilis is characterized by serpiginous ulcers, typically of the tonsil and soft palate (Fig. 5.3). Another characteristic feature is the "Gumma." It is in the stage of infiltration with granulomatous inflammation and may get ulcerated with regional lymphadenopathy mimicking malignancy. It is single or multiple within the oral cavity, including the tongue or palate [13]. Perforations leading to oronasal, oroantral fistula, and adhesions in the oropharynx may occur in this stage.

The oral cavity is commonly affected by congenital syphilis. Mucous patches on tongue, palate, and lips may become fissured and hemorrhagic [14]. Other typical feature of congenital syphilis is "Hutchinson's teeth" (Fig. 5.4). In this, teeth are notched, hypoplastic, and lack enamel. These children are also at risk for gummata, which may be present anywhere in the upper aerodigestive tract [14–16].

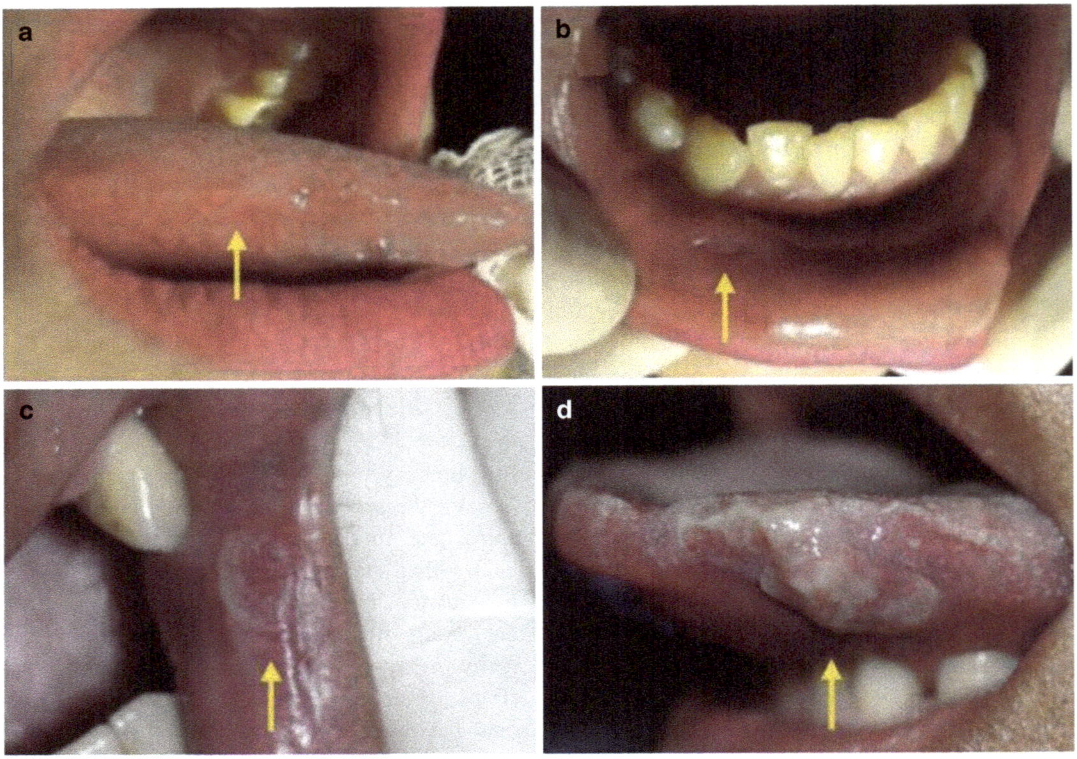

Fig. 5.1 Different patterns of clinical presentation of secondary syphilis. (**a**) Grayish white lesion on the lateral border of the right tongue. (**b**) Circular ulcer and well delimited in asymptomatic lower labial mucosa (**c**) Ulcerated lesion with fibrinous borders at the commissure of the lips. (**d**) Exuberant mucous plate present on the tongue (left) caused volume increase and remodeling on the superficial relief of the tongue [27]

5.4.3 The Larynx and Hypopharyngeal Manifestations

Primary syphilis may cause chancre involving epiglottis. Symptoms are limited to cough and foreign body sensation in the throat. It shows spontaneous recovery within weeks. Secondary syphilis involves the mucosa of the hypopharynx and larynx with resultant laryngitis and hoarseness. It is typically known as "syphilitic catarrh of larynx." Hoarseness may also occur in tertiary syphilis as a result of either laryngeal injury or damage to the recurrent laryngeal nerve. Tertiary syphilis- Gummata of the larynx may directly cause hoarseness, or they may scar and result in subglottic stenosis, adhesion between the vocal folds, or arytenoid fixation [13]. It may lead to airway obstruction and dyspnoea. Perichondritis and necrosis of laryngeal cartilages may occur. Dysfunction of the recurrent laryngeal nerve may be seen with neurosyphilis or with cardiovascular syphilis-induced aortic aneurysms that compress the recurrent laryngeal nerve [13].

5.4.4 The Nose and Nasopharyngeal Manifestations

Primary syphilis of the nose is rare but has been reported to occur commonly at the mucocutaneous junction in the nasal vestibule, however, it may involve the dorsum of the nose, too [12, 13]. Secondary syphilis may present as acute rhinitis with a thick discharge and irritation of the anterior nares.

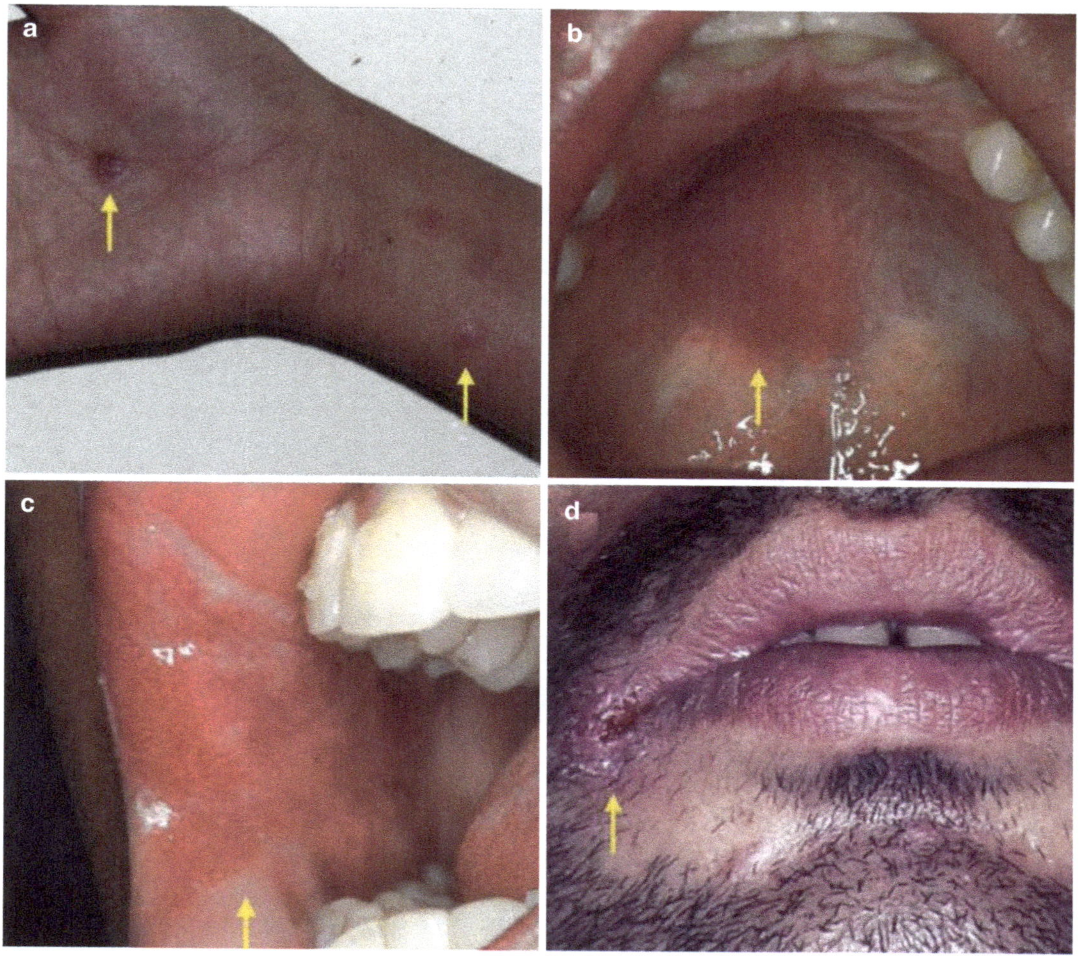

Fig. 5.2 Oral and cutaneous clinical aspect of secondary syphilis (**a**) Reddish macules present in the palms of the hands and brackets. (**b**) Erythematous lesion present on the hard palate. (**c**) Extensive mucosal plaque present with erythematous areas in the region of labial commissure and oral mucosa. (**d**) Ulcerated lesion present in labial commissure [27]

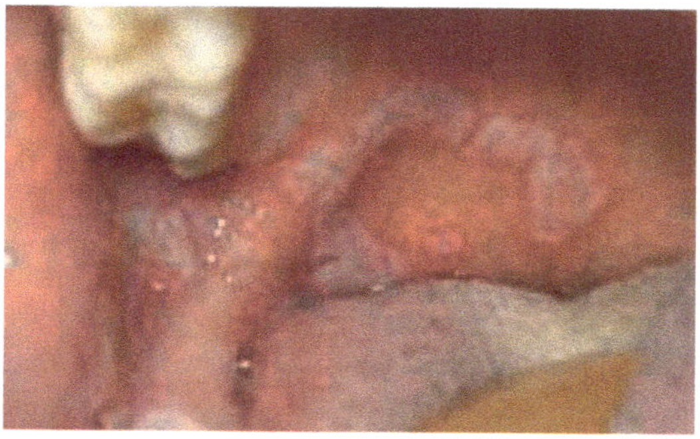

Fig. 5.3 Sepeginous (Snail Track) ulcer on the soft palate extending to the anterior pillar

Tertiary syphilis may develop gummata of the nose. The mucinous defense and the ciliary function of the nasal barrier are disturbed. Hyperallergic response to pathogens leads to the granulomatous reaction of the tissue with soft circumscribed swelling and inflammatory mucosa with ulceration (Fig. 5.5) [28]. The septal perichondritis with necrosis leading to septal perforation is common. Syphilitic ozoena with atrophic rhinitis may be seen. Destruction of the bony septum may lead to saddle nose deformity. Perichondritis, necrosis of lateral cartilages of the

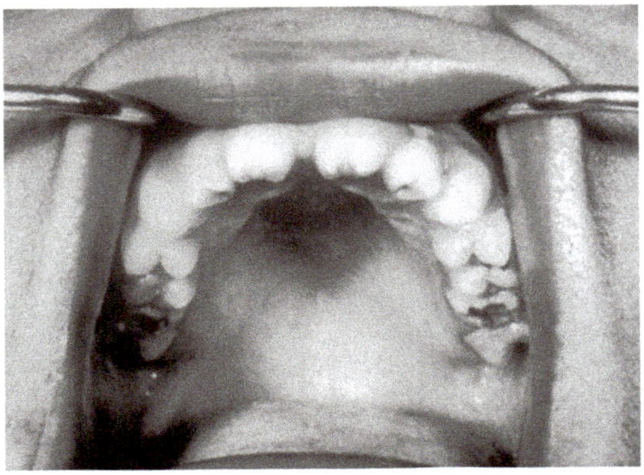

Fig. 5.4 Hutchinson's teeth: Notched incisors seen in congenital syphilis

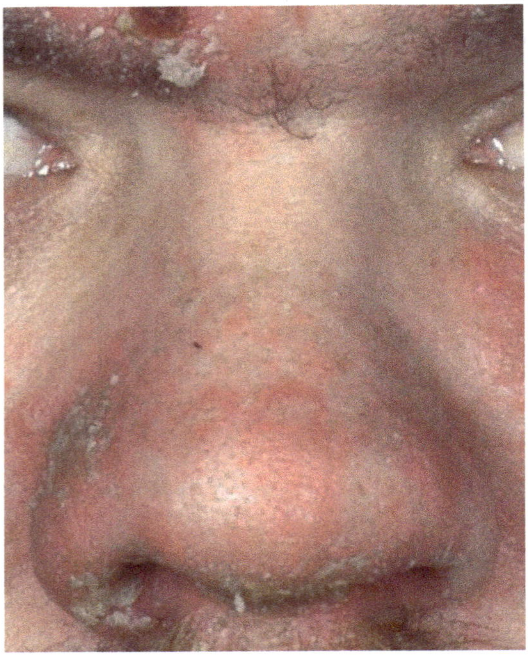

Fig. 5.5 Nasal gumma of tertiary syphilis [28]

nose and vestibular stenosis may also contribute to the external nasal deformity.

St. Clair Thomson states that "one of the first guiding principles to bear in mind is that necrosis in the nose is almost unknown except in connection with syphilis." [17, 28]

Congenital syphilis- The earliest symptom that occurs prior to age 2 years is rhinitis (snuffles) (Fig. 5.6), soon followed by cutaneous

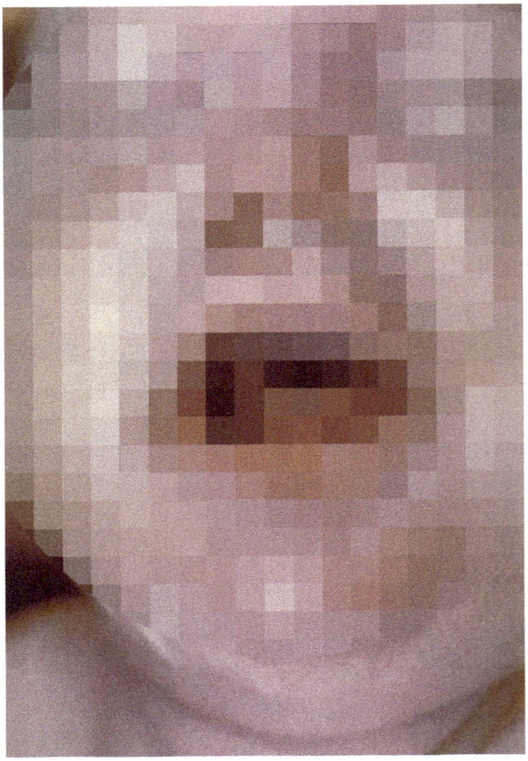

Fig. 5.6 "Snuffles" seen in congenital syphilis

lesions. Nasal discharge is the earliest sign, occurring 1–2 weeks before the rash. This watery discharge contains high concentrations of spirochetes. Over time the discharge becomes thick and purulent, then bloody. The resulting nasal obstruction may interfere with feeding. Erosion of the septal cartilage may occur, thus compromising nasal dorsum integrity. The incidence of the symptoms ranges from 10% to 75% in various series [14, 15].

Tertiary syphilis rarely affects the nasopharynx. A case of an extensive lesion resulting in ophthalmoplegia and blindness has been reported, along with stenosis of the nasopharynx from extensive scarring [16, 17].

Other system involvement: It is seen in secondary and tertiary syphilis. Hepatosplenomegaly, nephropathy, optic neuritis, and arthritis may occur. A small number of patients develop acute syphilitic meningitis and present with headaches, neck stiffness, facial numbness or weakness, and deafness.

Tertiary (late) syphilis is slowly progressive and may affect any organ. The disease is generally not thought to be infectious at this stage. Manifestations may include the following:

- Impaired balance, paresthesias, incontinence, and impotence
- Focal neurologic findings, including sensorineural hearing and vision loss
- Dementia
- Chest pain, back pain, stridor, or other symptoms related to aortic aneurysms

The lesions of gummatous tertiary syphilis usually develop within 3–10 years of infection. The patient complaints are usually secondary to bone pain, which is described as a deep pain characteristically worse at night. Trauma may predispose a specific site to gumma involvement.

Some patients may present up to 20 years after infection with behavioral changes and other signs of dementia, which is indicative of paresis [29].

5.5 Diagnosis

Syphilitic ulcer (Chancre) is to be differentiated from tubercular ulcer and the ulcer of Diphtheria. Diphtheria ulcer has the characteristic membrane. The syphilitic ulcer shows a typical "punched out" appearance (excavated ulcer) and the "wash leather" base and is usually not very painful. Tubercular ulcers lack these typical features and are usually very painful.

5.5.1 Clinical Diagnosis is Aided by the Following Diagnostic Tests [18]

Darkfield examination, serologic tests, and histopathologic studies.

5.5.2 Darkfield Examination

It is most useful when moist lesions with abundant spirochetes are available. Lesions of primary syphilis (chancres), secondary syphilis (mucous patches, condyloma lata), and of regional lymph nodes may also be used. Treponema is a very tiny organism that is invisible on light microscopy. Thus, it is identified by its distinct spiral movements on darkfield microscopy. Outside the body, it does not survive for long; hence the collected specimens must be evaluated immediately. The sensitivity of darkfield examination approaches 80%. Darkfield examination using fluorescent antibodies is also available and confers a higher sensitivity [19].

5.5.3 Serologic Tests

These include two categories, nontreponemal and treponemal.

Four nontreponemal tests are currently used. Venereal disease research laboratory (VDRL) slide test, unheated serum regain (USR), RPR (Rapid plasma reagin test), and toluidine red untreated serum test (TRUST). These tests measure antibody response to cellular particles released as a result of treponemal infection. Because other disease processes may cause the release of similar antigens, these tests are relatively nonspecific. Systemic lupus erythematosus, diseases with immunoglobulin abnormalities, leprosy, intravenous drug abuse, and malignancy may all cause chronic elevation of nontreponemal titers. Hepatitis, malaria, pregnancy, mononucleosis, and other viral infections have been noted to cause an acute elevation in nontreponemal titers. Despite these confounding factors, nontreponemal tests may be used either as qualitative screening examinations or as quantitative tests to follow treatment. Because of its nonspecific nature, a positive nontreponemal test does not confirm *T. pallidum* infection in the absence of other evidence for the diagnosis of syphilis. After successful treatment or eradication of the disease, nontreponemal tests are no longer positive [20].

Treponemal tests (FTA-ABS and microhemagglutination-*Treponema pallidum* [MHA-TP] use *T. pallidum* as the antigen and are based on the detection of antibodies against treponemal components. These tests are used primarily to verify the accuracy of nontreponemal tests. For nearly all syphilis patients, the treponemal tests remain positive for life even if the disease is eradicated. These tests are not quantified and may not be used to monitor disease progression [20].

Examination of the spinal fluid is useful in determining the presence of neurosyphilis. The VDRL test is most frequently used for the examination of cerebrospinal fluid. The FTA-ABS test should not be used with cerebrospinal fluid because trace amounts of blood in the cerebrospinal fluid may lead to a false-positive result in patients with seropositive syphilis [21, 31].

5.5.4 Histopathology

Histopathology reveals lichenoid superficial and deep perivascular and periadnexal lymphohistiocytic inflammation with admixed plasma cells. The marked proliferation of blood vessels can be seen. The characteristic feature of late secondary syphilis and tertiary syphilis is the gumma. Gumma is granulomatous inflammation with central necrosis flanked by plump or palisaded macrophages and fibrocytes surrounded by the large number of mononuclear leukocytes, including many plasma cells (Fig. 5.7) [13, 27].

Pathologic examination using silver staining has a sensitivity of 33–71%, however, immunohistochemistry directed against *T. Pallidum* improved both sensitivity and specificity [31].

5.5.5 Imaging

Primary syphilis and many manifestations of secondary syphilis do not exhibit any radiologic features.

CT scan—Bone lesions in late disease and bone destruction secondary to syphilitic gumma are best revealed by computed tomography (Fig. 5.8) [26].

MRI scan—It is particularly helpful in neurosyphilis where involvement of meninges, leptomeningeal vessels, brain parenchyma and spinal cord tracts is better delineated [26].

In the vast majority of cases, gummas have a very varied appearance across CT and MRI and are often mistaken for malignancy [26].

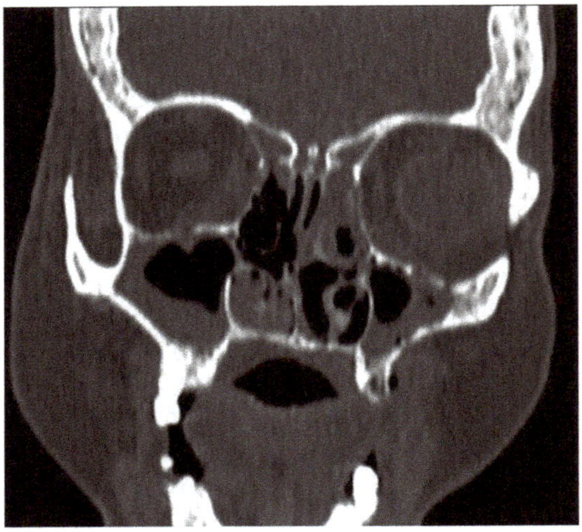

Fig. 5.8 CT PNS (Coronal view) showing complete destruction of bony and cartilaginous nasal septum

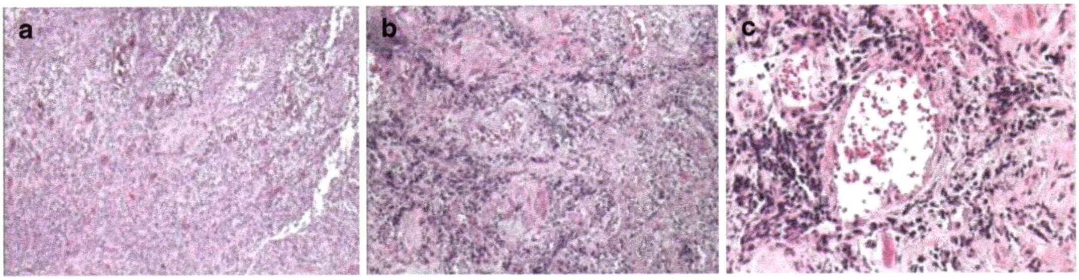

Fig. 5.7 Histopathological aspects of oral syphilis. (**a**) Hyperplasia of the epithelium. (**b**) A dense and diffuse chronic inflammatory infiltrate, composed mainly of lymphocytes and plasma cells, in the lamina propria. (**c**) The inflammatory infiltrates extended to the deeper area of the lamina propria showing a perivascular pattern [27]

Chest X-ray is helpful in tertiary syphilis to screen for aortic dilatation. Angiography may be useful to distinguish between abdominal aneurysms of syphilitic vs. arteriosclerotic origin [30].

Slit-lamp examination and ophthalmic assessment can be used to differentiate between acquired and congenital syphilis (presence of interstitial keratitis) in patients with latent infection of uncertain duration [30].

The diagnosis of congenital syphilis is complicated by the ability of maternal antibodies to cross the placenta and confound immunologic testing of the infant. Identification of spirochetes on darkfield microscopy, silver stain, or by immunofluorescence of suspicious lesions or body fluids (bullous rash or nasal discharge) represents the only true confirmation of congenital syphilis [14–16].

5.6 Treatment

Treatment is with penicillin and steroids. Benzathine Penicillin G, given parenterally, is the Gold standard treatment for syphilis. The preparation of penicillin used, dose, and duration of treatment depend on the manifestations. Several authors have demonstrated that intramuscular penicillin does not achieve treponemicidal levels in the cerebrospinal fluid or perilymph; thus, intravenous penicillin is recommended for patients with Otosyphilis and neurosyphilis [22, 23].

Treatment may result in the Jarish-Herxheimer reaction, an acute febrile illness that may occur in the first 24 h following treatment. Myalgias, headache, and other constitutional symptoms may manifest. Fetal distress in pregnant patients has been reported. All patients being treated with syphilis should be warned of these symptoms and may be treated with antipyretics [24].

5.6.1 Primary, Secondary, and Early Tertiary Disease

5.6.1.1 First-Line Treatment

- Benzathine Penicillin G 2.4 × 10^6 units, single intramuscular dose.
- Doxycycline 100 mg, taken twice a day orally for 14 days. Alternate treatment.
- Ceftriaxone 1gm, intravenous/intramuscular once a day for 10 days.
- Procaine Penicillin G 1.2 × 10^6 units, intramuscular once a day for 10 days.
- Azithromycin 2 gm single oral dose.

5.6.2 Late Tertiary Disease

5.6.2.1 First-Line Treatment

- Benzathine Penicillin G 2.4 × 10^6 units, intramuscular once weekly for 3 weeks.
- Doxycycline 100 mg, taken orally twice a day for 28 days.

5.6.2.2 Alternate Treatment

- Ceftriaxone 1gm, intravenous/intramuscular once a day for 10 days.
- Procaine Penicillin G 1.2 × 10^6 units, intramuscular once a day for 14–21 days [25].

Jarisch Herxheimer Reaction—Following treatment with penicillin, the dying organisms often release inflammatory cytokines that lead to the Jarisch Herxheimer reaction. The symptoms include headache, muscle pain, fever, tachycardia, and malaise. The reaction usually appears within 24 h of starting treatment. The treatment is supportive. Pregnant women who develop this reaction need to be observed closely, as it can lead to obstetric complications [31].

5.6.3 Surgical Management

- Ear—Incudomalleolar joint fixation may be corrected by ossiculoplasty.
- Nose—After completion of pharmacotherapy, correction of septal perforation and rhinoplasty for correction of the external nasal deformity is considered.
- Larynx—Acute airway obstruction may warrant tracheostomy till the completion of pharmacotherapy.
- Surgical closure of oronasal or oroantral fistula and adhesiolysis [23, 24].

5.7 Essential Features

- Syphilis is an infectious disease caused by the spirochete *Treponema pallidum*. The causative agent is pathogenic only for humans, and it is transmitted through sexual contact or vertically across the placenta.
- The disease progresses in three stages. Staging is important because it is the basis of management (treatment, prognosis, follow-up, and partner screening).
- Primary Stage: The characteristic feature is painless open sore "chancre" Because syphilis is usually spread with sexual contact, chancres are found in the mouth, anus, or in the genital area.
- Secondary Stage: Secondary syphilis is characterized by widespread clinical manifestations resulting from hematogenous spirochete dissemination. Condyloma lata and cutaneous manifestations are common presentations.
- Tertiary Syphilis: It is characterized by destructive granulomatous lesions (gummata) that involve epithelial, skeletal, or visceral tissue throughout the body.
- Congenital Syphilis: The earliest symptom is snuffles followed by a cutaneous rash. Mucous patches on tongue, palate, and lips may occur. Other typical feature of congenital syphilis is "Hutchinson's teeth."
- High index of suspicion for syphilis in any sexually active patient with genital lesions or rashes. Co-infection with HIV is common (30–60%).
- Diagnosis is usually based on serology using combination of treponemal and nontreponemal tests.
- Benzathine penicillin G still remains the gold standard treatment. Surgical management is in the form of excision of gumma or reconstruction.

References

1. Cates W, et al. Syphilis control. The historic context and epidemiologic basis for interrupting sexual transmission of Treponema pallidum. Sex Transm Dis. 1996;23(1):68–75.
2. Peeling RW, Hook EW. The pathogenesis of syphilis: the great mimicker, revisited. J Pathol. 2006 Jan;208(2):224–32.
3. Quinn TC, et al. The association of syphilis with risk of human immunodeficiency virus infection in patients attending sexually transmitted disease clinics. Arch Intern Med. 1990;150:1297.
4. Hutchinson CM, et al. Characteristics of patients with syphilis attending Baltimore STD clinics: multiple high-risk subgroups and interactions with human immunodeficiency virus infections. Arch Intern Med. 1991;141:511.
5. Smith ME, Canalis RF. Otologic manifestations of AIDS: the otosyphilis connection. Laryngoscope. 1989;99:365–72.
6. Kearns G, et al. Intraoral tertiary syphilis (Gumma) in a human immunodeficiency virus-positive man: a case report. J Oral Maxillofac Surg. 1993;51:85.
7. Sule RR, et al. Late cutaneous syphilis. Cutis. 1997;59:135.
8. Kasmin F, et al. Syphilitic gastritis in an HIV infected individual. Am J Gastroenterol. 1992;87:1820.
9. Wilcox RR, Goodwin PG. Nerve deafness in early syphilis. Br J Vener Dis. 1971;47:401.
10. Belal A, Stewart TJ. Pathological changes in the middle ear joints. Ann Otol Rhinol Laryngol. 1974;83(5):158–67.
11. Nadol JB. Positive "fistula sign" with an intact tympanic membrane. Arch Otolaryngol. 1974;100:273–8.
12. Fiumara NJ. Venereal diseases of the oral cavity. J Oral Med. 1976;31:36–40.
13. McNulty JS, Fassett RL. Syphilis: an otolaryngologic perspective. Laryngoscope. 1981;91:889–905.
14. Nabarro D. Congenital syphilis. London: E. Arnold; 1954.
15. Platou RV. Treatment of congenital syphilis with penicillin. Adv Pediatr Infect Dis. 1949;4:39.
16. Bowen V, et al. Increase in incidence of congenital syphilis – United States, 2012–2014. MMWR Morb Mortal Wkly Rep. 2015 Nov 13;64:1241–5.
17. Gager WE, et al. Nasopharyngeal syphilis with blindness. Arch Otolaryngol. 1969;90(11):125–30.
18. Ramstadt T. And Traaholt L destruction of the soft palate by tertiary "benign" syphilis: a case report. J Oral Rehab. 1980;7:111–5.
19. Daniels KC, Ferneyhough HS. Specific direct fluorescent antibody detection of Treponema pallidum. Health Lab Sci. 1977;14:164–71.
20. Schroeter AL, et al. Treatment of early syphilis and reactivity of serologic tests. JAMA. 1972;221:471–6.
21. Davis LE, Sperry S. The CSF-FTA test and significance of blood contamination. Ann Neurol. 1979;6:68–9.
22. Wiet RJ, Milko DM. Isolation of spirochetes in the perilymph despite prior antisyphilitic therapy. Arch Otolaryngol. 1975;101:104–6.
23. Dunlop EM, et al. Penicillin levels in blood and CSF achieved by treatment of syphilis. JAMA. 1979;241:2538–40.

24. Workowski KA, Levine WL. Sexually transmitted diseases treatment guilines 2002. MMWR Morb Mortal Wkly Rept. 2002;51(RR-6):18–29.
25. O'Byrne P, MacPherson P. Syphilis. BMJ. 2019;365:l4159. https://doi.org/10.1136/bmj.l4159.
26. Dr. Bahman Rasuli et.al. Syphilis. Radiopaedia. https://radiopaedia.org/articles/syphilis.
27. de Andrade R.-S. et al. Oral findings in secondary syphilis. Med Oral Patol Oral Cir Bucal. 2018 Mar; 23(2): e138–e143. Published online 2018 Feb 25. https://doi.org/10.4317/medoral.22196.
28. Laudien M. Orphan diseases of the nose and paranasal sinuses: Pathogenesis – clinic – therapy. GMS Curr Top Otorhinolaryngol Head Neck Surg. 2015; 14: Doc04. Published online 2015 Dec 22. https://doi.org/10.3205/cto000119
29. CDC. Primary and secondary syphilis--United States, 2003–2004. MMWR Morb mortal Wkly Rep. 2006 Mar 17;55(10):269–73.
30. Buffet M, Dupin N. Diagnosing Treponema pallidum in secondary syphilis by PCR and immunohistochemistry. J Investig Dermatol. October 2007;127(10):2345–50.
31. Clement ME, et al. Treatment of syphilis: a systematic review. JAMA. 2014 Nov 12;312(18):1905–17.

6 Leprosy

Abstract

Hansen's disease, commonly known as leprosy, is a chronic, granulo matous, infectious disease primarily affecting the skin, mucous membranes, and peripheral nervous system. It is caused by *Mycobacterium leprae*, an intracellular, acid-fast bacterium. The disease is clinically characterized by one or more of the three cardinal signs: hypopigmented or erythematous skin patches with definite loss of sensation, thickened peripheral nerves, and acid-fast bacilli detected on skin smears or biopsy material. Ridley–Jopling classification is most widely used and includes three major forms. Tuberculoid leprosy occurs in individuals with good cell-mediated immunity; patients develop a granulomatous response. Lepromatous leprosy occurs in individuals with poor cell-mediated immunity; do not develop a granulomatous response and borderline leprosy is an intermediate form between tuberculoid and lepromatous leprosy. Head–neck manifestations vary from cutaneous involvement to mucosal ulcers, granulomas, destruction with deformity in the upper airway. Otological manifestations are in the form of recurrent otitis externa and auricular perichondritis and deformity. Detection of acid-fast bacilli on skin biopsy, nasal smears, or both; serologic assays detecting phenolic glycolipid, lipoarabinomannan, and 16S ribosomal RNA gene PCR assay are diagnostic. Multidrug therapy recommended by the WHO includes Rifampicin, Dapsone, Clofazimine, Ofloxacin, and Minocycline.

Synonyms
Hansen's disease.

6.1 Background

Leprosy is a long-term infection by the bacteria *Mycobacterium leprae* or *Mycobacterium lepromatosis*. The disease takes its name from the Greek word "lepra," meaning "scale," while the term "Hansen's disease" is named after the Norwegian physician "Gerhard Armauer Hansen." The person who is infected does not have symptoms for 5–20 years. Gradually, the infection can lead to damage of the nerves, respiratory tract, skin, and eyes. Leprosy is curable with multidrug therapy. Leprosy has historically been associated with social stigma, which continues to be a barrier to self-reporting and early treatment [1, 2].

6.2 Epidemiology

At the end of 2016, there were 173,000 leprosy cases globally, down from 5.2 million in the 1980s. The number of new cases in 2016 was

S. V. Nemade, K. J. Shinde, *Granulomatous diseases in Otorhinolaryngology, Head and Neck*,
https://doi.org/10.1007/978-981-16-4047-6_6

216,000. Most new cases occur in 14 countries, with India accounting for more than half [3]. Every year, more than 200,000 new leprosy cases are registered globally. The number has been fairly stable over the past 8 years. WHO has set a target to interrupt the transmission of leprosy globally by 2020. In 2020, the country-level leprosy incidence has decreased to 6.2, 6.1, and 3.3 per 100,000 in India, Brazil, and Indonesia, respectively, meeting the elimination target of less than 10 per 100,000 [3, 4].

It has worldwide distribution due to travel and migration but is endemic in tropics. Leprosy is generally more common in males than in females, with a male-to-female ratio of 2:1. In some areas in Africa, the prevalence of leprosy among females is equal to or greater than that in males. Leprosy can occur at any age, but in developing countries, the age-specific incidence of leprosy peaks in children younger than 10 years, who account for 20% of leprosy cases. Leprosy is very rare in infants; however, they are at a relatively high risk of acquiring leprosy from the mother, especially in cases of lepromatous leprosy or borderline leprosy [3, 4].

6.3 Etiopathogenesis

M. leprae and *M. lepromatosis* are the mycobacteria that cause leprosy. *M. leprae* is an intracellular, acid-fast bacterium that is aerobic and rod shaped. *M. leprae* is surrounded by the waxy cell membrane coating characteristic of the genus Mycobacterium.

Spread occurs through cough or contact with fluid from the nose of a person infected by leprosy. Leprosy is not spread during pregnancy to the unborn children or through sexual contact. Leprosy occurs more commonly among people living in poverty. Genetic factors and immune function play a role in how easily a person catches the disease.

Two exit routes of *M. leprae* from the human body often described are the skin and the nasal mucosa, although their relative importance is not clear. Lepromatous cases show large numbers of organisms deep in the dermis, but whether they reach the skin surface in sufficient numbers is doubtful [5, 6]. The quantity of bacilli from nasal mucosal lesions in lepromatous leprosy ranges from 10,000 to 10,000,000. The majority of lepromatous patients show leprosy bacilli in their nasal secretions as collected through blowing the nose. Nasal secretions from lepromatous patients could yield as much as 10 million viable organisms per day [5].

Due to the wide spectrum of clinical findings in Leprosy, various classification protocols have been created to categorize patients within a particular zone of the spectrum and facilitate treatment directives. There are two main classifications:

(a) WHO classification: It divides the disease into three groups based on the number of cutaneous lesions [7]:
   - Single-lesion leprosy (one skin lesion)
   - Paucibacillary leprosy (2–5 skin lesions)
   - Multibacillary leprosy (>5 skin lesions)

(b) The Ridley–Jopling classification: It divides the spectrum into five groups based on the immunologic response. This classification is more commonly used [4, 7]:
   - Early and indeterminate leprosy (an early stage of the disease with insufficient clinical or histological features to fulfill a definitive category).
   - Tuberculoid (TT) at the mild end. It occurs in individuals with good cell-mediated immunity. Patients develop a granulomatous response to the infection.
   - Borderline tuberculoid (BT). It is an intermediate form between tuberculoid and lepromatous leprosy.
   - Borderline-borderline (BB, in the middle)
   - Borderline lepromatous (BL)
   - Lepromatous (LL) at the severe end. Lepromatous leprosy occurs in individuals with poor cell-mediated immunity; do not develop a granulomatous response [4, 7].

Conditions that reduce immune function, such as malnutrition, other illnesses, or genetic mutations, may increase the risk of developing leprosy [4, 7, 8]. The complexity of presentation is related to the varied immunologic responses. The incubation period is usually 3–5 years. In general, Hansen's disease primarily involves the skin and nervous system. In addition to cutaneous changes in pigmentation with possible anesthesia of the lesions, peripheral nerves can become enlarged and palpable [4].

6.4 Clinical Features

The first noticeable sign of leprosy is often the development of pale- or pink-colored patches of skin that may be insensitive to temperature or pain. Skin lesions can be single or many, and usually hypopigmented, although occasionally reddish or copper-colored (Fig. 6.1). The lesions may be flat (macules), raised (papules), or solid elevated areas (nodular) [4, 7, 10].

Skin lesions are accompanied or preceded by nerve problems including thickened nerves and numbness or tenderness in the hands or feet, muscle weakness, and joint deformities [9, 10].

Secondary infections (additional bacterial or viral infections) can result in tissue loss, causing fingers and toes to become shortened and deformed, as cartilage is absorbed into the body [11].

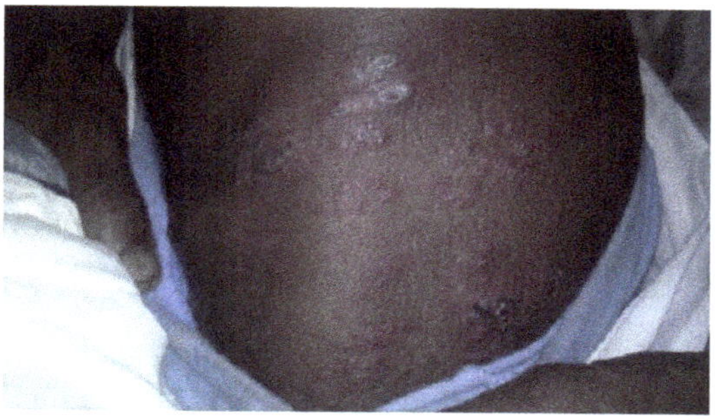

Fig. 6.1 Erythematous, scaly, and ulcerative rash with irregular margins present over the elbow [9]

6.5 ENT Manifestations

Nose The skin is always affected before the nose, and the nose (if at all) before the pharynx and larynx. The septum, turbinates, and anterior nasal spine are the most involved nasal structures [12]. Nose manifestations can be early, intermediate, and late ones. In the early stage, there is infiltration of the mucosa and abnormal drying leading to rhinorrhea. In the intermediate manifestation, infiltration grows causing nasal obstruction with an increase in nasal secretion then raising crusts, epistaxis, and plaque-like gray infiltration in the Little's area. Sinusitis, especially of the maxillary sinus, may complicate nasal leprosy. It commonly involves ethmoid air cells (80%) followed by the maxillary sinus (48%). In the late manifestation, there is the development of nodules that may ulcerate, deep ulcers with secondary infection, perichondritis involving cartilaginous septum, which can lead to septal perforation, anosmia/hyposmia. Destruction of lateral nasal cartilages can lead to external nasal deformity. Atrophic rhinitis and loosening of upper incisors may also occur in the late stage. This is due to osteolysis and osteoporosis leading to the destruction of turbinates and the anterior nasal spine [11–14].

Changes in the nasal mucosa can be found in a high proportion of patients (more than 90%). Specifically, those are initially:

- Pale, yellowish thickened mucosa
- Nodular infiltrates (Fig. 6.2)
- Flat plaques or nodules up to 5 mm

Symptoms include:

- Nasal obstruction
- Ulceration
- Crusts
- Sensory disturbances
- Hyposmia
- Destruction of cartilage and bone (with deformity of the external nose and chronic atrophic rhinitis)
- Epistaxis [14]

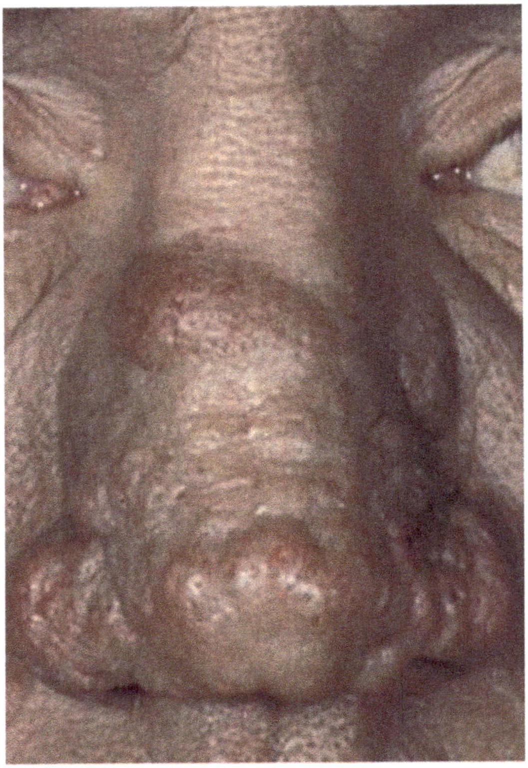

Fig. 6.2 Tuberculoid leprosy causing multiple nodular lesions of nose [15]

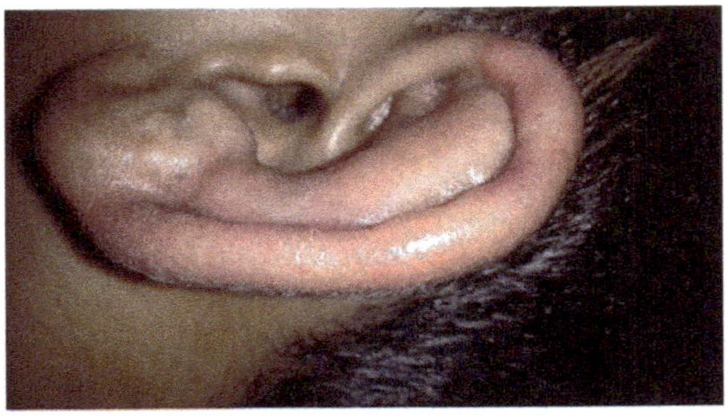

Fig. 6.3 Redness and swelling of cartilaginous upper two-thirds of the external ear [9]

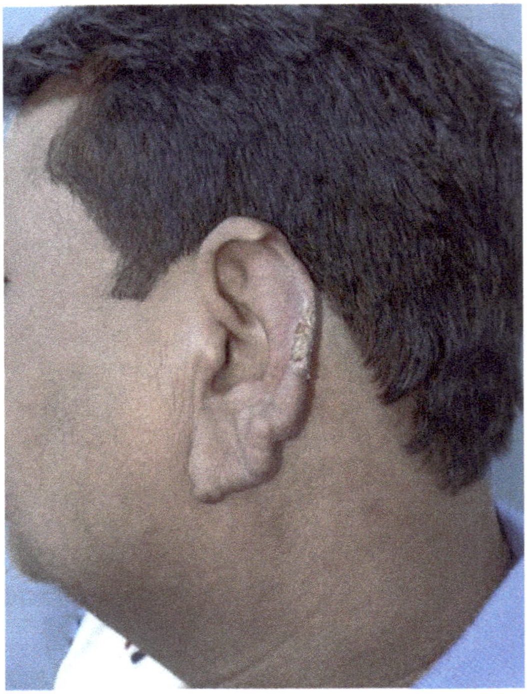

Fig. 6.4 Moth eaten appearance of pinna due to cartilage destruction [16]

Pharynx and Larynx The palate, the faucial pillars, and the uvula are locations of preference, and the tongue also can be affected. Specific infections of the dental pulp and periapical granulomata have been described. Diffuse stomatitis and oral ulcers are common [11]. Laryngeal lesions are rare but severe. The most frequent location of leprosy in the larynx is the epiglottis, which may be destroyed by perichondritis and cartilage destruction. Leprous affection of the epiglottis may lead to difficult inspection of vocal cords. The vocal cord lesions are either fibrotic leading to immobilization of vocal folds and dysphonia, or ulcerative, which are even more severe leading to pain, dysphonia, and dyspnea [13, 14].

Ear Otological manifestations are in the form of recurrent otitis externa and auricular perichondritis, ulcers. (Fig. 6.3). Recurrent ulcers healing with fibrosis leads to the destruction of cartilage giving characteristic moth-eaten deformity of the pinna (Fig. 6.4). Specific leprous changes of the middle ear, the inner ear, and the eighth nerve are not known [9, 14, 17].

Lucio Phenomenon It is seen in Mexican and Central American patients. It is a rare and severe form of multibacillary leprosy that is marked by blue hemorrhagic plaques and necrotic ulcerations. The bacilli may extend to endothelial cells along with the appearance of necrotic epidermis and vasculitis with thrombus formation and endothelial proliferation. The patient presents with purpuric macules with multiple and extensive areas of ulceration with bizarre-patterned, angulated borders mainly affecting extremities [18].

6.6 Diagnosis

The diagnostic evaluation for leprosy includes a complete physical examination with thorough skin observation, neurological examination and skin smears, and/or biopsies.

In 1997, the WHO Expert Committee on Leprosy established that a person is considered to have leprosy if they have one of the following three cardinal signs [4, 10, 11]:

- Hypopigmented, erythematous, or hyperpigmented skin lesions with sensory loss.
- Nerve enlargement (predominantly great auricular nerve in the neck, median and superficial radial cutaneous nerves at the wrist, ulnar nerve at the elbow, and common peroneal nerve at the popliteal fossa)
- The presence of acid-fast bacilli on a skin smear

At the present time, diagnosis is based on clinical criteria plus skin smears or biopsy, since it is known that multibacillary leprosy may not present with sensory loss and paucibacillary leprosy may be negative in skin smears [4, 9]. Skin smears that demonstrate acid-fast bacilli with Ziehl–Neelsen stain or Wade Fite stain (modified Ziehl–Neelsen stain) strongly suggest a diagnosis of leprosy (Fig.6.5); however, the bacilli may not be demonstrable in tuberculoid (paucibacillary) leprosy [16].

6.6.1 Histopathology

Biopsy of skin lesions or nasal, pharyngeal, laryngeal lesions may reveal acid-fast bacilli [4, 11].

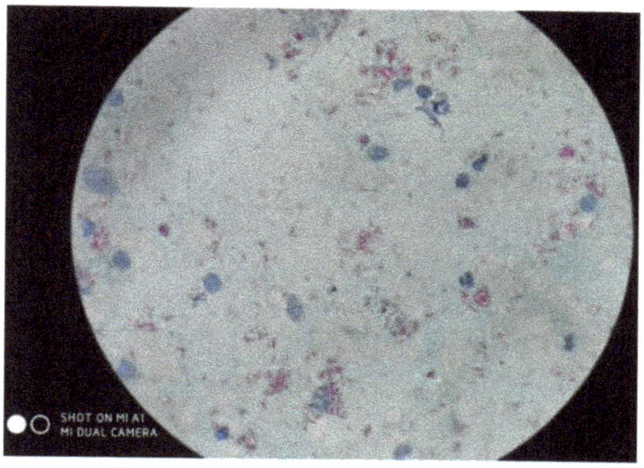

Fig. 6.5 Slit-skin smear from the ear lobule showing acid-fast bacilli [16]

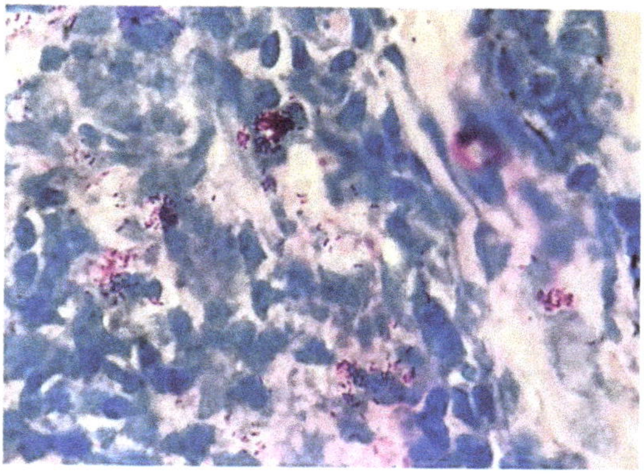

Fig. 6.6 Photomicrograph showing several clusters of lepra bacilli (Wade Fite stain; × 1000) [13]

Tissue samples stained with hematoxylin-eosin and Wade Fite stain are the primary basis for laboratory diagnosis and categorization. Wade Fite stain is the modified Ziehl–Neelsen stain used to demonstrate *Mycobacterium leprae*, which is much less acid and alcohol fast than the tubercle bacilli (Fig. 6.6) [13]. A full-thickness skin biopsy sample should be taken from an advancing border of an active lesion and should include dermis and epidermis [12, 13, 17]. A nerve biopsy can be beneficial in ruling out diseases such as hereditary neuropathies or polyarteritis nodosa. Nerve biopsies may also help identify abnormalities in patients with subclinical leprosy and maybe the only way to definitively diagnose completely neuropathic forms of leprosy. If a nerve biopsy is needed to confirm diagnosis, a purely sensory nerve (e.g., sural or radial cutaneous nerve) should be used. This procedure is rarely necessary [17].

Findings vary but can include dermatitis, giant cells, infiltration of nerve bundles with mononuclear cells, and granulomas (Figs. 6.7 and 6.8). Lepromatous lesions generally contain numerous acid-fast bacilli and fat-laden macrophages with a paucity of lymphocytes. In contrast, tuberculoid lesions contain few-to-no acid-fast bacilli but manifest granulomatous changes with epithelial cells and lymphocytes [17, 19, 20].

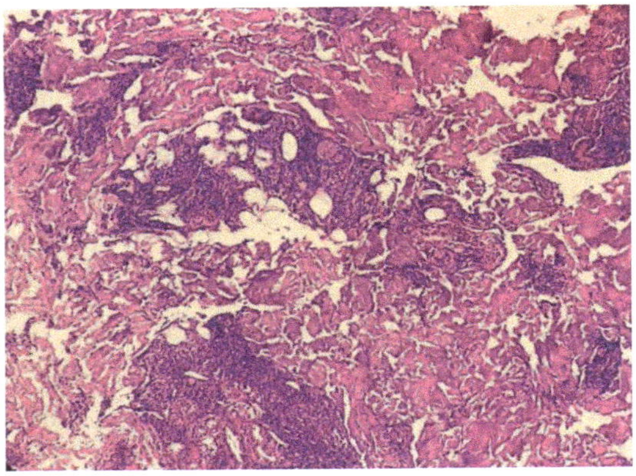

Fig. 6.7 Photomicrograph showing patchy infiltration by epithelioid cells and lymphoid population along with foam cells and neutrophils. The infiltration is mainly limited to perineural and around the sweat glands and arrector pili muscles (Hematoxylin stain; × 100) [13]

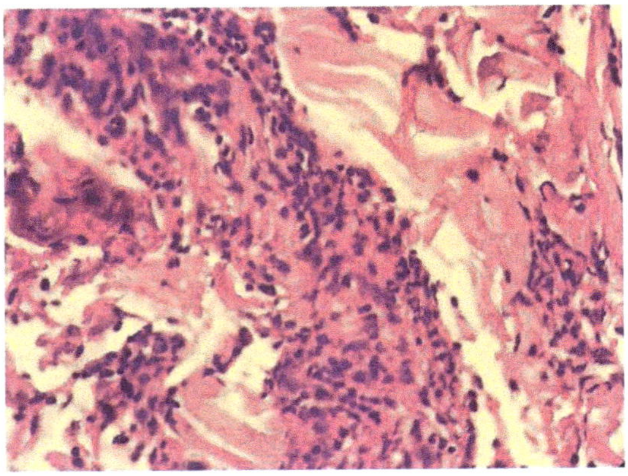

Fig. 6.8 High-power view showing perineural infiltration by inflammatory cells. (Hematoxylin stain, × 400) [13]

6.6.2 Serology

- Serologic assays can be used to detect phenolic glycolipid-1(PGL-1) and lipoarabinomannan (LAM-commonly seen in mycobacteria) [13]. Phenolic glycolipid-1 is a specific serologic test based on the detection of antibodies to phenolic glycolipid-1. This test yields a sensitivity of 95% for the detection of lepromatous leprosy but only 30% for tuberculoid leprosy.
- The use of the anti-45-kd and modified anti-PGL-1 antibody assays in combination may be more sensitive in detecting cases of paucibacillary leprosy than either assay individually [21].
- A combination of the NDO-LID test and the Smart-Reader system (a cellphone-based test reader platform) has demonstrated 87% sensitivity on multibacillary patients and 32.3% on paucibacillary patients, with a specificity of 97.4% in detecting specific antibodies of *M. leprae*, IgM and IgG [22].
- Rapid diagnostic tests and enzyme-linked immunosorbent assay (ELISA) systems continue to evolve and be highly sensitive and specific [21].

6.6.3 Molecular Assay

- Polymerase chain reaction (PCR) with recombinant DNA technology, 16S ribosomal RNA gene PCR assay (can use paraffin block) have allowed for the development of gene probes with *M. leprae*-specific sequences. This technology can be used to identify the mycobacterium in biopsy samples, skin and nasal smears, and blood [17].
- Molecular probes detect 40–50% of cases missed on prior histologic evaluation. Since probes require a minimum amount of genetic material (i.e., 10^4 DNA copies), they can fail to identify paucibacillary leprosy.
- The development of a one-step reverse transcriptase PCR assay may be more sensitive in detecting bacilli in slit smears and skin biopsy specimens. This RNA-based assay is also effective for monitoring bacteria clearance during therapy [23].

6.6.4 Other Tests

- Lymphocyte migration inhibition test (LMIT): As determined by a lymphocyte.
- transformation and LMIT, cell-mediated immunity to *M. leprae* is absent in patients with lepromatous leprosy but present in those with tuberculoid leprosy [24–26].
- Lepromin skin test: Although not diagnostic of exposure to or infection with *M. leprae*, this test assesses a patient's ability to mount a granulomatous response against a skin injection of killed *M. leprae*. Bacillary suspension is injected into the forearm. An assessment of the reaction at 48 hours is called the Fernandez reaction, and a positive result indicates delayed hypersensitivity to antigens of *M. leprae* or mycobacteria that cross-react with *M. leprae*. When the reaction is read at 3–4 weeks, it is called the Mitsuda reaction, and a positive result indicates that the immune system is capable of mounting an efficient cell-mediated response [24–26].

6.6.5 Interpretation

- Tuberculoid leprosy has a hypopigmented center and raised erythematous border (>5 mm).
- Lepromatous leprosy has no response or macules, papules, and plaques (<5 mm).
- Borderline leprosy has hypopigmented macules (>5 mm).

Patients with tuberculoid leprosy or borderline lepromatous leprosy typically have a positive response. A negative finding suggests a lack of resistance to disease and is observed in patients with lepromatous leprosy [24–26]. The results do not confirm diagnosis, but they are useful in determining the type of leprosy. A negative result also indicates a worse prognosis [24–26].

- Contact or family screening for a history of leprosy is also important.

6.6.6 Imaging

Doppler Ultrasonography and MR imaging are able to detect nerves abnormalities in leprosy. Active reversal reactions are indicated by endoneurial color flow signals as well as by an increased T2 signal and Gd enhancement. These signs would suggest rapid progression of nerve damage and a poor prognosis unless antireactional treatment is started [17, 19, 20]. CT PNS better delineates the extent of granuloma, cartilage, and bone destruction.

6.7 Treatment

Leprosy is curable with multidrug therapy. These treatments are provided free of charge by the World Health Organization. Multidrug therapy (MDT) remains highly effective, and people are no longer infectious after the first monthly dose.

6.7.1 WHO Recommendations for Treatment of Leprosy [14]

- Single skin lesion: Single dose of rifampin 600 mg + ofloxacin 400 mg + minocycline 100 mg (Abbreviated as ROM treatment)
- Paucibacillary: Dapsone 100 mg daily + rifampin 600 mg once a month (6 cycles in 9 months)
- Multibacillary: Dapsone 100 mg daily + rifampin 600 mg once a month + clofazimine 300 mg once a month + clofazimine 50 mg daily (for 1 year)

6.7.2 United States Recommendations for Treatment of Leprosy [14]

- Paucibacillary: Dapsone 100 mg daily + rifampin 600 mg once a month (for 1 year)
- Multibacillary: Dapsone 100 mg daily + rifampin 600 mg daily + clofazimine 50 mg daily (for 2 years)

People with rifampicin-resistant leprosy may be treated with second-line drugs such as Fluoroquinolones, Minocycline, or Clarithromycin, but the treatment duration is 24 months due to their lower bactericidal activity [27, 28].

- Local treatment such as nasal irrigation, removal of nasal crusts is helpful.
- Oral antihistaminics, decongestants, local application of antiseptic lubricating ointments, antibiotics in secondary infection may be necessary.
- Vitamin B 12 supplements, antioxidants are helpful in the healing process and to boost immunity.

6.7.2.1 Surgical Management

In case of acute airway obstruction by laryngeal lesions, temporary tracheostomy may be required till the completion of pharmacotherapy.

Reconstruction surgery is considered after the completion of the pharmacotherapy. It includes [27, 29]:

- Closure of septal perforation
- Rhinoplasty
- Removal of excess skin
- Replacement of eyebrows using transplants of scalp hair

6.8 Essential features

- Leprosy, also called Hansen disease, is a chronic granulomatous disease caused by *Mycobacterium leprae* and *Mycobacterium lepromatosis*.
- The complexity of the presentation is related to the varied immunologic responses.
- The incubation period is usually 3–5 years.
- Tuberculoid leprosy occurs in individuals with good cell-mediated immunity; patients develop a granulomatous response.
- Lepromatous leprosy occurs in individuals with poor cell-mediated immunity; do not develop a granulomatous response.
- Borderline leprosy is an intermediate form between tuberculoid and lepromatous leprosy.
- Transmitted by nasal discharge and digital impregnation of skin, as bacilli can be carried under nails and are inoculated under the skin by scratching.
- Lucio phenomenon is seen in Mexican and Central American patients who present with untreated, diffuse, nonnodular lepromatous leprosy with hemorrhagic infarct.
- Head–neck manifestations vary from cutaneous involvement to mucosal ulcers, granulomas, destruction with deformity in the upper airway.
- Otological manifestations are in the form of recurrent otitis externa and auricular perichondritis and deformity.
- Skin biopsy, nasal smears, or both are used to assess for acid-fast bacilli using Wade Fite stain (modified Ziehl–Neelsen stain).
- Serologic assays to detect phenolic glycolipid-1 (specific for *M. leprae*) and lipoarabinomannan (LAM—commonly seen in mycobacteria).
- 16S ribosomal RNA gene PCR assay (can use paraffin block): used to identify the mycobacterium in biopsy samples, skin and nasal smears, and blood
- Mitsuda reaction: intradermal injection of an armadillo-derived lepra bacilli, is useful for classification.
- Histopathology reveals dermatitis, giant cells, infiltration of nerve bundles with mononuclear cells, and granulomas. Lepromatous lesions contain numerous acid-fast bacilli and fat-laden macrophages with a paucity of lymphocytes. In contrast, tuberculoid lesions contain few-to-no acid-fast bacilli but manifest granulomatous changes with epithelial cells and lymphocytes.
- Multidrug Therapy Plan Recommended by the WHO includes Rifampin, Dapsone, Clofazimine, Ofloxacin, and Minocycline.
- Surgical correction of septal perforation and external nasal deformity is considered after completion of the pharmacotherapy.

- It is important to make an early diagnosis in order to control the epidemic process, case handling, and disability prevention. Besides, such diseases should be efficiently diagnosed and treated before patients become stigmatized.

References

1. Sotiriou MC, et al. Two cases of leprosy in siblings caused by mycobacterium lepromatosis and review of the literature. Am Jo Trop Med Hyg. 2016;95(3):522–7.
2. Barton RP, Davey TF. Early leprosy of the nose and throat. J Laryngol Otol. 1976;90:953–61.
3. Suzuki K, et al. Current status of leprosy: epidemiology, basic science and clinical perspectives. J Dermatol. 2012;39(2):121–9.
4. Moschella S. An update on the diagnosis and treatment of leprosy. J Am Acad Dermatol. 2004;5(3):417–26.
5. Bhat RM, Prakash C. Leprosy: an overview of pathophysiology. Interdiscip Perspect Infect Dis. 2012;2012:6. https://doi.org/10.1155/2012/181089. Article id: 181089
6. McMurray DN. Mycobacteria and Nocardia. In: Baron S, et al., editors. Baron's medical microbiology. 4th ed. Galveston: Univ of Texas Medical Branch; 1996. isbn 978-0-9631172-1-2.
7. World Health Organization. A guide to leprosy control. 2nd ed. Geneva: World Health Organization; 1988. p. 28.
8. World Health Organization. Guidelines for the diagnosis, treatment and prevention of leprosy. Geneva: World Health Organization; 2018. p. xiii. isbn 978-92-9022-638-3
9. Pruthi P, et al. Leprosy with atypical Skin lesions masquerading as relapsing polychondritis. Case Rep Infect Dis. 2016; 2016:7802423. Published online 2016 Dec 26. https://doi.org/10.1155/2016/7802423
10. James WD, et al. Andrews' diseases of the Skin: clinical dermatology. London: Saunders Elsevier; 2006. isbn 978-0-7216-2921-6
11. Mishra B, et al. Neuritic leprosy: further progression and significance. Acta Leprol. 1995;9(4):187–94.
12. WHO WHO Expert committee on leprosy – eight report (PDF). World Health Organization. Geneva, 2012. pp. 11–12. isbn 9789241209687.
13. Shiva Raj KC, et al. Leprosy – eliminated and forgotten: a case report. J Med Case Rep. 2019; 13:276. Published online 2019 Sep 1. https://doi.org/10.1186/s13256-019-2198-1
14. Yoder L, Guerra I. Hansen's disease: a guide to management in the united States 2. Carville: Hansen's Disease Foundation; 2001. p. 1–43.
15. Laudien M. Orphan diseases of the nose and paranasal sinuses: Pathogenesis – clinic – therapy. GMS Curr Top Otorhinolaryngol Head Neck Surg. 2015; 14: Doc04. Published online 2015 Dec 22. https://doi.org/10.3205/cto000119
16. Kaushik A, et al. "Rat-Bitten" Ulcer on the Pinna. Am J Trop Med Hyg. 2019 Nov;101(5):957. https://doi.org/10.4269/ajtmh.19-0495.
17. Bucci F Jr, et al. Oral lesions in lepromatous leprosy. J Oral Med. 1987;42:4–6.
18. Shrama P, et al. Lucio phenomenon: A rare presentation of Hansen's disease. J Clin Aesthet Dermatol. 2019;12(12):35–8.
19. Shrinivasan S, et al. CT findings in involvement of the paranasal sinuses by lepromatous leprosy. Br J Radiol. 1999;72:271–3.
20. Soni N. Leprosy of the larynx. J Laryngol Otol. 1992;106:518–20.
21. Duthie MS, et al. Rapid quantitative serological test for detection of infection with Mycobacterium leprae, the causative agent of leprosy. J Clin Microbiol. 2014 Feb.;52(2):613–9.
22. Duthie MS, et al. Rapid quantitative serological test for detection of infection with Mycobacterium leprae, the causative agent of leprosy. J Clin Microbiol. 2014;52(2):613–9.
23. Phetsuksiri B, et al. A simplified reverse transcriptase PCR for rapid detection of Mycobacterium leprae in skin specimens. FEMS Immunol Med Microbiol. 2006 Dec.;48(3):319–28.
24. Pinkweron FJ. Leprosy of the eye, ear, nose and throat. Trans Pac Coast Otoophthalmol Soc Annu Meet. 1954;35:179–88.
25. Bhushan P, et al. Diagnosing multibacillary leprosy: a comparative evaluation of diagnostic accuracy of slit-skin smear, bacterial index of granuloma and WHO operational classification. Indian J Dermatol Venereol Leprol. 2008 Jul–Aug.;74(4):322–6.
26. Reibel F, et al. Update on the epidemiology, diagnosis, and treatment of leprosy. Med Mal Infect. 2015;45(9):383–93.
27. Walker SL, Lockwood DN. Leprosy. Clin Dermatol. 2007 Mar–Apr.;25(2):165–72.
28. Anderson H, et al. Hansen disease in the United States in the 21st century: a review of the literature. Arch Pathol Lab Med. 2007 Jun.;131(6):982–6.
29. Martinez AN, et al. PCR-based techniques for leprosy diagnosis: from the laboratory to the clinic. PLoS Negl Trop Dis. 2014 Apr.;8(4):e2655.

Actinomycosis

7

Abstract

Actinomycosis is a subacute to chronic bacterial infection caused by filamentous, Gram-positive, non-acid-fast, anaerobic-to-microaerophilic bacteria. It is characterized by contiguous spread, suppurative and granulomatous inflammation, and the formation of multiple abscesses and sinus tracts that may discharge sulfur granules. The most common clinical forms of actinomycosis are cervicofacial (lumpy jaw), thoracic, and abdominal. In women, pelvic actinomycosis is possible. Differential diagnosis includes carcinoma, abscess, congenital anomalies, tuberculosis, fungal diseases, and osteomyelitis. Because of its complex presentation, actinomycosis may be termed "the masquerader of the head and neck." Bacterial cultures and pathology is the cornerstone of diagnosis. Prolonged bacterial culture in anaerobic conditions is necessary to identify the bacterium and typical microscopic findings include necrosis with yellowish sulfur granules and filamentous Gram-positive fungal-like pathogens. Patients with actinomycosis require prolonged (6- to 12-month) high doses of penicillin G or amoxicillin to facilitate the drug penetration in abscess and in infected tissues, but the duration of antimicrobial therapy could be shortened to 3 months in patients in whom optimal surgical resection of infected tissues has been performed.

7.1 Background

Actinomycosis is a suppurative and granulomatous chronic infectious disease that usually spreads into adjacent soft tissues without regard for tissue planes or lymphatic drainage; it may [1–3] also be associated with a draining sinus tract. It is a bacterial infection caused by Actinomyces species. In 1890, "Eugen Bostroem" isolated the causative organism from a culture of grain, grasses, and soil. After Bostroem's discovery, a general misconception was considering actinomycosis as a mycotic infection. Bergey's Manual of Systematic Bacteriology classified the organism as bacteria in 1939. In 1938, "Cope" classified actinomycosis infection into three distinct clinical forms: cervicofacial (50%), pulmonothoracic (30%), and abdomino-pelvic (20%) [4].

7.2 Epidemiology

Global incidence varies between 20,000 and 350,000 people/year. Disease incidence is greater in males than in females and is common between the ages of 20 and 60 years [5].

S. V. Nemade, K. J. Shinde, *Granulomatous diseases in Otorhinolaryngology, Head and Neck*,
https://doi.org/10.1007/978-981-16-4047-6_7

7.3 Etiopathogenesis

Actinomyces are Gram-positive, non-acid fast, anaerobic or microaerophilic filamentous branched bacteria that are very difficult to grow in culture. Culture is positive in less than 30% of cases. The pathogenic Actinomyces most frequently isolated is *A. Israelii*; less commonly, infection is caused by *A. Propionica*, *A. Naeslundii*, *A. Viscosus*, and *A. Odontolyticus*. These bacteria are all normal commensals of the human oral cavity [5–7].

They are also normal commensals among the gut flora of the caecum; thus, abdominal actinomycosis can occur following removal of the appendix. The three most common sites of infection are decayed teeth, the lungs, and the intestines. Actinomycosis does not occur in isolation, it is almost always accompanied by other bacterial infections. Actinomyces depend on other bacteria (Gram-positive, Gram-negative, and cocci) to aid in the invasion of tissue. Actinomycosis bacillus invades when, through a mucosal lesion, it gains access to the subcutaneous tissue. Thus, the infection is likely to be polymicrobial aerobic and anaerobic [8].

In cervicofacial actinomycosis, which is the most frequent manifestation, infection is frequently the result of oromaxillofacial trauma, dental manipulation, or dental caries [9]. Predisposing factors include poor oral hygiene, trauma, male gender, diabetes mellitus, immunosuppression, alcoholism, and malnutrition. Differential diagnosis includes carcinoma, abscess, congenital anomalies, tuberculosis, fungal diseases, and osteomyelitis. Because of its complex presentation, actinomycosis may be termed "the masquerader of the head and neck" [10].

7.4 Clinical Features

The disease is characterized by painful large ulcers and abscesses in the floor of the mouth and gingiva.

Cervicofacial actinomycosis, which is the most common type (50–60%) presents with:

- Neck mass: The mass is often located at the border of the mandible, firm but often fluctuant in late presentation (due to central necrosis), gradually progressive in size within weeks or months. The overlying skin may be erythematous and warm showing the signs of inflammation (Fig. 7.1) [7].
- Spontaneous sinus tracts formation: This is the classical presentation. Sinus tract draining purulent material is observed in approximately 40% of cases, and, when present, may be helpful in the differential diagnosis (Fig. 7.2) [9, 12].
- "Lumpy jaw syndrome": Large unilateral abscess located on the head and neck, usually following dental infection and mandibular osteomyelitis. It can be associated with fistula formation [13].
- Oral actinomycosis usually presents with painful large (>2 cm) oral and oropharyngeal ulcers, abscesses in the floor of the mouth. It is almost always associated with dental caries and gingival abscesses. In the oropharynx, tonsils are commonly involved. Involvement of the larynx is very rare (Fig. 7.3) and usually involves the pyriform sinus and aryepiglottic folds (Fig. 7.4).

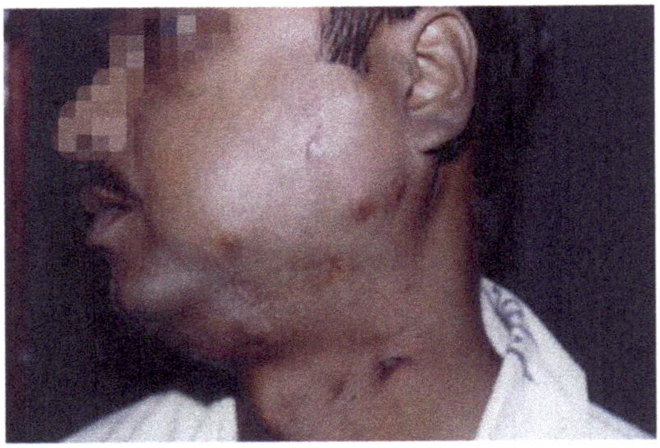

Fig. 7.1 Case of cervicofacial actinomycosis with parotid swelling and the draining sinuses [11]

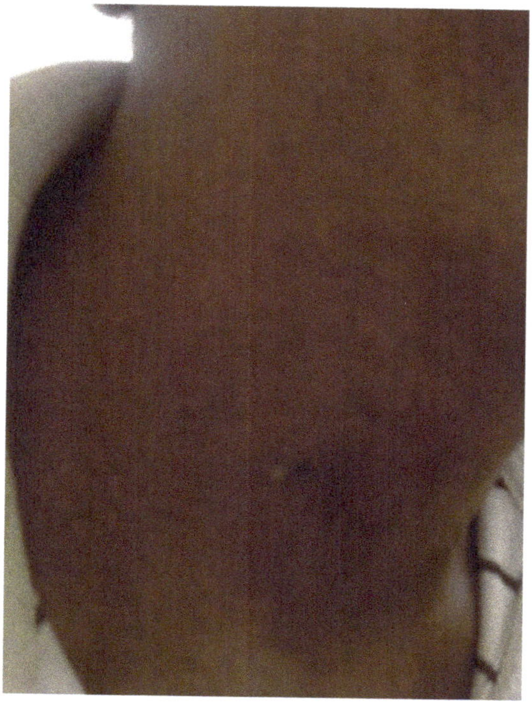

Fig. 7.2 Sinus tract with tiny abscess formation around the sinus opening and surrounding erythematous skin

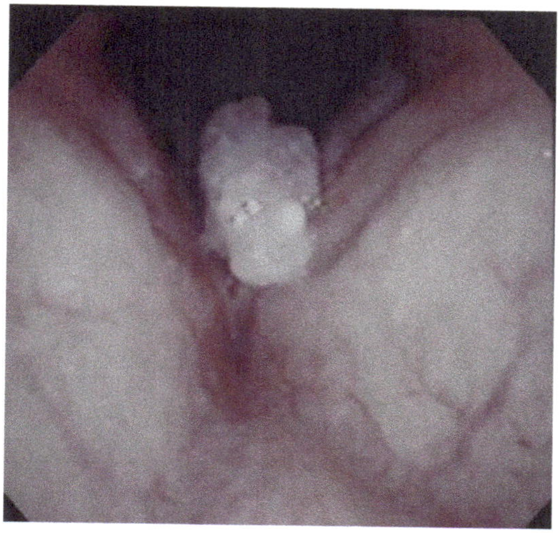

Fig. 7.3 Actinomycosis granuloma in the anterior one-third part of the left vocal cord [10]

- Rarely regional lymphadenopathy is associated.
- Constitutional symptoms such as fever, malaise, and headache [9, 12].

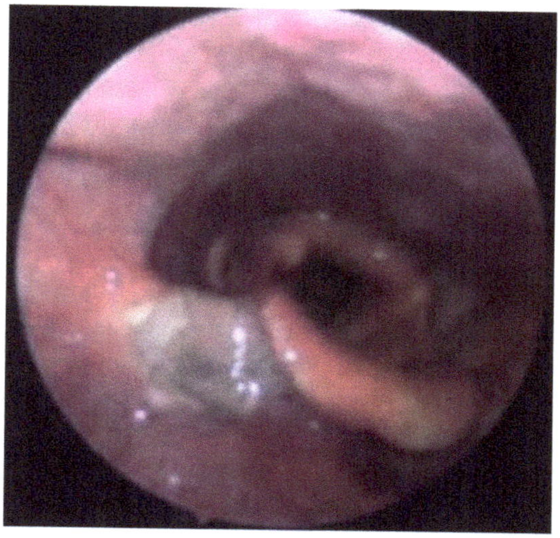

Fig. 7.4 Endoscopic view showing ulcerative lesion on the right pharyngo-epiglottic ligament, vallecula, and the right pyriform sinus [10]

7.4.1 Other Features

Pulmonary abscess, breast abscess, or gastrointestinal tract ulcers may occur [14, 15].

7.5 Diagnosis

Actinomycosis shows a wide variety of symptoms and a characteristic ability to mimic many other diseases. Because of its peculiarity, it can be considered a "great pretender." Only 10% of Actinomyces infections are correctly diagnosed on initial presentation. In the past, surgery has been used both to diagnose and to treat this pathology with its removal. Nowadays with the advent of FNAC, the diagnosis has become easier and less invasive [10].

7.5.1 Cytology

Fine-needle aspiration (FNA) not only allows morphologic identification, comparable to that obtained by incisional biopsy but is also an effective means of collecting material for microbiologic identification [16, 17].

7.5.2 Culture

When positive, it is 100% sensitive and specific. However, Actinomyces' growth is very difficult. Even on appropriate anaerobic media, the rate of positive culture is less than 50% [10]. Thus, microbiological identification of this organism is often impossible. The macroscopic presence of the classic sulfur granules in tissue specimens or drained fluid may be of some help when making diagnosis, even if these features are not pathognomic, since nocardiosis may also present with sulfur granules [16–18].

7.5.3 Histopathology

Incisional biopsy is of great help in the diagnosis of actinomycosis, since microscopic examination reveals a typical finding of an outer zone of granulation and a central zone of necrosis which contains multiple basophilic sulfur granules that represent lobulated micro-colonies of Actinomyces (Figs. 7.5, 7.6 and 7.7) [18].

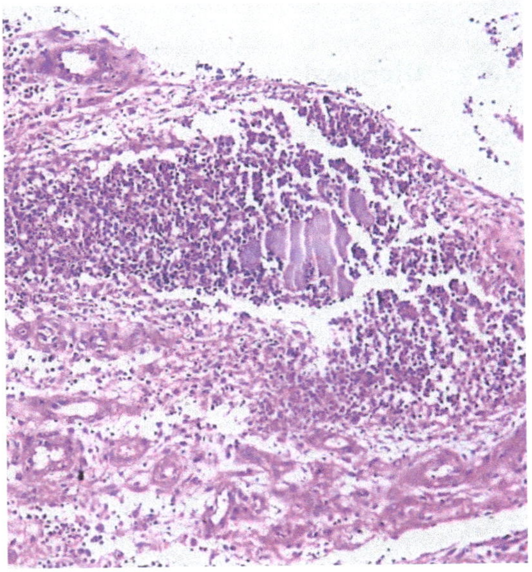

Fig. 7.5 Histopathology showing ulcerated epidermis with underlying neutrophilic microabscess surrounded by granulation tissues consisting of plasma cell, macrophage, and fibroblast infiltration (H&E * 10) [19]

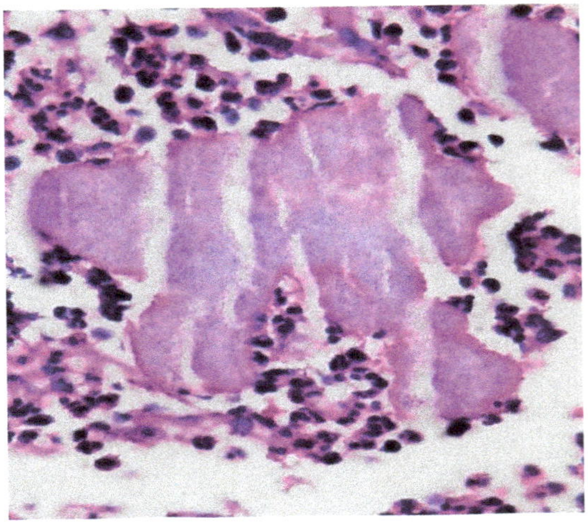

Fig. 7.6 Sulfur granules are found at the center of the inflammatory reactions as filamentous basophilic radiating fungal-like structures in the dermis (H&E * 40) [19]

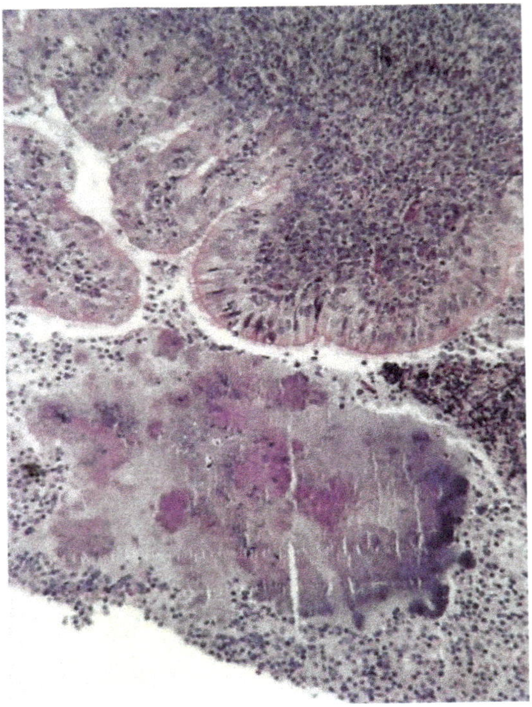

Fig. 7.7 Chronic inflammation and presence of actinomyces [20]

7.5.4 Imaging

It shows ill-defined infiltrative lesions with the tendency to cross-tissue planes and extend into different neck spaces that may be associated with fistulous tract. Computed tomography (CT) shows an enhancing soft-tissue mass with a low-attenuating center associated with inflammatory change in the adjacent soft tissue and invasion of the adjacent soft tissue (Figs. 7.8, 7.9, 7.10, and 7.11). MR imaging delineates the lesions with low intensity on T1-weighed images and intermediate intensity on T2-weighted images with moderate to marked contrast enhancement. Central suppurative necrosis may appear as non-enhancing region within the mass. Regional reactive lymphadenopathy may develop late in 40% of patients. Popcorn-like dystrophic calcifications are only rarely seen [20–22].

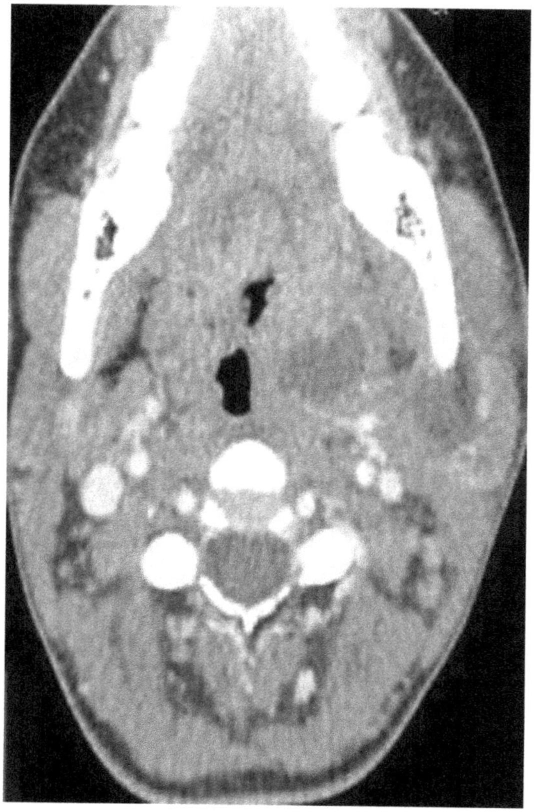

Fig. 7.8 Actinomycosis infection involving left tonsil causing abscess formation

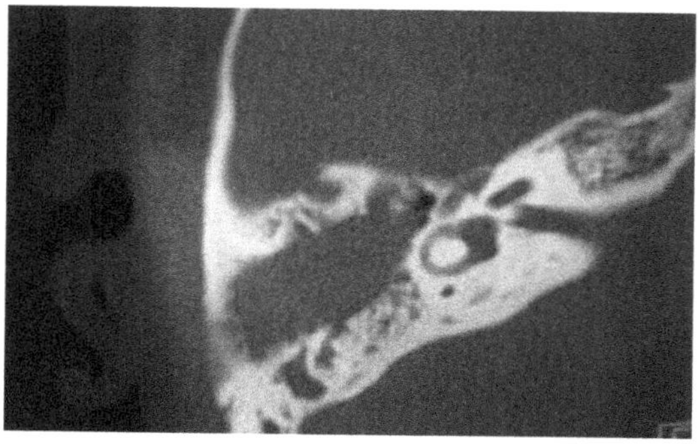

Fig. 7.9 CT scan showing middle ear and mastoid opacification

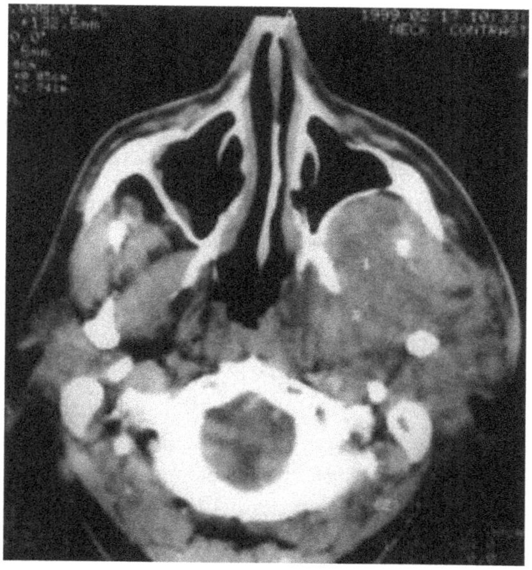

Fig. 7.10 CT scan showing the mass lesion in the parotid region with extension into left parapharyngeal space and thinning of the lateral wall of maxilla [11]

7.5.5 Serology

Fluorescence immunoassay of antibodies to, and surface antigens of, Actinomyces is highly sensitive and specific, but not readily available for all Actinomyces strains [23].

7.5.6 Molecular Assay

The classification of Actinomyces species that use genotypic methods such as comparative 16S

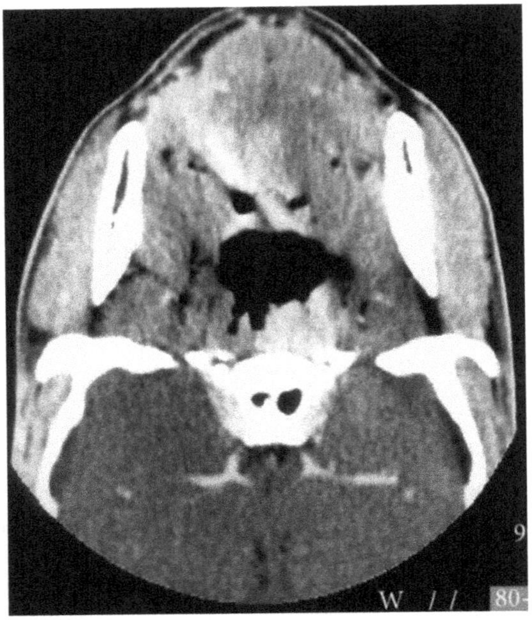

Fig. 7.11 CT skull base (Axial view) showing thickening of the left side of the nasopharynx [20]

ribosomal RNA (rRNA) gene sequencing is very useful. Therefore, nowadays, molecular techniques such as 16S rRNA sequencing serve as the reference for identification. Besides 16S rRNA sequencing, a practical identification method consists of 16S ribosomal DNA restriction analysis. Polymerase chain reaction with specific primers can also be used for direct detection of Actinomyces in clinical material. Finally, matrix-assisted laser desorption ionization time-of-flight (MALDI-TOF) should be a quicker and accurate tool for Actinomyces identification in the future [24].

7.6 Treatment

- Actinomyces bacteria are generally sensitive to penicillin G.
- Prolonged high doses of antimicrobial therapy with beta lactum antibiotics and penicillin G is recommended.
- The preferred therapy is IV 18–24 million units per day of Penicillin G over 2–6 weeks, followed by oral therapy with Amoxycillin-clavulanic acid for 6–12 months.
- In cases of penicillin allergy, Doxycycline (200 mg/day) is used. Sulfonamides such as Sulfamethoxazole may be used as an alternative regimen at a total daily dosage of 2–4 grams. Response to therapy is slow and may take months [9, 12]. In the acute phase of treatment, Penicillin can be replaced by Cephalosporins which are also effective if a co-infection with other bacteria not responding to penicillin and may cause persistence of symptoms due to Actinomyces [25–27].
- Surgical excision is necessary to make a definitive diagnosis, particularly in those cases presenting with abscess, unresponsive to antimicrobial therapy, or when FNA/biopsy is non-diagnostic [9].
- Hyperbaric oxygen therapy may also be used as an adjunct to conventional therapy when the disease is refractory to antibiotics and surgical treatment [9, 20].

7.7 Essential Features

- Rare suppurative and granulomatous infectious disease.
- Caused by a group of anaerobic, Gram-positive, filamentous bacteria, which are normal flora in the oral cavity, gastrointestinal tract, and female genital tract. The most common causative agent is *Actinomyces israelii*.
- Clinically presents with abscess formation, tissue fibrosis, draining fistulas, and occasionally a soft tissue mass mimicking a tumor.
- Cervicofacial (post-dental infection), skin (post-traumatic injury creating an anaerobic environment), pelvic (post intrauterine device placement), abdominal (post ruptured appendix or bowel perforation), and pulmonary (smokers with poor dental hygiene, aspiration of infective material) are the various forms of the disease.
- "Lumpy jaw syndrome": large unilateral abscess located on the head and neck, usually

following dental infection and mandibular osteomyelitis.

- GMS stain highlights the filamentous bacteria, which are not visualized by H&E stain.
- Histopathology reveals "Sulfur granules": small yellow granules found within the abscesses formed by Actinomyces infection.
- Polymerase chain reaction (PCR) and nucleic acid probes are being developed for faster and more accurate identification.
- High-dose penicillin G is necessary to penetrate areas of fibrosis and suppuration/ granules.
- Drainage of abscesses or radical excision of sinus tracts is necessary.
- Hyperbaric oxygen therapy is used as an adjunct to conventional therapy.

References

1. Bennhoff DF. Actinomycosis: diagnostic and therapeutic considerations and a review of 32 cases. Laryngoscope. 1984;94:1198–217.
2. Maurizi M, et al. L'actinomicosi cervico-facciale. Bollettino delle Malattie dell'Orecchio, della Gola, del Naso. Pisa: Pacini Editore; 1978. p. 1–43.
3. Smego RA Jr, Foglia G. Actinomycosis. Clin Infect Dis. 1998;26:1255–61.
4. Brook I. Actinomycosis: diagnosis and management. South Med J. Oct 2008;101(10):1019–23.
5. Belmont MJ, et al. Atypical presentations of actinomycosis. Head Neck. 1999;21:264–8.
6. Aguirrebengoa K, et al. Oral and cervicofacial actinomycosis. Presentation of five cases. Enferm Infecc Microbiol Clin. 2002;20:53.
7. Stewart MG, Sulek M. Pediatric actinomycosis of the head and neck. Ear Nose Throat J. 1993;72:614–9.
8. Bowden GHW. In: Baron S, et al., editors. Actinomycosis in: Baron's medical microbiology. 4th ed. Galveston: University of Texas Medical Branch; 1996. isbn 978-0-9631172-1-2.
9. Bartels LJ, Vrabec DP. Cervicofacial actinomycosis. Arch Otolaryngol. 1978;104:705–8.
10. Yoshihama K, et al. Vocal cord Actinomycosis mimicking a laryngeal tumor. Case Rep Otolaryngol. 2013;2013:2. https://doi.org/10.1155/2013/361986. Article ID: 361986
11. Varghese BT, et al. Actinomycosis of the parotid masquerading as malignant neoplasm. BMC Cancer. 2004; 4:7. Published online 2004 Mar 4. https://doi.org/10.1186/1471-2407-4-7
12. Becker DG, et al. Abscess with sulfur granules with organisms consistent with Actinomyces species. Arch Otolaryngol Head Neck Surg. 1992;118:1359–60.
13. Valour F, et al. A 22 year old woman with right lumpy jaw syndrome and fistula. BMJ Case Rep. 2015;2015:bcr2014206557. https://doi.org/10.1136/bcr-2014-206557.
14. Mabeza GF, Macfarlane J. Pulmonary actinomycosis. Eur Respir J 2003, March. 21(3):545–551. https://doi.org/10.1183/09031936.03.00089103. PMID 12662015.
15. Opeyemi AG, Gateley CA. Primary actinomycosis of the breast caused by Actinomyces turicensis with associated Peptoniphilus harei. Breast Dis. 2015, January 1;35(1):45–7.
16. Yadav SP, et al. Actinomycosis of tonsil masquerading as tumour in a 12-year-old child. Int J Pediatr Otorhinolaryngol. 2002;63:73–5.
17. Graybill JR, Silverman BD. Sulfur granules. Second thoughts. Arch Intern Med. 1969;123:430–2.
18. Silverman PM, et al. CT diagnosis of actinomycosis of the neck. J Comput Assist Tomogr. 1984;8:793–4.
19. Robati RM, et al. Primary cutaneous Actinomycosis along with the surgical scar on the hand. Case Rep Infect Dis. 2016; 2016: 5943932. Published online 2016 Nov 9. https://doi.org/10.1155/2016/5943932
20. Ouertatani L, et al. Nasopharyngeal Actinomycosis. Case Rep Otolaryngol. 2011, 2011:4. https://doi.org/10.1155/2011/367364. Article ID 367364
21. Park JK, et al. Cervicofacial actinomycosis: CT and MR imaging findings in 7 patients. Am J Neuroradiol. 2003;24:331–5.
22. Miller M, Haddad AJ. Cervicofacial actinomycosis. Oral Surg Oral Med Oral Pathol Radiol Endod. 1998;85:496–508.
23. Gillis TP, Thomsom JJ. Quantitative fluorescent immunoassay of antibodies to, and surface antigens of, Actinomyces Viscosus. J Clin Microbiol. 1978 Feb;7(2):202–8.
24. Valour F, et al. Actinomycosis: etiology, clinical features, diagnosis, treatment, and management. Infect Drug Resist. 2014; 7:183–197. Published online 2014 Jul 5. https://doi.org/10.2147/IDR.S39601
25. Hamed KA. Successful treatment of primary actinomyces viscosus endocarditis with third- generation cephalosporins. Clin Infect Dis. 1998;26:211–2.
26. Paludetti G, Rosignoli M. Su di un caso di actinomicosis cervico-facciale complicato da grave emorragia. Il Valsalva. Roma: Casa Editrice Luigi Pozzi. 1977;LIII:160–71.
27. Skoutelis A, et al. Successful treatment of thoracic actinomycosis with ceftriaxone. Clin Infect Dis. 1994;19:161–2.

8 Rhinoscleroma

Abstract

Rhinoscleroma is a chronic granulomatous infectious disease that affects the nose and other parts of the respiratory tract down to the trachea. It is caused by the Gram-negative bacterium *Klebsiella pneumoniae subsp. Rhinoscleromatis*. The disease progresses clinically and pathologically into three overlapping stages: catarrhal stage, proliferative stage, and sclerotic stage. Catarrhal stage causes nonspecific rhinitis lasting for weeks to months and often evolves into purulent and fetid rhinorrhea with crusting. The granulomatous stage results in the development of a bluish red nasal mucosa and intranasal rubbery nodules or polyps. Epistaxis, nasal deformity, and destruction of the nasal cartilage may also be noted (Hebra nose). The sclerotic stage is characterized by extensive fibrosis leading to scarring and possible nasal/laryngeal stenosis. Histology shows the appearance of Mikulicz cells, a hallmark of rhinoscleroma. These cells are large foamy macrophages with numerous enlarged vacuoles containing viable or non-viable bacteria. A delay in the diagnosis can lead to complications such as physical deformity, upper airway obstruction, and sepsis. Treatment includes surgery and a prolonged course of antibiotics to avoid relapses. Ciprofloxacin proves to be the most effective due to their increased penetrance. Surgical debridement or carbon dioxide laser are used to reduce symptoms of airway obstruction.

Synonyms
Scleroma.

8.1 Background

Rhinoscleroma is a chronic granulomatous, slowly progressing, and disfiguring infection predominantly affecting the upper respiratory tract.

This infection was first described in 1870 by "Von Hebra," 7 years later, "Mikulicz" described the histology and the characteristic foam cells [1]. In 1882, "Von Frisch" identified the causal agent now known as Klebsiella rhinoscleromatis [2]. The Polish surgeon "Johann von Mikulich" in Wroclaw described the histologic features in 1877. "Von Frisch" identified the organism in 1882. In 1932, "Belinov" proposed the use of the term "scleroma respiratorium" because the pathologic process in rhinosclerosis may involve not only the upper airways but also the lower airways [1–3]. Diagnosis depends on the identification of the pathognomonic Mickulicz cells (MCs) which are most prominent during the granulomatous phase but scanty or absent during catarrhal or sclerotic phases of the disease.

S. V. Nemade, K. J. Shinde, *Granulomatous diseases in Otorhinolaryngology, Head and Neck*,
https://doi.org/10.1007/978-981-16-4047-6_8

8.2 Epidemiology

Rhinoscleroma is a rare disease without accurate national or international incidence data. More than 16,000 cases have been reported since 1960. It is endemic to poor regions of Africa (Egypt, tropical areas), Southeast Asia, Mexico, Central and South America, and Central and Eastern Europe, it has been infrequent in the United States. Patients of all races can be affected. Females are affected more than males with an age preponderance of 10–30 years [4, 5].

8.3 Etiopathogenesis

Rhinoscleroma is acquired by inhalation of droplets or contaminated material, but it is probably through contaminated airborne particles, which are expelled by coughing and sneezing or by contact with fomites. Disease probably begins in areas of epithelial transition such as the vestibule of the nose, the subglottic area of the larynx, or the area between the nasopharynx and oropharynx. Cellular immunity is impaired in patients with rhinoscleroma; however, their humoral immunity is preserved.

The CD4/CD8 cell ratio in the lesion is altered with decreased levels of CD4 lymphocytes; this change possibly induces a diminished T cell response. Macrophages are not fully activated. Likewise, a genetic pattern (nicotinamide adenine dinucleotide phosphate oxidase complex, HLA-DQA1*0311-DQB*0301 haplotype) may contribute to disease exacerbation [6]. Rhinoscleroma usually affects the nasal cavity, but lesions associated with rhinoscleroma may also affect the larynx; nasopharynx; oral cavity; paranasal sinuses; or soft tissues of the lips, nose, trachea, and bronchi.

Although it is usually caused by the Gram-negative coccobacillus Klebsiella rhinoscleromatis (*K. pneumoniae* subspecies-rhinoscleromatis), *K. pneumoniae* subspecies-ozaenae is occasionally isolated. Crowded conditions, poor hygiene, and poor nutrition are the risk factors for transmission of the infectious agent [4, 5].

8.4 Clinical Features

Rhinoscleroma affects most areas of the upper respiratory tract, of which the nose is involved in 95–100% of cases [7]. Clinically the disease progresses in three stages:

1. The catarrhal stage/exudative stage: symptoms of rhinitis that progress to foul-smelling purulent rhinorrhea, crusting, and nasal obstruction which may last for months [7, 8].
2. The hypertrophic stage: formation of granulation tissue causing deformity and enlargement of the nose, upper lip, and adjacent structures. This lesion appears as a rubbery bluish-purple granuloma that evolves to a pale-indurated mass. Most cases are diagnosed in this stage because of complaints of epistaxis, anosmia, nasal obstruction, anesthesia of soft palate, hoarseness of voice, and dyspnoea. Bilateral nasal cavities full of granulomas give typical "Hebra nose" deformity, and destruction of the nasal cartilage (Fig. 8.1) [7, 8].
3. The sclerotic stage: fibrotic tissue surrounds the granulomatous area with extensive scarring and laryngeal, nasal stenosis. The gothic palate is the characteristic feature of this phase [7, 10, 11].

    These stages usually do not exist independently. In many cases of rhinoscleroma, the presence of all three stages can be found at the time of diagnosis [12]. The initial nodule is often intranasal and small in size. Rarely, if neglected, it can grow into an exophytic giant

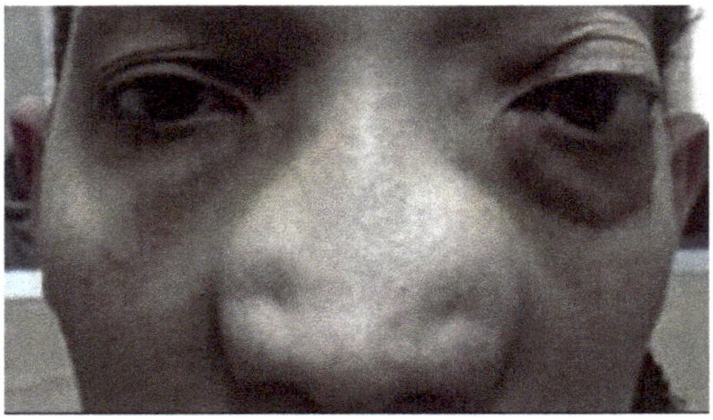

Fig. 8.1 Photograph demonstrates nasal enlargement and proptosis due to rhinoscleroma nodules [9]

tumor, which may obstruct the entire respiratory tract. Rarely, rhinoscleroma of the nasal cavity may extrude into the oral cavity. Rhinoscleroma may also extend into the orbit, to the base of the skull, and into the brain. It may enter the brain through the cribriform plate [11, 13].

Following the nose and nasopharynx in descending order of frequency, the pharynx (18–40%) (Figs. 8.2 and 8.3), the larynx (5%) (Fig. 8.4), the trachea (30%), and bronchi (2–7%) are affected. In rare cases, there may be a manifestation of the skin, the nasolacrimal duct, or the premaxilla. In most cases, the lymphatic system is not affected [6].

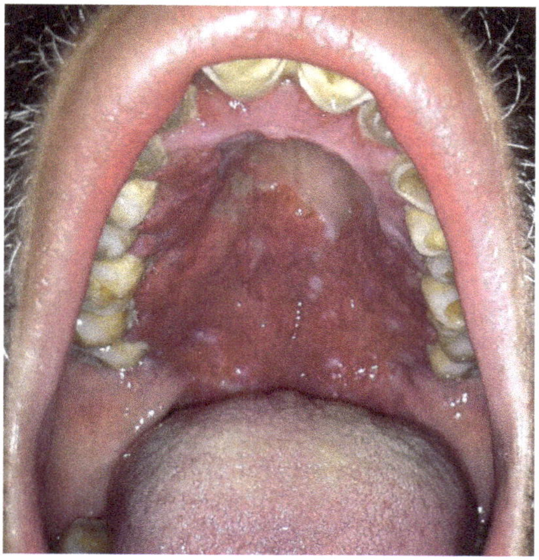

Fig. 8.2 Oral cavity showing a plaque-like erythematous mass involving the gingiva, hard and soft palates [14]

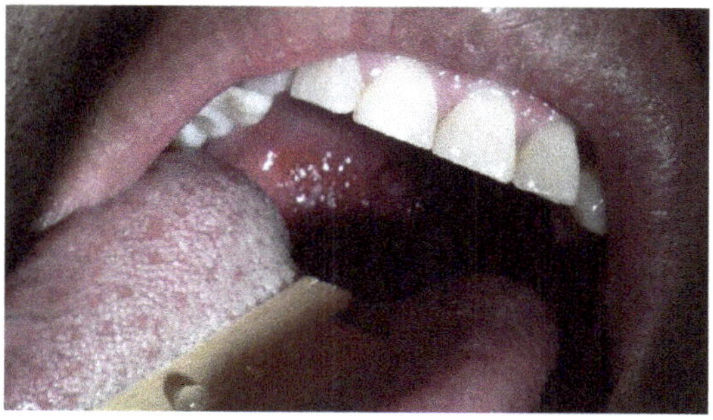

Fig. 8.3 Erythematous tissue with white exudates covering the oropharynx [15]

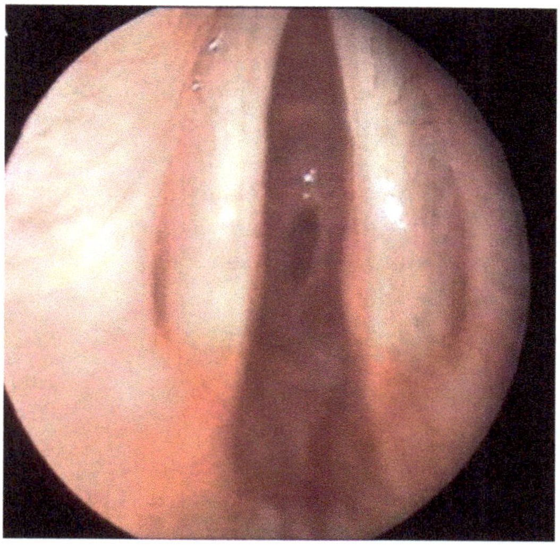

Fig. 8.4 Subglottic stenosis due to rhinoscleroma

8.5 Complications

Rhinoscleroma is a rare cause of upper airway obstruction. Subglottic stenosis may be a late sequelae of rhinoscleroma (Fig. 8.4). Scleroma is known to cause slowly progressive asphyxia [13, 16].

8.6 Diagnosis

8.6.1 Endoscopy

Nasal endoscopy usually reveals signs of all three stages of scleroma: catarrhal, granulomatous, and sclerotic. Blue-reddish granulomatous lesions are the most common presentation. In advanced disease, it is associated with increasing deformities of the nose such as the collapse of the bridge of nose and palatal perforation [6, 16, 17]. Bronchoscopy has a role in the early diagnosis of rhinoscleroma [18].

8.6.2 Microscopy and Culture

Bacteriological analyses with PAS, Giemsa, and Warthin-Starry stains confirm the diagnosis [8, 16, 17].

A positive result with culture in MacConkey agar is diagnostic of rhinoscleroma. However, culture results are positive in only 50–60% of patients [16, 17].

8.6.3 Histopathology

Histopathologic analysis has a definite role in the diagnosis of rhinoscleroma. Classic histopathologic findings include large vacuolated Mikulicz cells and transformed plasma cells with Russell bodies. The Mikulicz cell is a large macrophage with clear cytoplasm that contains the bacilli; this cell is specific to the lesions in rhinoscleroma. The disease is most commonly diagnosed during the proliferative phase, in which the clinical and histologic presentations are most easily recognized [17, 19].

8.6.3.1 The Histologic Findings Correspond to the Three Clinical Stages [7, 8]

Catarrhal (or atrophic) stage: Squamous metaplasia and a nonspecific subepithelial infiltrate of polymorphonuclear leukocytes with granulation tissue are observed.

Granulomatous stage: The diagnostic features include chronic inflammatory cells, Russell bodies, pseudoepitheliomatous hyperplasia, and groups of large vacuolated histiocytes that contain K rhinoscleromatis organisms (Mikulicz cells) (Fig. 8.5). If numerous, these bacteria can be seen with Hematoxylin and Eosin staining (Fig. 8.6), but Periodic Acid-Schiff, Silver impregnation, Steiner stain (Fig. 8.7), or immunohistochemical staining may be required to confirm their presence and identity.

Sclerotic stage: Extensive fibrous tissue is seen. Mikulicz's cells and Russell bodies are difficult to see at this stage.

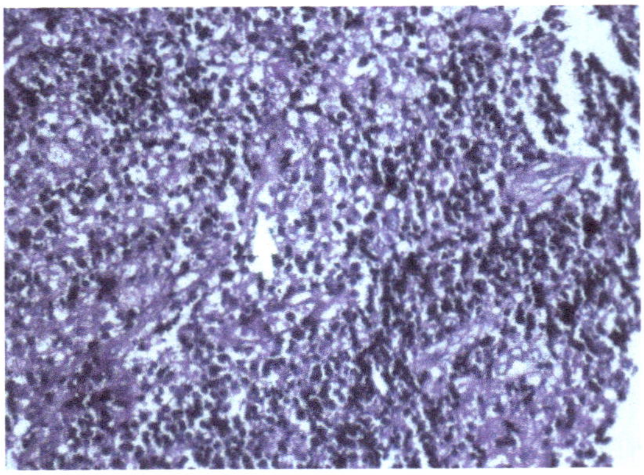

Fig. 8.5 PAS stain- the inflammatory infiltrate consists of an admixture of plasma cells and vacuolated macrophages (Mikulicz cells) (white arrow)

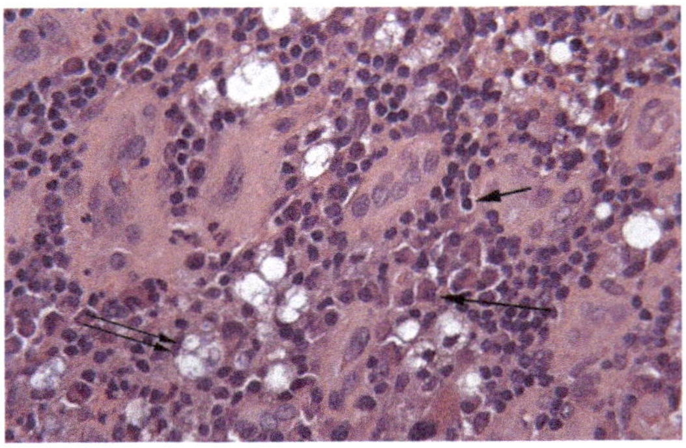

Fig. 8.6 H&E stain (400×) demonstrating a mixture of plasma cells (arrow), lymphocytes (short arrow), and vacuolated macrophages (Mikulicz cells) (double arrow) [14]

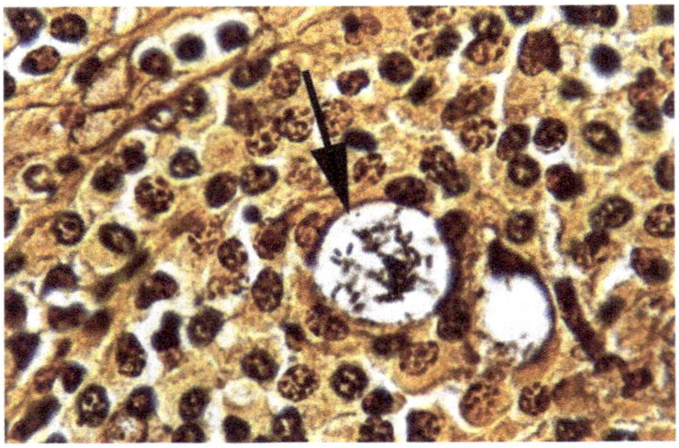

Fig. 8.7 Steiner stain, (1000×) with rod-shaped bacilli within a vacuolated macrophage (Mikulicz cell) (arrow) [14]

- Electron microscopy reveals large phagosomes filled with bacilli and surrounded by a finely granular or fibrillar material that is arranged in a radial pattern. This finding represents the accumulation of antibodies on the bacterial surface (type A granules), as well as the aggregation of bacterial mucopolysaccharides surrounded by antibodies (type B granules) [16, 20].

8.6.4 Imaging

Radiographic studies are of value in assessing the extension of disease.

- CT findings in primary nasal and nasopharyngeal rhinoscleroma include soft-tissue masses of variable sizes. The lesions are characteristically homogeneous and nonenhancing, and they have distinct edge definition (Fig. 8.8). Adjacent fascial planes are not invaded. The subglottic area is involved in laryngeal and tracheal scleroma. The lesions primarily cause concentric irregular narrowing of the airway. In the trachea, cryptlike irregularities are diagnostic of scleroma. Findings also include calcifications, luminal stenosis, wall thickening, and nodules (Fig. 8.9). Radiological imaging facilitates distinction from other granulomatous and malignant disorders [19, 20].
- MRI should be performed in patients with rhinoscleroma. Nasal mass can obstruct the ostiomeatal units, and secretions may be retained in the related sinuses. In the hypertrophic stage of rhinoscleroma, both T1- and T2-weighted images show characteristic mild-to-marked high signal intensity (Fig. 8.10) [20].

8.7 Treatment

- The treatment of both rhinoscleroma and ozena involves antibiotics coupled with surgical debridement in cases of airway obstruction or cosmetic deformity.
- Klebsiella rhinoscleromatis is an intracellular bacterium, so theoretically it responds best to antibiotics that can achieve high concentrations in macrophages. In vivo, the antibiotics that have shown activity include streptomycin, doxycycline, tetracycline, rifampin, second- and third-generation cephalosporins, sulfonamides, clofazimine, ciprofloxacin, and ofloxacin [21].

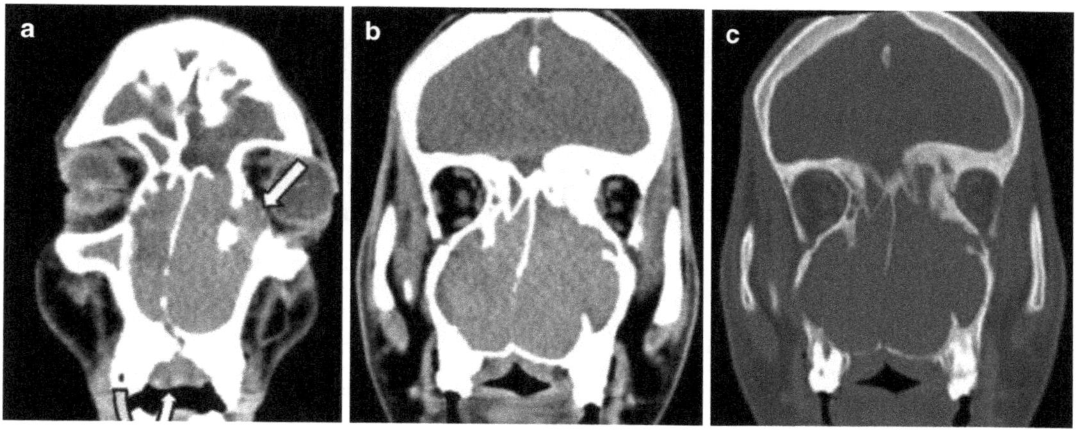

Fig. 8.8 Contrast-enhanced CT scan of the paranasal sinuses, (Left) coronal image of the paranasal sinuses showing large mass within nasal fossae with a small extension into the left orbital cavity (block arrow), also note the hard palatal mass (curved arrow), (Middle) coronal image of the paranasal sinuses showing large masses within nasal fossae, both maxillary antra and ethmoidal air cells, (Right) coronal image bone window showing areas of bone sclerosis and areas of bone thinning (pressure atrophy) [9]

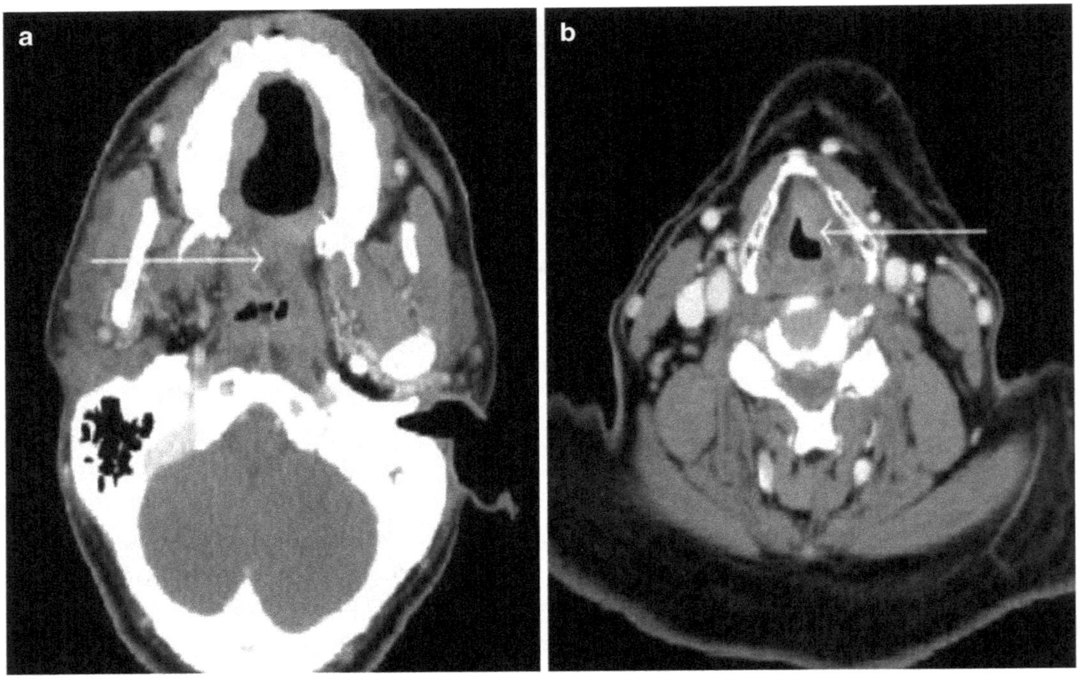

Fig. 8.9 CT neck axial view showing (**a**) mass involving the soft palate significantly narrowing the nasopharynx. (**b**) lesion along the anterior aspect of the left false vocal cord [15]

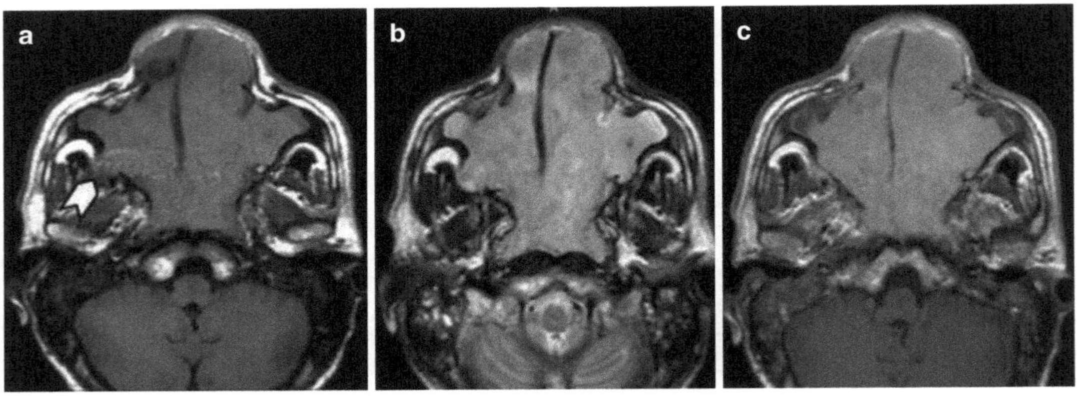

Fig. 8.10 Contrast-enhanced MRI examination of the paranasal sinuses; (**a**) The axial T1 weighted image showing bilateral large masses of intermediate signal intensity within nasal cavities, nasopharynx, both maxillary antra, with small right extramaxillary sinus extension (chevron), (**b**) Axial T2 weighted image showing diffuse high signal intensity of the masses, (**c**) axial T1 weighted image post-gadolinium contrast administration showing diffuse homogeneous post-contrast enhancement [9]

- Historically, treatment of rhinoscleroma was with tetracyclines and aminoglycosides such as streptomycin. Ciprofloxacin appears to be consistently more active than other quinolones against K. pneumonia due to their increased penetrance. Rhinoscleroma lesions respond well to treatment with Ciprofloxacin (500 mg twice a day).
- Long-term antibiotic therapy often eradicates this infection [22–24]. Repeat biopsy can be

performed to help determine the appropriate duration of the antibiotic therapy. The recommended duration of therapy varies from 2 months to 1 year [22–24]. Corticosteroids are also useful in the early stages to reduce inflammatory symptoms [7, 8].

8.7.1 Surgical Management

- Surgery (excision of granuloma) combined with antibiotic therapy is beneficial in patients with a nasal or pharyngeal obstruction or nasal sinus involvement due to the proliferation of lesions [25].
- Tracheotomy should be considered in patients with laryngeal obstruction of the second stage (granulomatous stage) and above (sclerotic stage) [25, 26]. Extensive laryngeal granulomatous lesions are treated by means of open excision by using the laryngofissure approach, which is the best method for a quick recovery in patients without evidence of subglottic stenosis [7, 8].
- Treatment of the advanced cicatrix with carbon dioxide laser vaporization gives excellent results. Obstructive lesions of the larynx and subglottic space are always a challenging problem for the endoscopist and anesthetist. At this level of the obstruction, the effectiveness and innocuous nature of carbon dioxide laser treatment are related to the degree of endoscopic exposure. Because of the transtracheal high-frequency jet ventilator, ensuring a free laryngeal endoscopic operative field is now possible [7, 8, 26].
- Palatal sclerosis with obstruction at velopharyngeal region may be relieved by means of uvulopalatopharyngoplasty [25].

One of the main difficulties in treating rhinoscleroma is the high rate of disease relapse, reaching 26% in some case series. According to Fawaz et al., such a high rate of recurrence may be attributed to noncompliance, short duration of therapy, extensiveness of the lesions, or progression to a cicatricial stage, which has a poor response to medications due to poor vascularity in the affected tissues [23]. Extensive disfigurement of the face may result from erosions over the infection. Damage may be widespread enough to cause complete obstruction of the airways resulting in death.

8.8 Essential Features

- Rhinoscleroma is a chronic granulomatous condition of the upper respiratory tract primarily involving nose, caused by the Gram-negative coccobacillus Klebsiella rhinoscleromatis or Klebsiella ozaena.
- Disease progresses in three stages. At the time of diagnosis, usually, all three stages coexist.
- Catarrhal phase- associated with rhinitis and mucopurulent discharge.
- Granulomatous phase- Granulomas form in the upper respiratory tract causing deformity (Hebra nose).
- Cicatricial/sclerotic phase- Granulomas heal with diffuse scarring with fibrosis and stenosis (Gothic palate, subglottic stenosis).
- Culture: Organism cultured on MacConkey agar gives positive results in 50–60% cases. Special stains Periodic Acid-Schiff, Giemsa, Gram, and Silver stains are used.
- CT and MRI imaging help to delineate calcifications, luminal stenosis, wall thickening, and nodules.
- Nasal endoscopy and bronchoscopy help in the early diagnosis of disease.
- Biopsy of the nodules reveals classic histopathologic findings of large vacuolated Mikulicz cells and transformed plasma cells with Russell bodies.
- Treatment consists of prolonged antibiotic therapy (2 months to 1 year). Ciprofloxacin proves to be the most effective due to its increased penetrance. Surgical debridement or carbon dioxide laser is used to reduce symptoms of airway obstruction if necessary. Corticosteroids are also useful in the early stages to reduce inflammatory symptoms.

References

1. von Hebra H. Ueber ein eigenthümliches Neugebilde an der Nase; Rhinosclerom; nebst histologischem Befunde vom Dr. M. Kohn. Wiener Medizinische Wochenschrift. 1870;20:1–5.
2. von Frisch A. Zur Aetiologie des Rhinoskleroms. Wiener Medizinische Wochenschrift. 1882;32:969–72.
3. Bartolomeo D, Joseph R. Scleroma of the nose and pharynx. West J Med. 1976;124:13–7.
4. Fawaz S, et al. Clinical, radiological and pathological study of 88 cases of typical and complicated scleroma. Clin Respir J. 2011;5(2):112–21.
5. Efared B, et al. Rhinoscleroma: a chronic infectious disease of poor areas with characteristic histological features – report of a series of six cases. Trop Dr. 2018 Jan.;48(1):33–5.
6. Laudien M. Orphan diseases of the nose and paranasal sinuses: Pathogenesis – clinic – therapy. GMS Curr Top Otorhinolaryngol Head Neck Surg. 2015; 14: Doc04. Published online 2015 Dec 22. doi: https://doi.org/10.3205/cto000119
7. Hart C. Rhinoscleroma. J Med Microbiol. 1990;48:395–6.
8. Simons M, et al. Rhinoscleroma: case report. Rev Bras Otorrinolaringol. 2006;72(4):568–71.
9. Ibrahim D, Fayed A. Report of a case of giant rhinoscleroma: CT and MRI. BJR Case Rep. 2018 Dec; 4(4):20180027. Published online 2018 Jul 10. https://doi.org/10.1259/bjrcr.20180027
10. Nayak P, et al. Rhinoscleroma of nose extruding into oral cavity. J Coll Physicians Surg Pak. 2015 Apr.;25(11):S27–9.
11. Ghosh SN, et al. Rhinoscleroma with intracranial extension: a rare case. Neurol India. 2016 May–Jun.;64(3):549–52.
12. Domanski MC, et al. Rhinoscleroma presenting as a nasal-palatal mass with airway obstruction. Version 1. F1000Res. 2013; 2:124. Published online 2013 May 9. https://doi.org/10.12688/f1000research.2-124.v1
13. Ibrahim D, Fayed A. Report of a case of giant rhinoscleroma: CT and MRI. BJR Case Rep. 2018 Dec.;4(4):20180027.
14. Domanski MC, et al. Rhinoscleroma presenting as a nasal-palatal mass with airway obstruction. Version 1. F1000Res. 2013; 2:124. Published online 2013 May 9. https://doi.org/10.12688/f1000research.2-124.v1
15. Gonzales Zamora J, Murali AR. Rhinoscleroma with Pharyngolaryngeal Involvement Caused by Klebsiella ozaenae. Case Rep Infect Dis. 2016; 2016: 6536275. Published online 2016 May 12. https://doi.org/10.1155/2016/6536275
16. Sood N, et al. Cytohistological features of rhinoscleroma. Indian J Pathol Microbiol. 2011 Oct–Dec.;54(4):806–8.
17. Maru YK, et al. Brush cytology and its comparison with histopathological examination in cases of diseases of the nose. J Laryngol Otol. 1999 Nov.;113(11):983–7.
18. Soni NK. Scleroma of the lower respiratory tract: a bronchoscopic study. J Laryngol Otol. 1994 Jun.;108(6):484–5.
19. Ahmed AR, et al. Rhinoscleroma: a detailed histopathological diagnostic insight. Int J Clin Exp Pathol. 2015;8(7):8438–45.
20. Zhong Q, et al. Rhinoscleroma: a retrospective study of pathologic and clinical features. J Otolaryngol Head Neck Surg. 2011 Apr.;40(2):167–74.
21. Maguiña C, et al. Rhinoscleroma: eight Peruvian cases. Revista do Instituto de Medicina Tropical de São Paulo. 2006;48(5):295–9. https://doi.org/10.1590/s0036-46652006000500011.
22. Suchanova PP, et al. Rhinoscleroma in an urban nonendemic setting. Otolaryngol Head Neck Surg. 2012;147(1):173–4.
23. Perkins BA, et al. In vitro activities of streptomycin and 11 oral antimicrobial agents against clinical isolates of Klebsiella rhinoscleromatis. Antimicrob Gents Chemother. 1992;36(8):1785–7.
24. Renois JJ, et al. Preliminary investigation of a mice model of *Klebsiella pneumoniae subsp. ozaenae* induced pneumonia. Microbes Infect. 2011;13(12–13):1045–51.
25. Sun Y, et al. Clinical analysis of 19 cases of scleroma respiratorium treated surgically. Lin Chuang Er Bi Yan Hou Ke Za Zhi. 1998 Jul.;12(7):314–6.
26. Divatia JV, et al. Fibreoptic intubation in cicatricial membranes of the pharynx. Anaesthesia. 1992 Jun.;47(6):486–9.

9 Cat Scratch Disease

Abstract

Cat scratch disease (CSD) is a zoonosis caused by *Bartonella henselae*, a fastidious, hemotropic, Gram-negative bacterium. *B. henselae* is spread among cats—the principal mammal reservoir species—by the cat flea (Ctenocephalides felis); transmission to humans occurs via scratches, and possibly bites, from cats. The predominant clinical feature of CSD is lymphadenopathy proximal to the site of a cat scratch or bite; in many patients, a papule develops at the initial wound site before the onset of lymphadenopathy. Some patients with *B. henselae* infection experience more serious manifestations, such as neuroretinitis, Parinaud oculoglandular syndrome, osteomyelitis, encephalitis, or endocarditis. *B. henselae* infection can be particularly severe for patients with immunocompromised conditions, such as AIDS, in whom vascular proliferative lesions (bacillary angiomatosis and bacillary peliosis) may develop. Lymph node biopsy is the major diagnostic modality. Special stains such as Brown–Hopp tissue Gram stain and Warthin–Starry silver stain can show clumps of small, curved, Gram-negative bacilli usually in the walls of blood vessels and in the microabscesses, which is characteristic of CSD. PCR of the lymph node aspirate is the most sensitive test and is able to differentiate between different Bartonella species. The preferred antibiotic for treatment is Azithromycin, Ciprofloxacin, or Trimethoprim/sulfamethoxazole (TMP-SMZ).

Synonyms

Cat scratch fever, Teeny's disease, inoculation lymphoreticulosis, subacute regional lymphadenitis [1, 2].

9.1 Background

Cat scratch disease is an infectious disease transmitted by young cats, in which the causative factor is *Bartonella henselae*. Parinaud first described conjunctival inflammation with preauricular adenopathy following animal contact more than 100 years ago. In 1931 Debre observed the occurrence of regional lymphadenopathy following cat scratches, then 20 years later published a report of "la maladie des griffe du chat," establishing CSD as a clinical entity [3]. The typical course of cat scratch disease is usually benign and self-limited and requires only supportive therapy. It causes a bump or blister at the site of bite or scratch followed by regional lymphadenopathy. The infection leads to granulomatous changes in the draining lymph nodes and may spread to involve CNS, eyes (neuroretinitis), skin (bacillary angiomatosis, erythema nodosum,

S. V. Nemade, K. J. Shinde, *Granulomatous diseases in Otorhinolaryngology, Head and Neck*,
https://doi.org/10.1007/978-981-16-4047-6_9

erythema multiforme), lungs, and bones (arthritis and osteomyelitis) [1, 2, 4].

9.2 Epidemiology

Cat scratch disease has a worldwide distribution, but public health data on this disease is inadequate. The incidence varies globally from 0.1 to 4.5 per 100000 population. An estimated 22,000 cases of CSD, with more than 2000 hospital admissions, are diagnosed every year in the United States, peaking in fall and winter. The incidence is between 1.8 and 9.3 cases per 100,000 population of USA [3]. Children and women are more prone to get an infection than men.

The association between cats and human infection with *B. henselae* was confirmed following the identification of the bacteriological cause of CSD. More than 90% of patients gave a history of cat contact [2–4].

9.3 Etiopathogenesis

Bartonella henselae, the causative organism is a fastidious, intracellular, Gram-negative bacterium. Formerly known as Rochalimaea henselae, the organism was reclassified as *B. henselae* in 1993, following 16S rRNA sequence analysis. Based on the high degree of relatedness with *Bartonella bacilliformis*, all Rochalimaea were reclassified into the genus Bartonella [3].

The cat was recognized as the natural reservoir of the disease in 1950 by "Robert Debre." However, fleas serve as a vector for transmission of *B. henselae* among cats. As a consequence, a likely means of transmission of *B. henselae* from cats to humans may be inoculation with flea feces containing *B. henselae* through a contaminated cat scratch wound or by cat saliva transmitted in a bite.

The characteristic feature of CSD is regional lymphadenopathy proximal to the site of inoculation. In immunocompetent patients, Bartonella infection causes a granulomatous and suppurative response. In immunocompromised patients, the response to Bartonella infection can be vasculoproliferative with neovascularization. Bartonella is able to promote angioproliferation through adhesin A, which is observed in bacillary angiomatosis [3, 4].

9.4 Clinical Features

Patients with CSD usually have a history of sustaining a scratch or bite from a cat (typically a kitten). The initial symptom is the formation of a papule at the inoculation site, followed by solitary or regional lymphadenopathy within 1–2 weeks. In most patients, the disease resolves spontaneously within 2–4 months. Lymph nodes are often tender and occasionally become fluctuant if suppuration supervene (Fig. 9.1).

Approximately 50% of patients also experience systemic symptoms such as malaise/fatigue, fever, anorexia, headache, sore throat, and arthralgia [5, 6].

Parinaud's oculoglandular syndrome (POGS): It refers to unilateral granulomatous follicular palpebral or bulbar conjunctivitis (Fig. 9.2) associated with ipsilateral preauricular and submandibular lymphadenopathy (Fig. 9.3). The lymphadenopathy may extend to the cervical or parotid lymph nodes and may develop concomitantly with conjunctivitis or its onset may be delayed by several weeks. The physiologic basis of POGS is that the lymphatic drainage of the eyelids leads to the preauricular and submandibu-

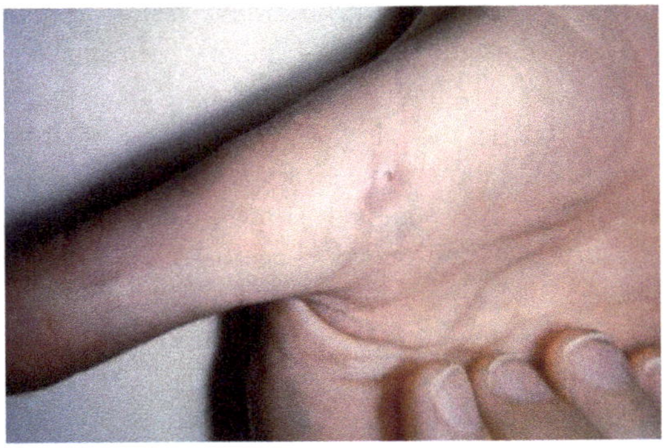

Fig. 9.1 A lesion on the hand of a person with cat scratch disease

lar lymph nodes. POGS has been observed in various bacterial, fungal, and viral infections, but most commonly in cat scratch disease. It is also reported in Tularemia infections [7].

Hematogenous spread of infection may affect other systems:

- Central nervous system

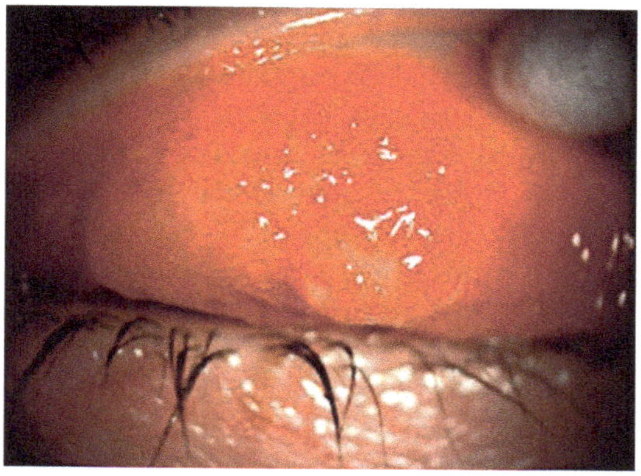

Fig. 9.2 Granuloma in upper tarsal conjunctiva with surrounding papillary reaction in a case of CSD POGS [7]

Encephalopathy is the most common neurologic manifestation, occurring in 2–3% of patients. The onset is usually abrupt and occurs 1–6 weeks after the lymphadenopathy becomes apparent. Fever, confusion, disorientation, and hemiparesis are common symptoms, and the condition can deteriorate to coma. Seizures, which occur in as many as 80% of patients with neurologic sequelae, are often prolonged and recurrent. Recovery is usually complete in 1 week or longer, but persistent neurologic deficits have been reported [8, 9].

- Neuroretinitis

Patients with neuroretinitis generally present with painless, unilateral visual loss. Examination reveals decreased visual acuity, decreased color vision, and centrocecal scotoma. The optic disc appears edematous, and exudates frequently surround the macula. Neuroretinitis is possibly due to a subretinal angiomatous nodule similar to that seen in bacillary angiomatosis [8, 10].

- Bacillary angiomatosis

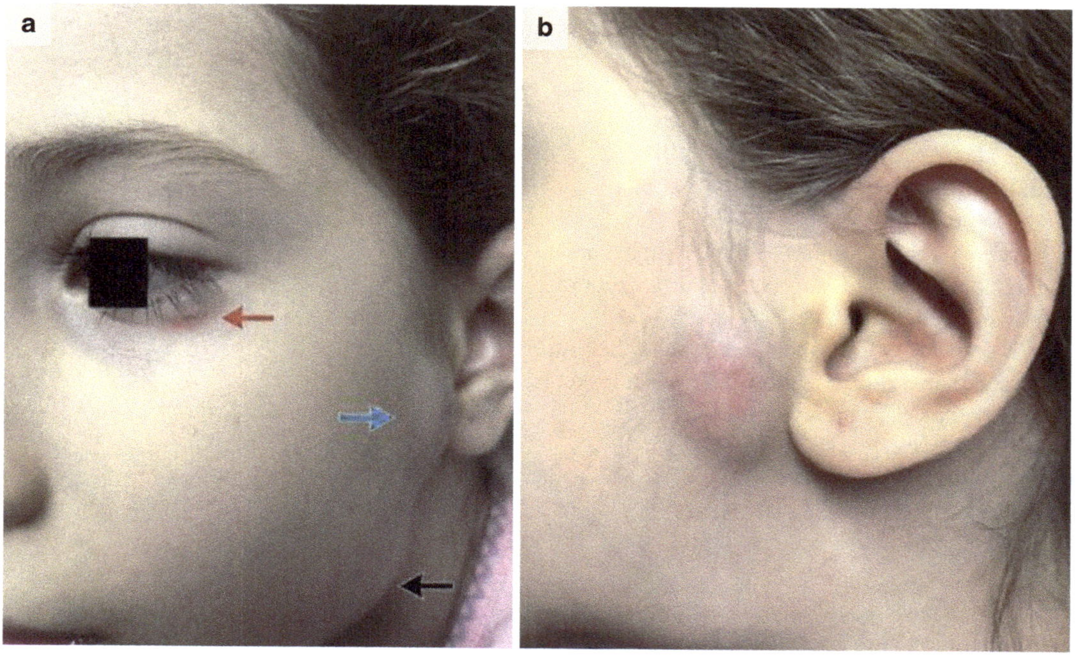

Fig. 9.3 (**a**) Preauricular (blue arrow) and submandibular (black arrow) lymphadenopathy and excoriation below the left eye (red arrow) in a 5-year-old girl with cat scratch disease Parinaud's oculoglandular syndrome (CSD POGS); (**b**) lateral view of preauricular and submandibular lymphadenopathy [7]

Bacillary angiomatosis almost exclusively occurs in immunocompromised patients. Skin lesions consisting of numerous brown to violaceous or colorless vascular tumors of the skin and the subcutaneous tissue are the most common manifestation. Disseminated disease may involve bone, liver, spleen, lymph nodes, gastrointestinal and respiratory tracts, and bone marrow [8, 11].

- Pulmonary

Pulmonary features develop 1–5 weeks after lymphadenopathy. Cough, hemoptysis, and pulmonary abscess are the common manifestations [12, 13].

- Vertebral osteomyelitis and splenic abscess [14, 15].
- Endocarditis

Bartonella endocarditis should be considered in patients with manifestations of endocarditis and negative blood culture results who have regular contact with cats [11, 16]. Possible risk factors include alcoholism and body louse infestation.

9.5 Diagnosis

9.5.1 Imaging

Ultrasonography confirms the lymph node enlargement and can also determine a suppurative lymph node [15].

CT scan and MRI scan are particularly helpful in disseminated disease with CNS, musculoskeletal and pulmonary involvement [17, 18].

9.5.2 Fine Needle Aspiration Cytology

It usually shows reactive lymphadenitis. In case of suppuration, pus should be sent for culture. Culturing Bartonella species is difficult, as the ideal medium has not been established. Blood agar is often used, and incubation for up to 6 weeks is frequently necessary; however, results are often negative [19–21].

9.5.3 Lymph Node Biopsy

It is usually not indicated in the typical cases of CSD, due to the risk of fistula formation. In cases of possible malignancy or in an unclear presentation in an immunocompromised host, it is preferred. Lymphoid hyperplasia with arteriolar proliferation and reticular cell hyperplasia is seen early in the disease. As the disease progresses, granulomas appear, with central necrosis surrounded by lymphocytes [11, 20]. Histiocytes and multinucleated giant cells are often present. Finally, stellate microabscesses form (Fig. 9.4). Histopathological features of lymph nodes are consistent but not pathognomonic for CSD. Special stains such as Brown–Hopp tissue Gram stain and Warthin–Starry silver stain can show clumps of small, curved, Gram-negative bacilli usually in the walls of blood vessels and in the microabscesses, which is characteristic of CSD (Fig. 9.5) [15, 22].

9.5.4 Serology

Indirect fluorescence assay (IFA) testing and Enzyme-linked immunoassay (ELISA) are used to detect serum antibody to *B. henselae*. An antibody titer that exceeds 1:64 suggests recent

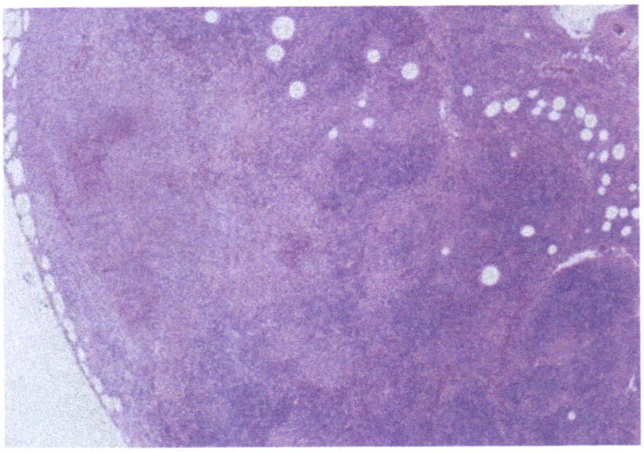

Fig. 9.4 The lymph node showing reactive follicular hyperplasia and multiple geographic microabscesses (H&E stain × 40) [22]

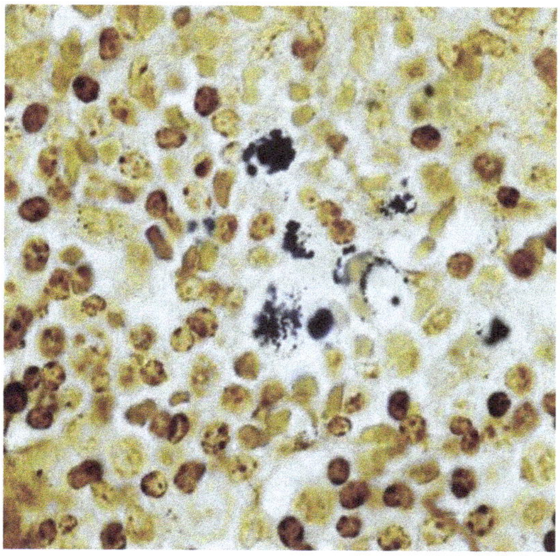

Fig. 9.5 Clumps of bacteria found in the lymph node (Warthin–Starry silver stain × 1000) [22]

Bartonella infection. The accuracy of IFA can be improved by concurrent use of both immunoglobulin G (IgG) and immunoglobulin M (IgM) testing. The specificity of IgM and IgG testing ranges from 88 to 98% and 50 to 62%, respectively. ELISA testing for IgM has a sensitivity of 95% and a specificity of 77%. ELISA for IgG has a sensitivity of only 18% [23–25].

9.5.5 Molecular Assay

Polymerase chain reaction (PCR) of the lymph node aspirate is the most sensitive test and is able to differentiate between different Bartonella species, as well as subspecies and strains. However, this test is not readily available [11, 19–21].

In CNS involvement, CSF examination shows mononuclear pleocytosis in 20–30% of patients. Electroencephalographs (EEGs) show nonspecific slowing.

9.6 Treatment

In immunocompetent patients, complete recovery without sequelae occurs in nearly all patients. Antibiotics are usually not indicated in most cases of CSD, but they may be considered for severe or systemic diseases. Lymphadenitis usually resolves spontaneously over 2–4 months, but 1–2 years may be required. One episode of cat scratch disease confers lifelong immunity.

Immunocompromised patients may experience a dramatic and potentially life-threatening course of the disease. However, with appropriate antibiotic use and management of complications, these patients also experience full resolution of disease.

The preferred antibiotic for treatment is Azithromycin (500 mg/day on the first day followed by 250 mg/day for next 9 days), Ciprofloxacin (500 mg 12 hrly for 10 days), or Trimethoprim/sulfamethoxazole (TMP-SMZ) (6–8 mg TMP/kg/day for 10 days) [18]. Azithromycin is preferably used in pregnancy. In case of disseminated or severe disease IV Gentamicin (5 mg/kg/day) may be used. However, Doxycycline (100 mg 12 hrly) is preferred to treat *B. henselae* infections with optic neuritis due to its ability to adequately penetrate the tissues of the eye and central nervous system. [26].The efficacy of antibiotics for patients with severe CSD: [27]

- Rifampin—Efficacy of 87%
- Ciprofloxacin—Efficacy of 84%
- Azithromycin—Efficacy of 80%
- Gentamicin intramuscularly—Efficacy of 73%
- Trimethoprim/sulfamethoxazole (TMP-SMZ) —Efficacy of 58%

Surgical treatment: In case of suppurative lymph node not responding to repeated aspirations, incision and drainage is necessary. Regular cleaning and dressing of the wound combined with antibiotic therapy prevent fistula formation [27].

Prevention- Cat scratch disease can be primarily prevented by taking flea control measures and washing hands after handling a cat or cat feces; since cats are mostly exposed to fleas when they are outside, keeping cats inside can help prevent infestation.

9.7 Essential Features

- Caused by Bartonella (formerly Rochalimaea) harbored by kittens and young cats; transmitted between cats by cat flea (but not from cats to humans).
- Cutaneous red papule 7–12 days after contact that may become crusted or pustular, with regional lymphadenopathy.
- May have necrotizing granulomas in liver, spleen, or bone
- Gram stain shows Pleomorphic, curved, Gram-negative coccobacillus. Catalase negative, oxidase negative.
- Characteristic histopathological changes in nodal biopsy—histiocytes and follicular hyperplasia in early stage. Also multinucleated giant cells, lymphocytes, and eosinophils. In late stages, associated with capsulitis and subcapsular granulomas and abscess.
- PCR of the lymph node aspirate is the most sensitive test and is able to differentiate between different Bartonella species, as well as subspecies and strains.
- Serologic Testing: Indirect fluorescence assay (IFA) testing and Enzyme-linked immunoassay (ELISA) are used to detect serum antibody to *B. henselae*.
- Usually resolves spontaneously. The preferred antibiotic for treatment is Azithromycin, Ciprofloxacin, or Trimethoprim/sulfamethoxazole (TMP-SMZ).
- Surgical treatment: In case of suppurative lymph node not responding to repeated aspirations, incision and drainage is necessary.

References

1. Klotz SA, et al. Cat-scratch disease. Am Fam Physician. 2011;83(2):152–5. PMID 21243990
2. Florin TA, et al. Beyond cat scratch disease: widening spectrum of Bartonella henselae infection. Pediatrics. 2008;121(5):e1413–25.
3. Opavsky MA. Cat scratch disease: the story continues. Can J Infect Dis. 1997 Jan–Feb;8(1):43–9. https://doi.org/10.1155/1997/982908.
4. Windsor JJ. Cat-scratch disease: epidemiology, etiology, and treatment. Br J Biomed Sci. 2001;58:101–10.
5. Regnery R, Tappero J. Unraveling mysteries associated with cat-scratch disease, bacillary angiomatosis, and related syndromes. Emerg Infect Dis. 1995 Jan-Mar.;1(1):16–21.
6. Carithers HA. Cat-scratch disease. An overview based on a study of 1,200 patients. Am J Dis Child. 1985 Nov.;139(11):1124–33.
7. Kevin Dixon M, et al. Parinaud's Oculoglandular syndrome: case in an dult with flea- borne typhus and a review. Trop Med Infect Dis. 2020 Sep;5(3):126. https://doi.org/10.3390/tropicalmed5030126.
8. Moriarty RA, Margileth AM. Cat scratch disease. Infect Dis Clin N Am. 1987 Sep.;1(3):575–90.
9. Marra CM. Neurologic complications of Bartonella henselae infection. Curr Opin Neurol. 1995 Jun.;8(3):164–9.
10. Chrousos GA, et al. Neuroretinitis in cat scratch disease. J Clin Neuroophthalmol. 1990 Jun.;10(2):92–4.
11. Margileth AW, et al. Cat-scratch disease. Bacteria in skin at the primary inoculation site. JAMA. 1984 Aug 17;252(7):928–31.
12. Gerd J. Ridder et al. cat-scratch disease: Otolaryngologic manifestations and management. Otolaryngology Head and Neck Surgery. 2005;132(3):353–8.
13. Abbasi S, Chesney PJ. Pulmonary manifestations of cat-scratch disease; a case report and review of the literature. Pediatr Infect Dis J. 1995 Jun;14(6):547–8.
14. De Kort JG, et al. Multifocal osteomyelitis in a child: a rare manifestation of cat scratch disease: a case report and systematic review of the literature. J Pediatr Orthop B. Jul 2006;15(4):285–8.
15. Rolain JM, et al. Lymph node biopsy specimens and diagnosis of catscratch disease: discussion. Emerg Infect Dis. Sep 2006;12(9):1338–44.
16. Walvogel K, et al. Disseminated catscratch disease: detection of R. henselae in affected tissue. Eur J Pediatr. 1994;153:23–7.
17. Avidor B, et al. Molecular diagnosis of cat scratch disease: a two-step approach. J Clin Microbiol. 1997 Aug.;35(8):1924–30.
18. Wang CW, et al. Computed tomography and magnetic resonance imaging of cat-scratch disease: a report of two cases. Clin Imaging. 2009 Jul–Aug.;33(4):318–21.
19. Margileth AM. The diagnostic challenge of cat scratch disease. Inf Med. 1987:57–75.
20. English CK, et al. Cat-scratch disease. Isolation and culture of the bacterial agent. JAMA. 1988 Mar 4;259(9):1347–52.
21. Cheung VW, Moxham JP. Cat scratch disease presenting as acute mastoiditis. Laryngoscope. 2010;120(Suppl 4):S222.
22. Shin OR, et al. A case report of seronegative cat scratch disease, emphasizing the histopathologic point of view. Diagn Pathol. 2014; 9:62. Published online 2014 Mar 19. https://doi.org/10.1186/1746-1596-9-62
23. Abarca K, et al. Accuracy and diagnostic utility of IgM in Bartonella henselae infections. Rev Chilena Infectol. 2013 Apr;30(2):125–8.

24. Vermeulen MJ, et al. Evaluation of sensitivity, specificity and cross -reactivity in Bartonella henselae serology. J Med Microbiol. 2010 Mar; 59:743–745. (Epub ahead of print)
25. Huang J, et al. Application of Warthin-starry stain, immunohistochemistry and transmission electron microscopy in diagnosis of cat scratch disease. Zhonghua Bing Li Xue Za Zhi. 2010 Apr.;39(4):225–9.
26. Bass JW, et al. Prospective randomized double blind placebo-controlled evaluation of azithromycin for treatment of cat-scratch disease. Pediatr Infect Dis J. 1998 Jun.;17(6):447–52.
27. Margileth AM. Antibiotic therapy for cat-scratch disease: clinical study of therapeutic outcome in 268 patients and a review of the literature. Pediatr Infect Dis J. 1992 Jun.;11(6):474–8.

10 Lyme Disease

Abstract

Lyme disease (Lyme borreliosis) is a tick-borne, zoonosis caused by genospecies of the Borrelia burgdorferi sensu lato complex. Clinical manifestations result from the inflammatory response elicited by the bacterium and its constituents. The deposition of spirochetes into human dermal tissue generates a local inflammatory response (early localized infection) that manifests as erythema chronicum migrans (ECM), the hallmark skin lesion. Seventy-five percent of patients with Lyme disease present with ENT and head neck manifestations. The early disseminated infection causes lymphadenopathy, mucocutaneous lesions in the upper respiratory tract, cardiovascular, and nervous system involvement. The late disseminated infection manifests as migratory polyarthritis, cutaneous lesions (Acrodermatitis chronica atrophicans) and peripheral nerve palsy. B burgdorferi can be isolated and cultivated in Barbour-Stoenner-Kelly II medium. It can be detected by light microscopy in tissue sections. Serological assay detecting IgG and IgM antibody by ELISA is highly sensitive, however less useful in early-stage disease. PCR of synovial fluid to detect the genetic material (DNA) of spirochete and CSF analysis is helpful in neuroborreliosis. Early infection is treated with antibiotics such as doxycycline, amoxicillin, azithromycin. For late infection, IV penicillin G or third-generation cephalosporins (ceftriaxone or cefotaxime) is considered the treatment of choice.

Synonyms
Lyme borreliosis.

10.1 Background

Lyme disease is caused by a tick-borne spirochete, Borrelia burgdorferi. It is transmitted to humans by the bite of Ixodes ricinus ticks. After the initial tick bite, a characteristic skin lesion, erythema migrans, occurs in most cases. A virus-like illness occurs as the bacteria spread throughout the body hematogenously and causes other system involvement. Lyme disease was diagnosed as a separate condition for the first time in 1975 in Old Lyme, Connecticut, New London County, USA. It was originally mistaken for juvenile rheumatoid arthritis. The bacterium involved was first described in 1981 by "Willy Burgdorfer" [1, 2].

10.2 Epidemiology

Lyme disease is the most common disease spread by ticks in the Northern Hemisphere [3]. It is estimated to affect 300,000 people a year in the USA

S. V. Nemade, K. J. Shinde, *Granulomatous diseases in Otorhinolaryngology, Head and Neck*,
https://doi.org/10.1007/978-981-16-4047-6_10

and 65,000 people a year in Europe. The global incidence is 365,000 per year. Infections are most common in the spring and early summer with no age and gender predilection [3–5]. In North America, *B. burgdorferi* causes nearly all infections; in Europe, *B. afzelii* and *B. garinii* are most associated with human disease.

10.3 Etiopathogenesis

Lyme disease is caused by spirochetes, spiral bacteria Borrelia burgdorferi sensu lato complex.

B. burgdorferi sensu lato is transmitted by ticks from the Ixodes ricinus complex. Spirochetes are surrounded by peptidoglycan and flagella, along with an outer membrane similar to other Gram-negative bacteria. Lyme disease is classified as a zoonosis, as it is transmitted to humans from a natural reservoir among small mammals and birds by ticks that feed on both sets of hosts. The spirochete's unusual fragmented genome encodes a plethora of differentially expressed outer surface lipoproteins that play a seminal role in the bacterium's ability to sustain itself within its enzootic cycle and cause disease when transmitted to its incidental human host.

B. burgdorferi can spread throughout the body during the course of the disease and has been found in the skin, heart, joints, peripheral nervous system, and central nervous system. Many of the signs and symptoms of Lyme disease are a consequence of the immune response to spirochete in those tissues [6]. Exposure to the Borrelia bacterium during Lyme disease possibly causes a long-lived and damaging inflammatory response, [7] a form of pathogen-induced autoimmune disease [8]. Chronic symptoms from an autoimmune reaction could explain why some symptoms persist even after the spirochetes have been eliminated from the body [6, 7].

10.4 Clinical Features

The incubation period from infection to the onset of symptoms is usually one to two weeks but can be much shorter (days) or much longer (months to years). Lyme symptoms most often occur from May to September because the nymphal stage of the tick is responsible for most cases [9].

10.4.1 Stages of Disease

10.4.1.1 Early Localized Infection

It presents with skin lesion (erythema chronicum migrans—ECM)). The disease starts as a papule in the area of the tick bite that expands slowly to an erythematous annular plaque that clears in the center creating a bull's-eye appearance known as erythema migrans (Fig. 10.1). The ECM rash is often accompanied by symptoms of a viral-like illness, including fatigue, headache, body ache, fever with chills, usually in the absence of upper respiratory symptoms [9, 11].

Morgellons disease (MD)—It is a contested dermopathy that is associated with Borrelia spirochetal infection. It is a dermatological condition characterized by multicolored filaments embedded within or projecting from skin Fig. 10.3d). It is predominantly associated with spirochetal infection caused by members of the genus Borrelia, as well as infection with other tick-borne and non-tick-borne pathogens including *Helicobacter pylori* and *Treponema denticola*. [13]

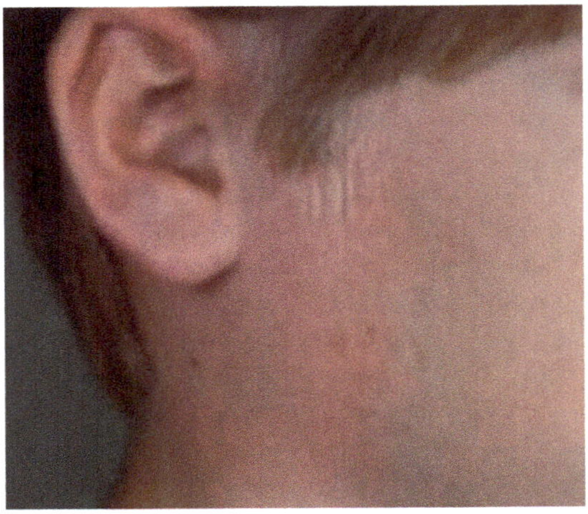

Fig. 10.1 Erythema migrans involving right pinna extending to preauricular and infra-auricular region. Ref—same as ear lobule [10]

10.4.1.2 Early Disseminated Infection

ENT and Head Neck involvement –75% of patients with Lyme disease present with ENT and head neck manifestations.

- Upper respiratory tract involvement: Mucocutaleous involvement in the upper respiratory tract is seen leading to odynophagia, head neck dysesthesia, otalgia, and dysgeusia.
- Borrelial lymphocytoma: It typically presents as a bluish-red plaque or nodule that varies from one to a few centimeters in diameter. The most common sites include the earlobe, preauricular region, nipple, and genital area (Fig. 10.2a, b). Lesions are typically noted 30–45 days after a tick bite [14].
- Regional lymphadenopathy: It manifests with pain and swelling. The commonest presentation is cervical lymphadenopathy secondary to upper respiratory tract involvement [15, 16].

Nervous System Involvement (Neuroborreliosis)

- Lymphocytic meningitis.
- Cranial neuritis—It is an inflammation of cranial nerves. Facial nerve palsy is the most typical presentation. Bilateral facial nerve paralysis is seen in 25% of patients. Dysphagia due to IX and X cranial nerve involvement, Diplopia due to VI nerve palsy, tinnitus, hearing loss, vertigo due to VIII cranial nerve involvement can be seen [9, 11, 17].
- Lyme radiculopathy—It is an inflammation of spinal nerve roots that often causes pain and less often weakness, numbness, or altered sensation in the areas of the body supplied by nerves connected to the affected roots, e.g., limb(s) or part(s) of the trunk [17].
- Mononeuritis multiplex is an inflammation-causing similar symptoms in one or more unrelated peripheral nerves [17].

Cardiovascular Involvement

- Lyme carditis [18]. Symptoms may include palpitations, (in 69% of people), dizziness, fainting, shortness of breath, and chest pain [19].
- Cardiomegaly, left ventricular dysfunction, or congestive heart failure [19].

10.4.1.3 Late Disseminated Infection

- Acrodermatitis chronica atrophicans is the most common presentation. It is evident on the extremities. It begins with an inflammatory stage characterized by bluish-red discoloration with cutaneous swelling and concludes several months or years later with an atrophic phase.

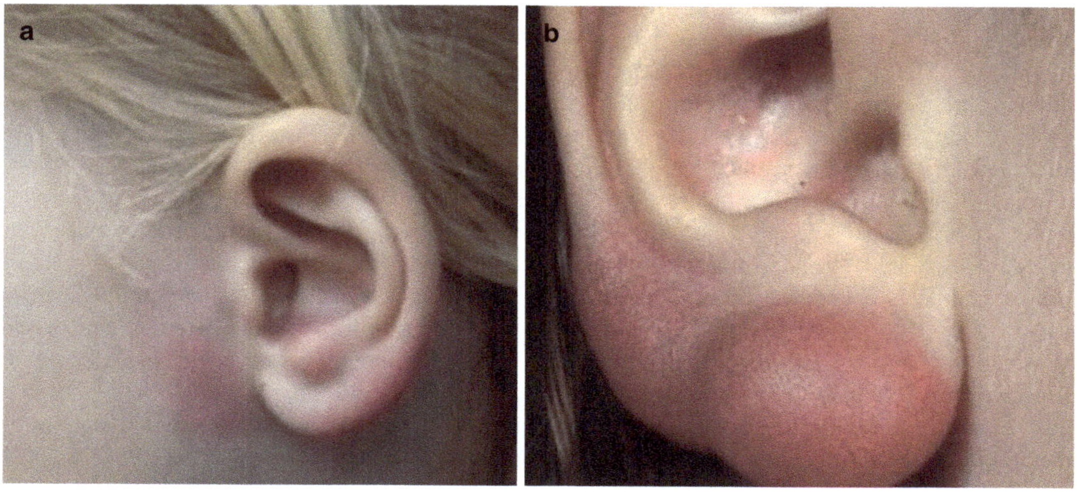

Fig. 10.2 Borrelial lymphocytoma in (**a**) Left preauricular region and (**b**) in the right ear lobule [10]

- Migratory polyarthritis. Temporomandibular joint involvement may lead to trismus.
- Chronic neurologic symptoms occur in up to 5% of untreated people [15]. A peripheral neuropathy or polyneuropathy may develop, causing abnormal sensations such as numbness, tingling, or burning starting at the feet or hands and over time possibly moving up the limbs [15]. It may manifest as peripheral facial nerve paralysis.

10.5 Diagnosis

Clinical diagnosis is suspected with history of tick bite, erythema migrans, fever, facial palsy and/or arthritis.

10.5.1 Microscopy and Culture

Direct detection of *B. burgdorferi* can be achieved by the culture of the infectious agent, by microscopy, and by the use of molecular methods for the detection of Borrelia nucleic acids. These methods vary in sensitivity and procedure complexity. They can provide evidence for the presence of intact spirochetes or spirochete components, such as DNA or protein, in tick vectors, reservoir hosts, or patients.

Microscopy—*Borrelia burgdorferi* detection by light microscopy is not feasible in clinical practice. It is almost never seen in peripheral blood smears. The low Borrelia load does not allow a direct recognition of the spirochetes in tissue slides for routine diagnostic procedures. However, for specific purposes, the Warthin–Starry's silver stain, darkfield microscopy and more recently the focus floating microscopy (FFM), which are light microscopy-based techniques, can be used to detect Borrelia in clinical tissues (Fig. 10.3) [12, 20, 21].

Culture—Although in vitro cultivation of Borrelia from clinical samples represents the gold standard for proving an active infection, this method cannot be routinely used for diagnosis as it is time consuming and has low clinical sensitivity. Borrelia burgdorferi culture can be obtained from various tissues and body fluids with variable yield using dedicated media, such as the modified Kelly-Pettenkofer medium (MKP), the Barbour-Stoenner-Kelly II (BSK-II) medium, and the commercially available BSK-H medium. Borrelia cultivation from clinical samples is mostly successful from skin biopsy when compared to blood and CSF cultures [20, 22].

10.5.2 Histopathology

Histopathology of lymph node reveals superficial and deep perivascular polymorphic infiltrate of neutrophils, lymphocytes, plasma cells, eosinophils, and mast cells (Fig. 10.4) [10, 23].

Erythema Migrans—Histologic findings in erythema migrans are nonspecific, usually showing a perivascular cellular infiltrate consisting of lymphocytes, plasma cells, and histiocytes. Occasionally, mast cells and neutrophils are seen. Central biopsies may show eosinophilic infiltrates consistent with a local reaction to an arthropod bite. Spirochetes occasionally may be identified using silver or antibody-labeled stains, although usually, a paucity of spirochetes is found in the tissues of patients with Lyme disease [23].

Borrelial Lymphocytoma—It shows a dense dermal lymphocytic infiltrate with lymphoid follicles and pseudogerminal centers. Lymphocytes with both B- and T-cell markers, occasional macrophages, plasma cells, and eosinophils are seen [14, 24].

Acrodermatitis Chronica Atrophicans—In acrodermatitis chronica atrophicans, biopsy specimens from early lesions show a lymphocytic dermal infiltrate, sometimes perivascular in location, with some vascular telangiectasia and lymphedema. Plasma cells also may be seen in the cellular infiltrate. Later lesions demonstrate epidermal thinning with loss of skin appendages. At this stage, plasma cells may be the only feature to distinguish acrodermatitis chronica atrophicans from morphea [23].

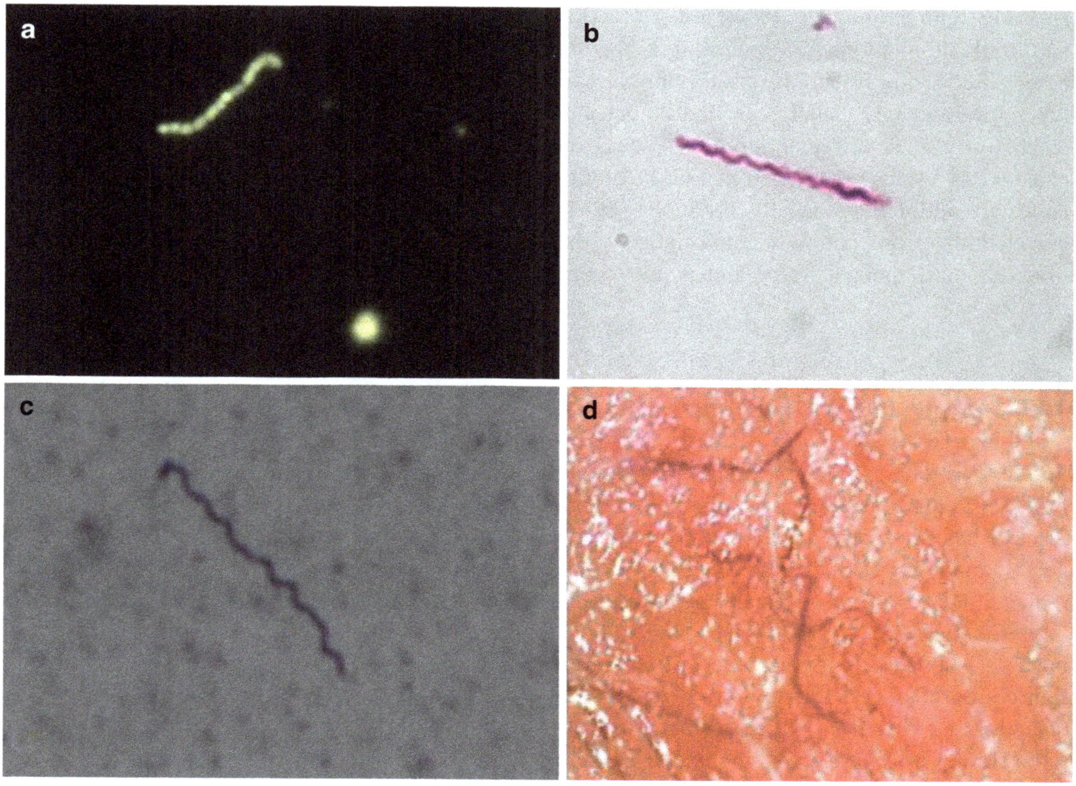

Fig. 10.3 (**a**) (Top left): Darkfield microscopy of blood culture showing live spirochete and spherules. Magnification 400×. (**b**) (Bottom left): Dieterle silver stain of culture fluid from Case 10 showing live spirochetes. Magnification 1000×. (**c**) (Top right): Borrelia immunostain of culture fluid from Case 9 showing live spirochetes. Magnification 1000×. (**d**) (Bottom right). Typical dermal filaments from a patient with Morgellons disease. Magnification 100× [12]

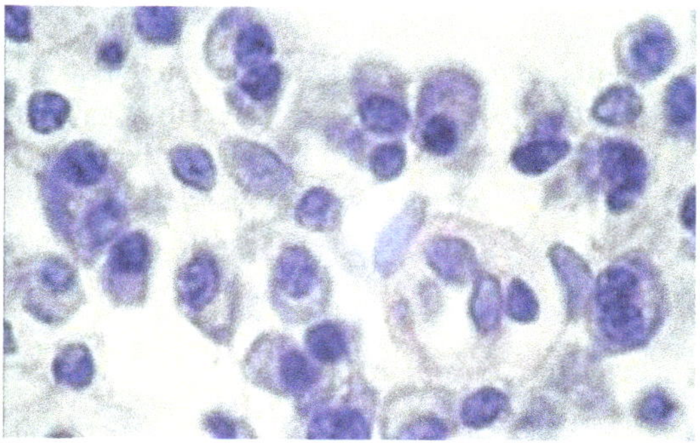

Fig. 10.4 Typical perivascular plasma-cellular infiltrate [10]

10.5.3 Immunohistochemistry

Immunohistochemical analysis shows positive stains for CD 20 and variable staining for CD 3 in the small lymphocytes.

10.5.4 Serology

Currently, serological tests (indirect immunofluorescence assay, enzyme-linked immunosorbent assay and Western immunoblot) for detection of

IgG and IgM antibodies are the most practical and available methods for confirming Lyme disease. After Lyme infection onset, antibodies of types IgM and IgG usually can first be detected respectively at 2–4 weeks and 4–6 weeks, and peak at 6–8 weeks [16]. When an ECM rash first appears, antibodies usually cannot yet be detected; therefore, antibody confirmation at that time has no diagnostic value and is not recommended [25].

10.5.5 Molecular Assay

Polymerase chain reaction (PCR) of synovial fluid/CSF/blood/respiratory secretions for Lyme disease has also been developed to detect the genetic material (DNA) of the Lyme disease spirochete. However, it is usually recommended only for synovial fluid. In other fluids, false-positive results are common due to contamination. Culture or PCR is the current means for detecting the presence of the organism, as serologic studies only test for antibodies of Borrelia [11, 17]. Detection of OspA lipoprotein, an outer surface protein of bacteria shed by live Borrelia bacteria into the urine, is a promising technique being studied [26].

10.5.6 Imaging

Magnetic resonance imaging (MRI) and single-photon emission computed tomography (SPECT) are two of the tests that can identify abnormalities in neuroborreliosis (Fig. 10.5). Neuroimaging findings in an MRI include granulomatous lesions in the periventricular white matter, as well as enlarged ventricles and cortical atrophy [15, 24].

10.5.7 Other Tests

- CSF Analysis: Spinal fluid levels of IgM and IgG antibodies to *B. burgdorferi* should be measured, and an index of cerebrospinal fluid (CSF) to serum antibody (immunoglobulin-to-albumin ratio) should be calculated. This is particularly true in patients who have no other signs of Lyme disease. Although CSF cultures are positive in fewer than 10% of Lyme disease patients with apparent meningitis, intrathecal antibodies and a lymphocytic pleocytosis (approximately 100 cells/μL) are present in more than 80%. Patients with meningitis typically have elevated protein concentrations (>50 mg/dL) but normal glucose levels (45–80 mg/dL). Oligoclonal bands specific for *B. burgdorferi* may be present [28].
- In Lyme carditis, electrocardiograms may show myocardial dysfunction [18].

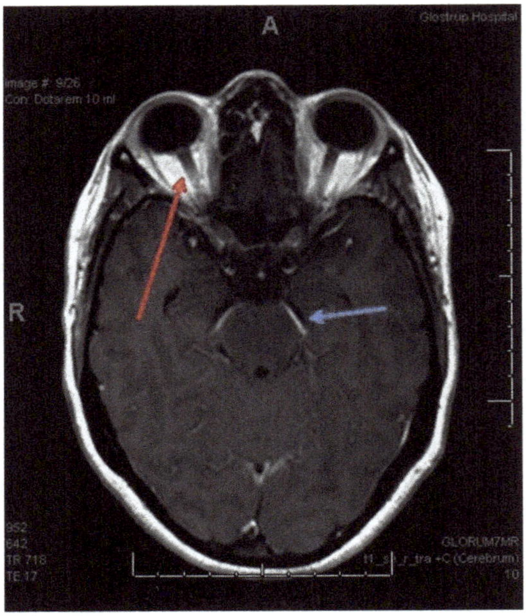

Fig. 10.5 MRI of cerebrum with gadolinium contrast, axial picture. Red arrow showing papilledema and blue arrow showing meningeal enhancement in neuroborreliosis [27]

10.6 Treatment

Oral administration of Doxycycline (100 mg twice a day) is widely recommended as the first choice, as it is effective against not only Borrelia bacteria but also a variety of other illnesses carried by ticks [24]. People taking Doxycycline should avoid sun exposure because of higher risk of sunburns [9]. Doxycycline is contraindicated in children younger than eight years of age and women who are pregnant or breastfeeding; [24] Alternatives to Doxycycline are Amoxicillin, Cefuroxime axetil, and Azithromycin [24, 29].

In Lyme carditis and neuritis, intravenous administration of Ceftriaxone is recommended as the first choice; Cefotaxime and Doxycycline are available as alternatives [10, 29].

The recommended duration of treatment is as follows:

- Early localized/disseminated infection should be treated for 10–21 days. The length of treatment depends on the duration and severity of the clinical symptoms; in the case of solitary erythema migrans without general symptoms, a 10 to 14 day treatment is sufficient [10].
- Late disseminated infection without neurological involvement should be treated with doxycycline or amoxicillin orally for 30 days. However, if there are associated neurological symptoms, intravenous treatment with penicillin G or third generation cephalosporins (ceftriaxone or cefotaxime) may be necessary [10].

In Lyme arthritis, symptomatic treatment with NSAIDs, disease-modifying antirheumatic drugs (DMARDs) is necessary along with antimicrobials. Arthroscopic synovectomy may be required in few cases. Physiotherapy plays an important role in cranial nerve palsy and arthritis [9, 29].

The cure rate is defined as the reinstatement of the body's original condition with regression of the disease-specific symptoms after successful treatment. It is between 95 and 100% when the localized and disseminated early manifestations are treated in time [10].

Post-treatment Lyme disease syndrome (PTLDS): It may occur after antibiotic treatment of any stage of Lyme disease and is associated with ongoing symptoms of fatigue, musculoskeletal pain, and cognitive complaints. These symptoms may wax, wane, and persist for years and may be mild or, in other cases, can result in a significant decline in health-related quality of life. The known risk factors for PTLDS include greater severity of initial disease, presence of initial neurologic involvement, delay in diagnosis and treatment, and the persistence of symptoms after the completion of initial antibiotic therapy [30].

10.7 Essential Features

- Lyme disease is caused by a tick-borne spirochete, Borrelia burgdorferi sensu lato complex.
- The bite of an infected Ixodes dammini tick causes the proliferation of spirochetes in the dermis. The host dermal inflammatory response causes a rash known as erythema chronicum migrans.
- Over days, the spirochetes spread to the regional lymph nodes, nervous system, cardiac tissue and joints via the bloodstream.
- Early localized infection: skin lesion (erythema chronicum migrans).
- Early disseminated infection: Lymphadenopathy, mucocutaneous lesions in the upper respiratory tract, cardiovascular, and nervous system involvement are seen.
- Late disseminated infection: arthritis stage characterized by migratory polyarthritis; however, cutaneous lesions (Acrodermatitis chronica atrophicans) and peripheral nervous system involvement are also encountered in this stage. May manifest as facial nerve paralysis.
- Lyme disease spirochetes are almost never seen in peripheral blood smears.
- Microscopy: Borrelia burgdorferi spirochete detection in the tissues by light microscopy with Warthin–Starry's silver stain, darkfield microscopy and more recently, the focus floating microscopy (FFM). B burgdorferi can be isolated and cultivated in Barbour-Stoenner-Kelly II medium.
- Histopathology of Lymph nodes: Superficial and deep perivascular polymorphic infiltrate of neutrophils, lymphocytes, plasma cells, eosinophils, and mast cells.
- Serology: IgG and IgM antibody detection by ELISA.
- Molecular assay: Polymerase chain reaction (PCR) of synovial fluid to detect the genetic

material (DNA) of the spirochete and CSF analysis in neuroborreliosis.

- Early infection: Antibiotics such as doxycycline, amoxicillin, or azithromycin are preferred.
- Late infection: IV penicillin G or third-generation cephalosporins (ceftriaxone or cefotaxime) is considered the treatment of choice.

References

1. Nelson KE, Williams CF. Infectious disease epidemiology: theory and practice. 2nd ed. Sudbury, Mass: Jones and Bartlett Publishers; 2007. p. 447. isbn 9780763728793
2. Willy Burgdorfer – obituary. Daily Telegraph. 1 December 2014.
3. Regional disease vector ecology profile: central Europe. Darby: DIANE Publishing. April 2001. p. 136. isbn 9781428911437.
4. Shapiro ED. "Clinical practice. Lyme disease" (PDF). N Engl J Med. May 2014;370(18):1724–31.
5. Berger SA. Lyme disease: Global status 2014 edition. Los Angeles: GIDEON Informatics; 2014. p. 7. isbn 9781498803434
6. Auwaerter PG, et al. Lyme borreliosis (Lyme disease): molecular and cellular pathobiology and prospects for prevention, diagnosis and treatment. Expert Rev Mol Med. 2004;6(2):1–22.
7. Ercolini AM, Miller SD. The role of infections in autoimmune disease. Clin Exp Immunol. 2009;155(1):1–15.
8. Singh SK, Girschick HJ. Lyme borreliosis: from infection to autoimmunity. Clin Microbiol Infect. 2004;10(7):598–614.
9. Wormser GP, et al. The clinical assessment, treatment, and prevention of lyme disease, human granulocytic anaplasmosis, and babesiosis: clinical practice guidelines by the Infectious Diseases Society of America (PDF). Clin Infect Dis. 2006;43(9):1089–134.
10. Hofmann H, et al. Cutaneous Lyme Borreliosis: guideline of the german dermatology society. Ger Med Sci. 2017; 15:Doc14. Published online 2017 Sep 5. https://doi.org/10.3205/000255
11. Pachner AR, Steere AC. Neurological findings of Lyme disease. Yale J Biol Med. 1984;57(4): 481–3.
12. Middelveen MJ, et al. Persistent Borrelia infection in patients with ongoing symptoms of Lyme disease. Healthcare (Basel). 2018 Jun; 6(2):33. Published online 2018 Apr 14. https://doi.org/10.3390/healthcare6020033
13. Middelveen MJ, et al. Classification and staging of Morgellons disease: lessons from Syphilis. Clin Cosmet Investig Dermatol. 2020; 13: 145–164. Published online 2020 Feb 7. https://doi.org/10.2147/CCID.S239840
14. Kandhari R, et al. Borrelial Lymphocytoma cutis: a diagnostic dilemma. Indian J Dermatol. 2014 Nov–Dec;59(6):595–7. https://doi.org/10.4103/0019-5154.143530.
15. Auwaerter PG, et al. Lyme borreliosis (Lyme disease): molecular and cellular pathobiology and prospects for prevention, diagnosis and treatment. Expert Rev Mol Med. 2004;6(2):1–22.
16. Depietropaolo DL, et al. Diagnosis of Lyme disease. Am Fam Physician. 2005;72(2):297–305.
17. Halperin JJ. Nervous system Lyme disease. Infect Dis Clin N Am. 2008;22(2):261–74.
18. Fish AE, et al. "Lyme carditis" (PDF). Infect Dis Clin N Am. 2008;22(2):275–88.
19. Stanek G, et al. Lyme borreliosis. Lancet. 2012;379(9814):461–73.
20. Trevisan G, et al. A practical approach to the diagnosis of Lyme Borreliosis: from clinical heterogeneity to laboratory methods. Front Med (Lausanne). 2020; 7:265. Published online 2020 Jul 23. https://doi.org/10.3389/fmed.2020.00265.
21. Veinovic G, et al. Influence of MKP medium stored for prolonged periods on growth and morphology of Borrelia afzelii, Borrelia garinii, and Borrelia burgdorferi sensu stricto. APMIS. 2014;122:230–5. https://doi.org/10.1111/apm.12129.
22. MacDonald AB. Borrelia burgdorferi tissue morphologies and imaging methodologies. Eur J Clin Microbiol Infect Dis. 2013;32:1077–82. https://doi.org/10.1007/s10096-013-1853-5.
23. Duray PH. Histopathology of clinical phases of human Lyme disease. Rheum Dis Clin N Am. 1989 Nov;15(4):691–710.
24. Wright WF, et al. Diagnosis and management of Lyme disease. Am Fam Physician. 2012;85(11):1086–93.
25. Centers for Disease Control and Prevention. Lyme disease: diagnosis and testing. CDC. Available at http://www.cdc.gov/lyme/diagnosistesting/LabTest/TwoStep/index.html. November 20, 2019; Accessed: March 30, 2021.
26. Hyde FW, et al. Detection of antigens in urine of mice and humans infected with Borrelia burgdorferi, etiologic agent of Lyme disease. J Clin Microbiol. 1989;27(1):58–61.
27. Gimsing LN, Larsen LSL. A rare case of pseudotumor cerebri in adult Lyme disease. Clin Case Rep. 2020 Jan; 8(1):116–119. Published online 2019 Dec 18. https://doi.org/10.1002/ccr3.2582.
28. Roos KL, Berger JR. Is the presence of antibodies in CSF sufficient to make a definitive diagnosis of Lyme disease? Neurology. 2007 Sep 4;69(10):949–50.
29. Wahlberg P, et al. Treatment of late Lyme borreliosis. J Infect. 1994 Nov.;29(3):255–61.
30. Novak C, et al. Early disseminated Lyme disease with Carditis complicated by posttreatment Lyme disease syndrome. Case Rep Infect Dis. 2017, 2017:4. https://doi.org/10.1155/2017/5847156. Article ID 5847156

11 Tularemia

Abstract

Tularemia is an acute bacterial infectious disease caused by zoonotic bacterium *Francisella tularensis*. This highly infectious microorganism is considered a potential biological threat agent. Humans are usually infected through direct contact with the animal reservoir and tick bites. Six major clinical forms of tularemia are classically recognized. The most frequent route of contamination is through the skin, through contact with an infected animal or arthropod bites. The ulceroglandular form of tularemia combines a skin ulcer at the site of *F. tularensis* inoculation and regional lymphadenopathy. The glandular form corresponds to regional lymphadenopathy without any visible skin lesion. Infection with *F. tularensis* through the conjunctiva or the oral cavity corresponds to the oculoglandular and oropharyngeal forms, respectively. Lung involvement through inhalation of infected aerosols or hematogenous spread of bacteria corresponds to the pneumonic form. Finally, whatever the portal of entry of bacteria, severe sepsis is often associated with confusion and *F. tularensis* bacteremia corresponds to the typhoidal form. Diagnosis of tularemia is based upon a high degree of clinical suspicion coupled with either serological testing or polymerase chain reaction (PCR) assays due to the difficulty of growing the organism on standard culture media. The mainstay of treatment for tularemia is aminoglycosides.

Synonyms
Rabbit fever, Hunters' disease, deer fly fever, tick fever, O'Hara's Disease, Francis' Disease and Pahvant Valley plague [1, 2].

11.1 Background

Tularemia is an acute bacterial infectious disease caused by a pleomorphic, non-mobile, non-capsulated, small Gram-negative coccobacillus and zoonotic bacterium, *Francisella tularensis*. This zoonotic bacteria has reportedly infected a wide range of wild animals (rabbits, hares, squirrels, and deer), some domestic animals (sheep, cattle, cats), birds, some amphibians and many invertebrates (ticks, deer flies, mosquitoes). The first report of *F. tularensis* infection was described in 1911 by "McCoy," who isolated the bacteria in rodents who had contracted a plague-like disease in Tulare County, California, USA. Though the first case of verified human tularemia was not until 1914, and it is considered to have existed in Anatolia for several thousand years [1–4].

S. V. Nemade, K. J. Shinde, *Granulomatous diseases in Otorhinolaryngology, Head and Neck*,
https://doi.org/10.1007/978-981-16-4047-6_11

11.2 Epidemiology

Tularemia is most common in the Northern Hemisphere, including North America and parts of Europe and Asia. It occurs between 30° and 71° north latitude. Males are affected more often than females. It occurs most frequently in the young and the middle aged. In the USA, most cases occur in the summer. The disease is named after Tulare County, California, where the disease was discovered in 1911. The global incidence varies between 0.5 and 2/100,000 population [3, 5].

11.3 Etiopathogenesis

Francisella tularensis is a Gram-negative, intracellular bacterium causing zoonosis tularemia. This highly infectious microorganism is considered a potential biological threat agent. The bacteria can penetrate into the body through damaged skin, mucous membranes, inhalation or ingestion. It can be transmitted to humans by insect vectors, such as ticks or deer flies, handling or ingestion of infected animal tissues, inhalation of infectious aerosol or the consumption of contaminated drinking water (the bacteria have been isolated from environmental sources such as the mud and water from streams and wells). Water-borne tularemia outbreaks and sporadic cases have occurred worldwide in the last decades, with specific clinical and epidemiological traits [6]. Groups of people at risk include foresters, hikers, hunters, people in contact with meat and animals, people living in rural areas, farmers, laboratory workers and veterinarians [6].

Francisella tularensis can live both within and outside the cells of the animal it infects, meaning it is a facultative intracellular bacterium. It primarily infects macrophages, a type of white blood cell, and thus is able to evade the immune system. The course of the disease involves the spread of the organism to multiple organ systems, including the lungs, liver, spleen, and lymphatic system [2, 4, 5].

11.4 Clinical Features

The incubation period for tularemia is 1–14 days; most human infections become apparent after 3–5 days. The constitutional symptoms include fever, lethargy, loss of appetite, signs of sepsis, and possibly death. Fever is moderate or very high, and tularemia bacilli can be isolated from blood cultures at this stage. The face and eyes become inflamed. Inflammation spreads to the lymph nodes, which enlarge and may be suppurating (mimicking bubonic plague). Lymph node involvement is accompanied by a high fever [6, 7].

Depending on the site of infection, tularemia has six characteristic clinical variants: ulceroglandular (the most common type representing 75% of all forms), glandular, oropharyngeal, pneumonic, oculoglandular, and typhoidal. The oropharyngeal form is the most common clinical presentation in the Eastern European region. The oculoglandular form (also known as tularemic POGS) is the least common. The severity of tularemia varies from self-limited to disseminated disease to life-threatening sepsis [8].

1. Ulceroglandular Form: The ulceroglandular form of tularemia combines a skin ulcer at the site of *F. tularensis* inoculation and regional lymphadenopathy. The disease is localized to the head and neck area and manifests with signs such as sore throat, fever, and neck mass (cervical lymphadenopathy) [2, 9, 10]. Cervical lymph nodes may be the seat of the typical granulomatous reaction when the site of the infection is the head neck [11, 12].
2. Oropharyngeal Form: Oropharyngeal tularemia is contracted through ingestion of infected food or water and can present with a painful exudative pharyngitis. Tularemia should be suspected in patients with tonsillopharyngitis and accompanying extensive necrotic cervical lymphadenitis not responding to penicillin treatment [9].
3. Glandular Form: It corresponds to regional lymphadenopathy without any visible skin lesion (Fig. 11.1).

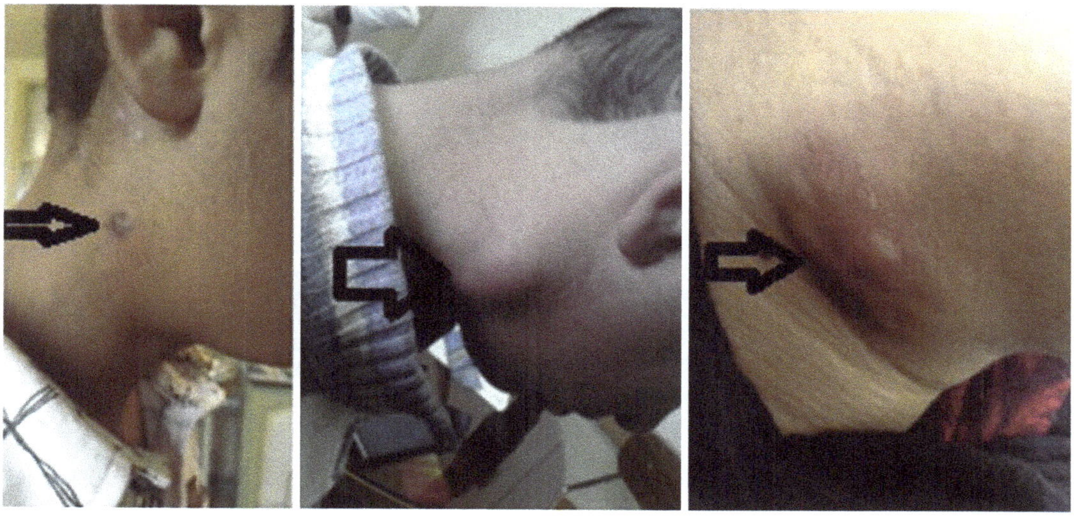

Fig. 11.1 Cervical adenopathy in glandular tularemia patients [2]

4. Oculoglandular Form/Tularemic Parinaud's Oculoglandular Syndrome (POGS): About 3–5% of cases of tularemia are the oculoglandular form [13]. Infection with *F. tularensis* is through the conjunctiva (hand to eye contamination). It is characterized by unilateral granulomatous follicular palpebral or bulbar conjunctivitis associated with ipsilateral preauricular and submandibular lymphadenopathy. The lymphadenopathy may extend to the cervical or parotid lymph nodes and may develop concomitantly with conjunctivitis, or its onset may be delayed by several weeks. The conjunctival granulomata usually measure 0.3–2 cm in diameter and typically involve the eyelids, but occasionally may be bulbar, forniceal, or medial canthal. Corneal involvement is rare and is typically limited to superficial punctate keratitis [14, 15].
5. Pneumonic Form: It can occur either through the inhalation of organisms or through the hematogenous spread from another site. It causes interstitial infiltrates, pleural effusion, or hilar lymphadenopathy [16].
6. Typhoidal Form: It carries a high morbidity and mortality. It can present with fever, prostration, vomiting, and diarrhea and can progress to renal failure, meningitis, pericarditis, and rhabdomyolysis [16].

11.5 Diagnosis

11.5.1 Culture

The laboratory isolation of *F. tularensis* requires special media such as buffered charcoal yeast extract agar. Because the culture medium is not readily available and because of high virulence and ability to spread via inhalation pose a risk for laboratory personnel. Therefore, routine isolation of the bacteria is not recommended [17–19].

11.5.2 Serology

It includes the detection of serum IgG and IgM antibodies. ELISA is widely used test with 99% sensitivity for both antibody types, and >99% specificity for IgM and 96.9% for IgG [20].

The VIRapid tularemia test (Vircell, Granada, Spain) is an immunochromatographic (ICT) test detecting both IgM and IgG type anti-*F. tularensis* antibodies. The sensitivity and specificity of

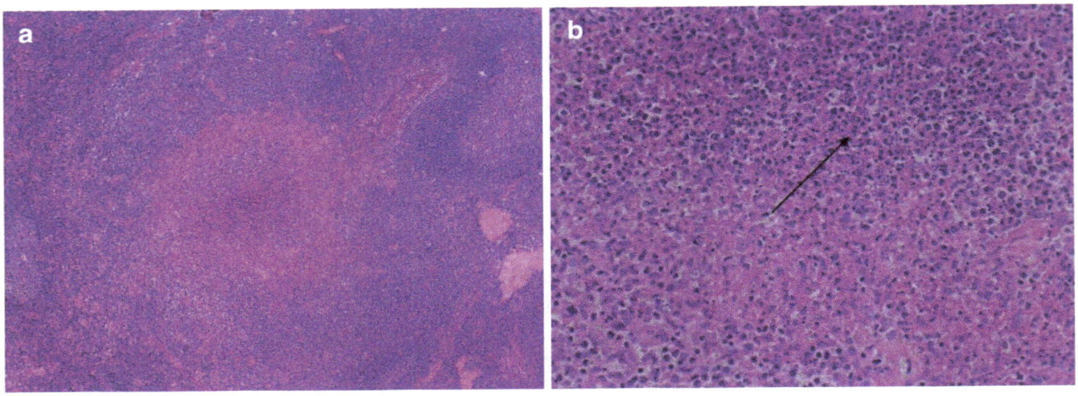

Fig. 11.2 (**a**) H&E stain, 4x: lymphadenitis with follicular hyperplasia and necrosis (arrow) surrounded by a histiocytic reaction. (**b**) H&E stain, 20x: necrotizing and granulomatous lymphadenitis, with numerous neutrophils cells (arrow) [24]

the VIRapid tularemia test were 90% and 83.6%, respectively [20].

A presumptive diagnosis of tularemia can be made if a single serum antibody titer is at least 1: 160 by tube agglutination (T) or at least 1: 128 by microagglutination (M); however, this can also represent past infection. Diagnosis is confirmed if there is a fourfold or higher increase in the titer between acute and convalescent serology with one specimen having a minimum titer of 1: 160 by T or 1: 128 by M However, it is important to remember that serology may remain negative for the first 7 to 14 Days of infection [21].

11.5.3 Molecular Assay

PCR assays for *Francisella tularensis* (targeting the insertion sequence ISFtu2 and the gene encoding the surface protein Tul4 are used. PCR, however, carries a sensitivity of 78% and a specificity of 96% in diagnosing tularemia [22, 23].

11.5.4 Histopathology

The lesion consists of a granulomatous reaction that may have a tuberculoid appearance, in particular in the more chronic lesions.

The necrosis is more liquefactive than caseous. The widespread necrosis with polymorphs, lymphocytes, and multinucleated giant cells is surrounded by radially arranged epithelioid cells and fibrosis (Fig. 11.2a, b) [2, 4, 19, 25].

11.5.5 Imaging

- The radiological imaging features of tularemia are not specific.
- The chest radiograph in pneumonic tularemia may show interstitial infiltrate, pleural effusion, or hilar lymphadenopathy.
- Enlarged lymph nodes with central necrosis may be well demonstrated by magnetic resonance imaging (MRI), associated with hypertrophy of the tonsils, adenoids, and lymph nodes in children [17].
- Endobronchial ultrasonography (EBUS): It is helpful to identify the hilar lymphadenopathy and to perform EBUS guided transbronchial fine-needle aspiration (TBNA) of the lesion [16].

11.6 Treatment

The antibiotic classes that are recommended for tularaemia treatment are aminoglycosides, fluoroquinolones, and tetracyclines. However, cure rates vary between 60 and 100% depending on the antibiotic used, the time to appropriate antibiotic therapy setup and its duration, and the presence of complications, such as lymph node suppuration. Thus, antibiotic susceptibility testing (AST) of *F. tularensis* strains remains of primary importance for detection of the emergence of antibiotic resistances to first-line drugs and to test new therapeutic alternatives [20, 24].

11.6.1 First-Line Therapy

Aminoglycosides- Streptomycin is the drug of choice for the treatment of tularemia, with gentamicin as an alternative.

- Intramuscular Streptomycin (10 mg/Kg twice daily for 14 days) has been considered the management of choice. *F. tularensis* is resistant to beta-lactam antibiotics, including ceftriaxone [26].
- According to the World Health Organization, however, gentamicin is now the preferred antibiotic for those with severe tularemia requiring hospitalization due to its bactericidal properties against *F. tularensis* and its widespread availability. Recommended gentamicin dosing is 5 mg/kg/day divided into dosing every 8–12 h with a desirable peak concentration ranging from 8 to 12 mcg/mL with treatment duration ranging between 7 and 10 days to minimize relapses [16].

11.6.2 Second-Line Therapy

- It includes tetracyclines or chloramphenicol for 14 days, but treatment failures and relapses occur at a higher rate with these agents as compared to the aminoglycosides [26].
- Immunotherapy for tularemia has shown strong promise in animal models and will presumably continue to be a focus for future studies, particularly due to the potential threat of weaponized antibiotic-resistant Francisella [27].

With antibiotic treatment, the overall case fatality rate of tularemia in the USA is less than 2% [26]. Indicators of poor response to treatment are persistent fever, suppuration, and drainage of the affected lymph nodes, an enlargement of the affected lymph nodes, and the appearance of new sites of lymphadenopathy [28].

Surgical drainage of any fluctuant abscess is also indicated. Ciprofloxacin was found to be effective in treating tularemia in immunosuppressed patients [13].

11.7 Essential Features

- Caused by *Francisella tularensis*, a Gram-negative coccobacilli found in rodents, rabbits, and hares, transmitted by ticks and deer flies.
- Commonly due to food and water contamination by rodents, hunting hares and mosquito bites
- The incubation period for tularemia is 1–14 days.
- Tularemia has six characteristic clinical variants: ulceroglandular (the most common type representing 75% of all forms), glandular, oropharyngeal, pneumonic, oculoglandular, and typhoidal.
- The ulceroglandular form combines a skin ulcer at the site of *F. tularensis* inoculation and regional lymphadenopathy.
- The glandular form corresponds to regional lymphadenopathy without any visible skin lesion.
- Infection with *F. tularensis* through the conjunctiva or the oral cavity corresponds to the oculoglandular and oropharyngeal forms, respectively.
- Lung involvement through inhalation of infected aerosols or hematogenous spread of bacteria corresponds to the pneumonic form.
- Severe sepsis and *F. tularensis* bacteremia correspond to the typhoidal form.
- Diagnosis of tularemia is based upon a high degree of clinical suspicion coupled with either serological testing or polymerase chain reaction (PCR) assays due to the difficulty of growing the organism on standard culture media.
- The mainstay of treatment for tularemia is aminoglycosides.

References

1. Gürcan Ş. Epidemiology of Tularemia. Balkan Med J. 2014 Mar; 31(1) 3–10. Published online 2014 Mar 1. https://doi.org/10.5152/balkanmedj.2014.13117.
2. Esmaeili S, et al. Francisella tularensis human infections in a village of northwest Iran. BMC Infect Dis. 2021; 21:310. Published online 2021 Mar 31. https://doi.org/10.1186/s12879-021-06004-y
3. Rapini, Ronald P et al. (2007). Dermatology: 2-volume set. St. Louis: Mosby. isbn: 978-1-4160-2999-1
4. Ellis J, et al. Tularemia. Clin Microbiol Rev. 2002;15:631–46.
5. Gürcan S. Epidemiology of Tularemia. Balkan Med J. 2014;31:3–10.
6. Hennebique A, et al. Tularemia as a waterborne disease: a review. Emerg Microbes Infect. 2019; 8(1):1027–1042. Published online 2019 Jul 9. https://doi.org/10.1080/22221751.2019.1638734
7. Wills PI, et al. Head and neck manifestations of tularemia. Laryngoscope. 1982;92:770–3.
8. Luotonen J, et al. Tularemia in Otolaryngologic PracticeAn analysis of 127 cases. Arch Otolaryngol Head Neck Surg. 1986;112(1):77–80.
9. Pikula J, et al. Ecological conditions of natural foci of tularaemia in the Czech Republic. Eur J Epidemiol. 2003;18:1091–5.
10. Nordahl SH, et al. Tularemia: a differential diagnosis in oto-rhino-laryngology. J Laryngol Otol. 1993;107:127–9.
11. Robson CD. Imaging of granulomatous lesions of the neck in children. Radiol Clin N Am. 2000;38:969–77.
12. Johansson A, et al. Comparative analysis of PCR versus culture for diagnosis of ulceroglandular tularemia. J Clin Microbiol. 2000;38:22–6.
13. Gok S.E et al. Evaluation of tularemia cases focusing on the oculoglandular form. J Infect Dev Ctries 2014;8:1277–1284. doi: https://doi.org/10.3855/jidc.3996.
14. Arjmand P, et al. Parinaud oculoglandular syndrome 2015: review of the literature and update on diagnosis and management. Clin Exp Ophthalmol. 2015;6:1000443. https://doi.org/10.4172/2155-9570.1000443.
15. Kevin Dixon M, et al. Parinaud's Oculoglandular syndrome: a case in an adult with flea-borne typhus and a review. Trop Med Infect Dis. 2020 Sep; 5(3):126. Published online 2020 Jul 29. https://doi.org/10.3390/tropicalmed5030126
16. Dietrich T, et al. Extended-interval gentamicin dosing for pulmonic Tularemia. Case Rep Infect Dis. 2019;2019:3. https://doi.org/10.1155/2019/9870510. Article ID 9870510
17. Umlas SL, Jaramillo D. Massive adenopathy in oropharyngeal tularemia; CT demonstrations. Pediatr Radiol. 1990;20:483–4.
18. Mair IWS, et al. Otolaryngological Manifestations of Tularemia. Arch Otolaryngol. 1973;98(3):156–8.
19. Hepburn MJ, Simpson AJ. Tularemia: current diagnosis and treatment options. Expert Rev Anti-Infect Ther. 2008;6(2):231–40.
20. Yanes H, et al. Evaluation of in-house and commercial serological tests for diagnosis of human Tularemia. J Clin Microbiol. 2018 Jan; 56(1): e01440-17. Published online 2017 Dec 26. Prepublished online 2017 Nov 8. https://doi.org/10.1128/JCM.01440-17.
21. Kumar R, et al. Difficulty in the clinical diagnosis of Tularemia: highlighting the importance of a physical exam. Case Rep Pediatr. 2018;2018:4. https://doi.org/10.1155/2018/9682815. Article ID 9682815
22. Grunow R, et al. Differential diagnosis of tularemia. Dtsch Med Wochenschr. 2001;126:408–13. (in German)
23. Faucher JF, et al. Typhoidal Tularemia: 2 familial cases. Case Rep Infect Dis. 2012, 2012:2. https://doi.org/10.1155/2012/214215. Article ID 214215
24. Longo MV, et al. Long-lasting fever and Lymphadenitis: think about F. Tularensis. Case Rep Med. 2015;2015., Article ID 191406:4. https://doi.org/10.1155/2015/191406.
25. Syrjälä HK, et al. Bronchial changes in airborne tularemia. J Laryngol Otol. 1986;100:1169–76.
26. Dennis DT, et al. Tularemia as a biological weapon: medical and public health management. JAMA. 2001;285:2763–73. https://doi.org/10.1001/jama.285.21.2763.
27. Skyberg JA. Immunotherapy for tularemia. Virulence. 2013 Nov 15; 4(8):859–870. Published online 2013 Jun 19. https://doi.org/10.4161/viru.25454
28. Kosker M, et al. A case of oculoglandular tularemia resistant to medical treatment. Scand J Infect Dis. 2013;45:725–7. https://doi.org/10.3109/00365548.2013.796089.

12 Aspergillosis

Abstract

Since Aspergillus species are ubiquitous in the environment and humans inhale Aspergillus spores on a daily basis, sinopulmonary diseases are the most common manifestations of aspergillosis. Depending on the underlying immune status of the host, Aspergillus species cause a wide spectrum of diseases in humans that can be roughly classified into three groups with distinct pathogenetic mechanisms, clinical manifestations, and overlapping features. These are saprophytic, allergic, and invasive. Saprophytic aspergillosis is commonly seen in immunocompetent individuals and includes aspergilloma and chronic pulmonary aspergillosis. Allergic aspergillosis includes allergic bronchopulmonary aspergillosis, allergic rhinosinusitis and bronchocentric granulomatosis. Invasive form usually occurs in immunocompromised individuals and includes pulmonary invasive aspergillosis, acute necrotizing rhinosinusitis, chronic invasive rhinosinusitis, granulomatous invasive aspergillosis and cutaneous aspergillosis. Microscopy, culture, and histopathology form the mainstay of diagnosis, demonstrating septate branching hyphae at an acute angle of 45. Serology and molecular assay aid the diagnosis. The current medical treatments for aggressive invasive aspergillosis include voriconazole and liposomal amphotericin B in combination with surgical debridement. For the less aggressive allergic bronchopulmonary aspergillosis, findings use of oral steroids for 6–9 months is preferred. Itraconazole is given with steroids, as it is considered to have a "steroid-sparing" effect.

12.1 Background

Aspergillosis refers to the diseases caused by infection by fungi of the genus Aspergillus. Depending on the underlying immune status of the host, Aspergillus diseases can be roughly classified into three groups with distinct pathogenetic mechanisms, clinical manifestations, and overlapping features, which are based on their relative clinical importance. These are saprophytic, allergic and invasive aspergillosis. Saprophytic aspergillosis is commonly seen in immunocompetent individuals and includes aspergilloma, chronic pulmonary aspergillosis (CPA). Allergic aspergillosis includes allergic bronchopulmonary aspergillosis (ABPA) and allergic rhinosinusitis. It is observed in patients with atopy, asthma, or cystic fibrosis. Since Aspergillus species are ubiquitous in the environment and humans inhale Aspergillus spores on a daily basis, sinopulmonary diseases are the most common manifestations of aspergillosis [1, 2]. Invasive form is seen in immunocompromised individuals [2]. Cutaneous aspergillosis is classi-

S. V. Nemade, K. J. Shinde, *Granulomatous diseases in Otorhinolaryngology, Head and Neck*,
https://doi.org/10.1007/978-981-16-4047-6_12

fied under invasive form and is subdivided into primary and secondary cutaneous aspergillosis. Mucocutaneous and subcutaneous forms of aspergillosis include otomycosis (ear infection), onychomycosis (nail bed infection), keratitis (eye infection) and Madura foot which follow traumatic inoculation of the spores directly into the affected tissues [3, 4]. These are less severe and curable with effective antifungal treatment.

12.2 Epidemiology

Aspergillosis affects more than 14 million people worldwide with allergic bronchopulmonary aspergillosis (ABPA, >4 million), severe asthma with fungal sensitization (>6.5 million), and chronic pulmonary aspergillosis (CPA, ~3 million) being considerably more prevalent than invasive aspergillosis (IA, >300,000) [5].

Other types are Aspergillus bronchitis, Aspergillus rhinosinusitis, otitis externa, and Aspergillus onychomycosis (10 million) [5, 6]. Pulmonary Aspergillosis is common in the old age group with female predominance. Aspergillus rhinosinusitis is common in the young age group with no gender predilection [6].

12.3 Etiopathogenesis

Aspergillus is one of the oldest known genera of fungi first described by a Roman Catholic clergyman and biologist, Pier Antonio Micheli, in 1729. To date, over 330 species of Aspergillus have been described. Of these, approximately 50 species are recognised to be pathogenic to humans, and the five most clinically relevant include Aspergillus fumigates (Fig. 12.1), *A. flavus*, *A. niger*, *A. terreus*, and *A. nidulans*, in order of frequency [4, 8].

Fungal spores are inhaled from the environment leading to fungal colonisation in the nasal or pulmonary cavities. Following their deposition in the tissue and recognition by phagocytes, an inflammatory response is triggered. Hemolytic toxins, as well as fungal protease and elastase, are released leading to tissue damage. In the case of cutaneous aspergillosis (as seen in the external ear canal), fungal spores are inoculated in the skin abrasion followed by colonisation, inflammatory response and dermonecrotic toxins causing tissue damage [4, 7].

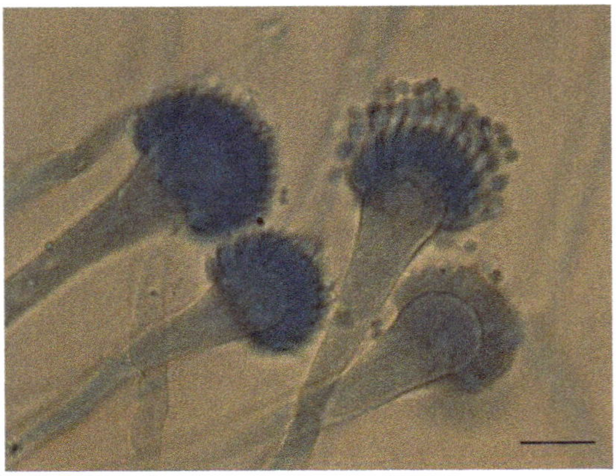

Fig. 12.1 *Aspergillus fumigatus* (bar is 10 um) [7]

12.4 Risk Factors

- Immunocompromised conditions—People taking immune-suppressing drugs after undergoing transplant surgery—especially bone marrow or stem cell transplants—or people who have certain hematological malignancy are at the highest risk of invasive aspergillosis. People in the later stages of AIDS also may be at increased risk.
- Leucopenia—People who have had chemotherapy, an organ transplant or leukemia have lower white cell levels, making them more susceptible to invasive aspergillosis. Lung cavities—People with lung cavities are at higher risk of developing aspergillomas.
- Asthma or cystic fibrosis—People with asthma or cystic fibrosis are more likely to have an allergic response to aspergillus mold.
- Long-term corticosteroid therapy—Long-term use of corticosteroids may increase the risk of aspergillosis and similar infections, depending on the underlying disease being treated and what other drugs are being used [2, 4–6].

12.5 Clinical Features

12.5.1 Saprophytic Aspergillosis

12.5.1.1 Aspergilloma (Fungal Ball)

It is seen in immunocompetent individuals. In particular, saprophytic colonization in a cavity by Aspergillus is referred to as aspergilloma and consists of both dead and living mycelial elements, inflammatory cells, fibrin, mucus, and components of degenerating blood and epithelia. The mycelial mass may lie free within the cavity or be attached to the cavity wall by inflammatory/granulomatous tissue [2].

Nose and Sinuses: Aspergilloma of the sinuses causes nasal obstruction, discharge, headache. The maxillary sinus is most commonly affected, followed by sphenoid sinus. It is characterized by sinus opacification, cheesy discharge, chronic inflammatory reaction without any tissue invasion by fungi. Bone erosion is reported in 4–17% of patients [9].

Pulmonary Involvement: Certain chronic lung (pulmonary) conditions, such as emphysema, tuberculosis or advanced sarcoidosis, can form cavities in the lungs. When people with lung cavities are also infected with aspergillus, fungus fibers may find their way into the cavities and grow into tangled masses (fungus balls) known as aspergillomas. Aspergillomas may produce no symptoms or cause only a mild cough initially [2, 4]. Over time and without treatment, however, aspergillomas can worsen the underlying disease and possibly cause:

- Hemoptysis
- Wheezing
- Dyspnoea
- Unintentional weight loss
- Fatigue

12.5.1.2 Chronic Pulmonary Aspergillosis (CPA)

This chronic, inflammatory form of Aspergillus infection of the lung has been recognized in patients with chronic cavitary lung disease, which is characterized by an indolent clinical course of a chronic inflammatory disease evolving over months to years. This disease is characterized by constitutional symptoms, serum IgG-positive antibodies (Abs) (precipitins) to *A. fumigatus*, elevated acute-phase markers of inflammation, and an immune status that ranges from normal to mild immunosuppression. This is a very complex and heterogenous syndrome, which has been subclassified in the past as chronic, necrotizing pulmonary aspergillosis (CNPA), chronic cavitary pulmonary aspergillosis (CCPA), and chronic fibrotic pulmonary aspergillosis (CFPA) [7, 10–12].

12.5.2 Allergic Aspergillosis

It is observed in patients with atopy, asthma, or cystic fibrosis. It is commonly seen in immunocompetent hosts.

1. Allergic Fungal Rhinosinusitis (AFRS): Allergic fungal rhinosinusitis (AFRS) is a unique variety of chronic polypoid rhinosinusitis, usually in atopic individuals, characterized by the presence of eosinophilic mucin and fungal hyphae in paranasal sinuses without invasion into surrounding mucosa. It is characterized by nasal polyposis, type I (raised IgE) and possibly type III hypersensitivity reaction, production of allergic mucin with abundant eosinophils and non-invading fungal hyphae. The fungi behave as allergens in atopic host, causing inflammation of sinuses, thereby obstructing the sinus ostia hampering drainage [9].
2. Allergic Bronchopulmonary Aspergillosis (ABPA): The most severe form of aspergillosis among atopic patients is allergic bronchopulmonary aspergillosis (ABPA), which develops the following sensitization to *A. fumigatus* allergens in a unique subset of atopic individuals: those patients with cystic fibrosis or individuals with genetic predisposition for ABPA. ABPA is a hypersensitivity disease of the lung that is almost always related to *A. fumigatus* [13].

   In fact, nearly all patients with ABPA have a history of chronic asthma. Clinically, ABPA symptoms include episodic wheezing, malaise, low-grade chronic fevers and cough, sputum containing brown mucus and plugs, chest pain, migrating pulmonary infiltrates, and sputum and blood eosinophilia. As ABPA progresses, central bronchiectasis becomes a dominant feature of the disease and may result in chronic pulmonary secretions and, occasionally, hemoptysis, as well as characteristic radiographic abnormalities.

Criteria for the diagnosis of ABPA have evolved and now consist of (i) clinical and/or pulmonary function deterioration from baseline status (ii) positive immediate cutaneous reaction to *A. fumigatus* antigens or elevated IgE *A. fumigatus* antibody serum level, (iii) elevated serum total IgE level of >1,000 U/ml, (iv) elevated serum IgG *A. fumigatus* antibody level or positive *A. fumigatus* precipitins, and (v) abnormal chest imaging findings or a change in baseline abnormalities [14].

3. Bronchocentric Granulomatosis

   It may be isolated or part of allergic bronchopulmonary aspergillosis. Cell-mediated reaction to aspergillus in the airway causes circumferential granulomatous inflammation surrounding small airways with mucus and cellular debris and loss of lining epithelium within the airway. Bronchocentric granulomas in asthmatics contain numerous eosinophils and noninvasive aspergillus organisms or other fungi. Patients have elevated IgE directed against aspergillus antigens, also thick mucus plugs. Impacted mucus may form the cast of airways (plastic bronchitis); over time, bronchi become dilated, causing bronchiectasis. Eventually, patients develop intractable bronchospasm [15].

12.5.3 Invasive Aspergillosis

1. Invasive Pulmonary Aspergillosis (IPA) : Invasive pulmonary aspergillosis occurs only in immunocompramised people as a result of chemotherapy, bone marrow transplantation or a disease of the immune system. Untreated, this form of aspergillosis may be fatal. The invasive disease usually shows targetoid granulomatous lesions with peripheral fibrosis and central thrombosed vessels due to angioinvasive fungi, variable bronchopneumonia or lobar pneumonia. Pleuritic chest pain and progression to pneumonia occur as a clinical manifestation of angioinvasion and tissue necrosis induced by invasive fungal growth [2, 10–12]. Poorly controlled aspergillosis can disseminate through the bloodstream to cause widespread disease causing renal failure, hepatic failure, shock, delirium, and seizures [2, 13].
2. Acute (Fulminant, Necrotizing) Fungal Rhinosinusitis (FRS): It is characterized by vascular invasion by fungal hyphae, necrotizing reaction with abundant hyphae. Aspergillus is the second most common fungus causing acute necrotizing fungal rhinosinusitis, the first being the Mucorale species.
3. Granulomatous Invasive Fungal Rhinosinusitis: This form of FRS is seen in immunocompetent patients from tropical regions from Sudan to India. The lesion typically presents with granuloma and sparse *A. flavus* hyphae with or without foreign body or giant cells. The duration of illness is more than 12 weeks and affects the cheek (Fig. 12.2), nose, orbit, and paranasal sinuses with predominant proptosis [9].
4. Chronic Invasive Fungal Rhinosinusitis: This condition is seen in mildly immunosuppressed patients (diabetes, steroid therapy) and lasts for more than 12 weeks, with progression at a relatively slow pace. It affects ethmoid and sphenoid sinuses commonly. Histologically, it presents abundant fungal hyphae (commonly *A. fumigatus*), mixed inflammatory reaction, and occasional vascular invasion. The disease spreads to the cheek; orbit-like chronic granulomatous type [8, 16].
5. Cutaneous Aspergillosis: It is divided in primary and secondary forms.
   - Primary cutaneous aspergillosis (PCA) usually involves sites of skin injury, namely, at or near intravenous access catheter sites, at sites of traumatic inoculation, and at sites

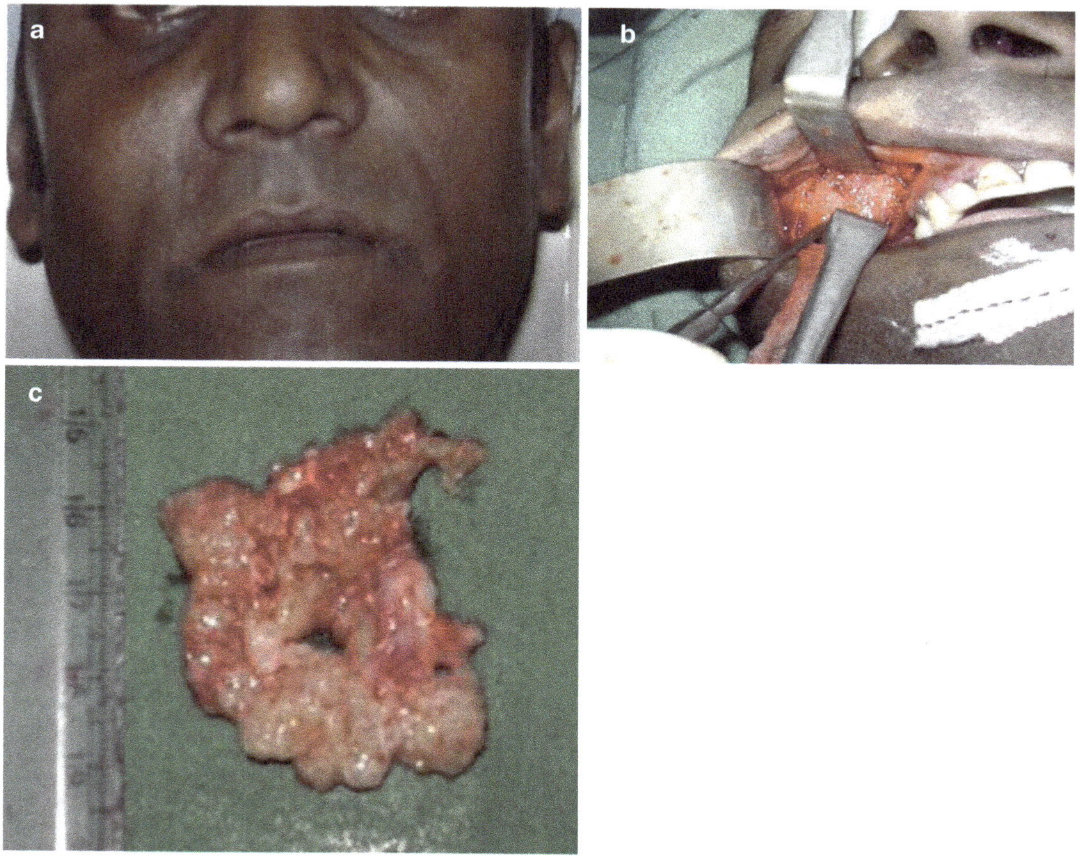

Fig. 12.2 (**a**) Patient with right cheek swelling due to granuloma. (**b**) Granulomatous invasive aspergillosis mass involving buccal space. (**c**) Excised aspergillus granuloma

associated with occlusive dressings, burns, or surgery. Mucocutaneous and subcutaneous forms of aspergillosis such as otomycosis (ear infection), onychomycosis (nail bed infection), keratitis (eye infection) and Madura foot which follow traumatic inoculation of the spores directly into the affected tissues. These are less severe and respond well to local and oral antifungal medications [4, 17].

- Fungal keratitis—Patient typically presents with a red, painful eye, together with reduced vision (Fig. 12.3a, b) [18].
- Otomycosis (fungal infection of the external auditory canal)—Pruritus, discharge, pain, and diminished hearing are the main complaints of the patients. Aspergillus niger and *Candida albicans* are the main causes of the disease.
- Secondary cutaneous aspergillosis (SCA) lesions result either from contiguous extension to the skin from infected underlying structures or from hematogenous spread of Aspergillus infection from a distal site (e.g., the lungs) to the skin. Particularly in immunocompromized patients, secondary cutaneous aspergillosis has the potential to progress to systemic infection (disease dissemination) and is frequently lethal [17].

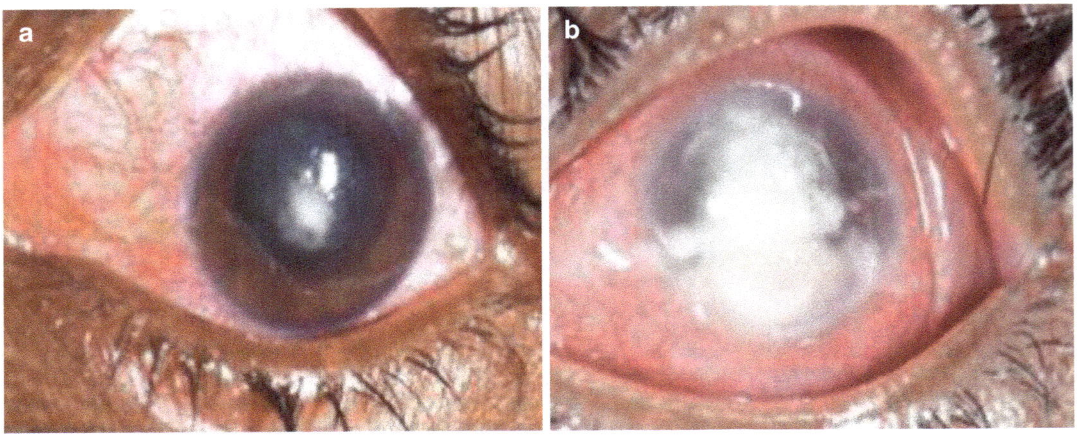

Fig. 12.3 The progression of a patient with fungal keratitis caused by Aspergillus sp. (**a**) Early in the course of the disease, a relatively small corneal ulcer, with serrated feathery margins to the corneal infiltrate is seen. (**b**) Despite intense, appropriate, prompt treatment with topical natamycin 5%, the corneal infiltrate increased in size [18]

12.6 Diagnosis

12.6.1 Microscopy and Culture

Direct microscopy of sinus secretions, sputum, skin lesions, bronchoalveolar lavage demonstrates fungal hyphae on direct KOH (Fig. 12.4) mount or more sensitive calcofluor white stain (Fig. 12.5) [16]. Gridley stain or Gomori methenamine-silver stains give the fungal walls a gray-black color [11]. The hyphae of Aspergillus species range in diameter from 2.5 to 6 μm. They have septate hyphae [12], but these are not always apparent, and in such cases, they may be mistaken for Zygomycota [11]. Aspergillus hyphae tend to have dichotomous branching that is progressive and primarily at acute angles of around 45° [7, 11].

Culture—most Aspergillus sp grow relatively rapidly (typically within 48 h) and on most microbiology media, including both mycological media such as Sabouraud's agar and blood agar used for general bacteriological culture. While the technique of culturing specimens is inherently simple and low cost, an enhanced method of sensitively, rapidly, and specifically detecting digitonin immobilized microcolonies of Aspergillus using the enzymatic cleavage of a fluorescent compound has been developed [19].

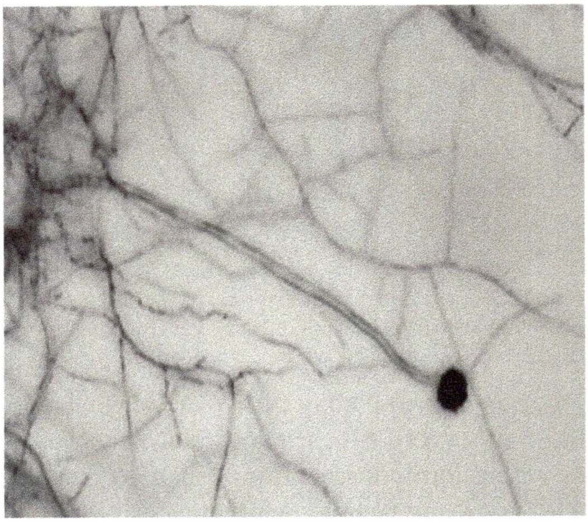

Fig. 12.4 *Aspergillus niger* seen on microscopy

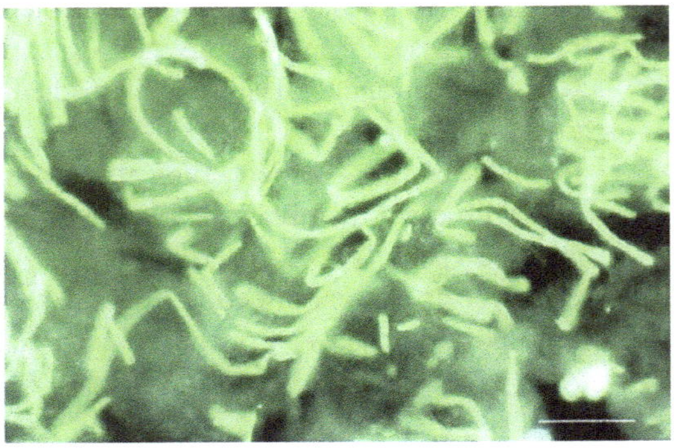

Fig. 12.5 Calcoflour stained tissue from a wound infection that grew *A. flavus*. Bar = 10 um [7]

12.6.2 Histopathology

Lung biopsy or tissue biopsy from paranasal sinuses may be necessary to confirm a diagnosis of invasive aspergillosis. Haematoxylin Eosin stain demonstrates the fungal hyphae along with granulomatous inflammation. Angioinvasion can be seen in the case of invasive aspergillosis (Fig. 12.6a). Special stains such as PAS and Gomori SM stain highlights the fungal sepatate branching hyphae (Fig. 12.6b, c).

12.6.3 Immunohistochemistry for Fungal Identification

It is a method of localizing specific antigens in tissues or cells based on antigen–antibody recognition. The use of an enzymatic label antibody such as horseradish peroxidase allows visualization of the labeled antibody using conventional light microscopy in the presence of a suitable chromogenic substrate system. It has the potential advantage of providing rapid and specific identification of several fungi, allowing pathologists to identify and accurately distinguish them from confounding artifacts [20].

12.6.4 Imaging

A chest X-ray (Fig. 12.7) or computerized tomography (CT) (Fig. 12.8a, b) scan usually reveal a fungal mass (aspergilloma), as well as characteristic signs of invasive and allergic bronchopulmonary aspergillosis In pulmonary aspergillosis, it classically manifests as a halo sign, and later, an air crescent sign [10, 21].

X-ray of paranasal sinuses shows haziness of multiple sinuses, thickened mucosal lining and bony erosions. This modality is the least specific.

CT scan nose and paranasal sinuses (PNS) may reveal fungal ball in the sinuses; bony walls expansion and remodeling in chronic infection or mucocele formation; destruction in invasive sinusitis, granuloma; and intracranial or intraorbital extension of the disease (Fig. 12.9a–e) [11, 23].

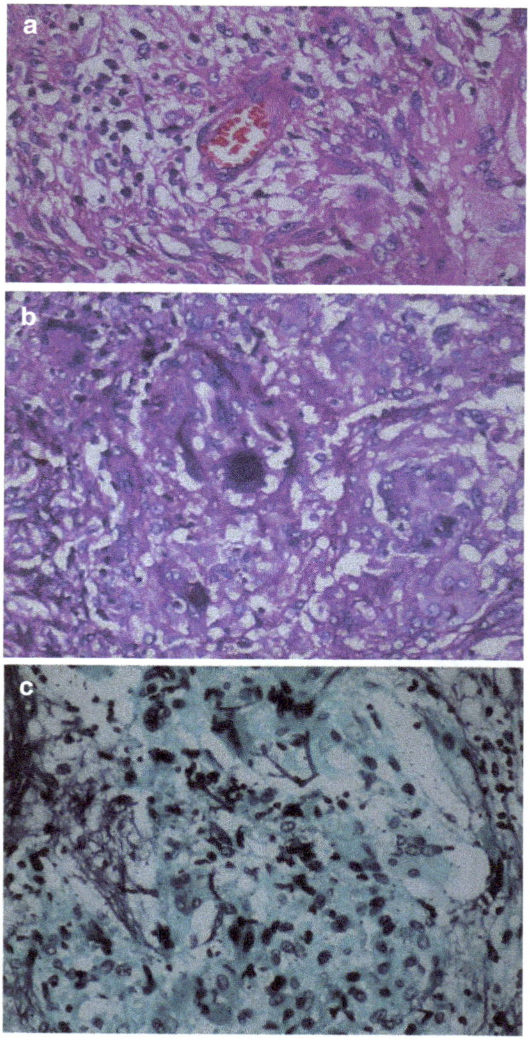

Fig. 12.6 (**a**) H&E stain shows fungal hyphae with inflammatory cell infiltrate (**b**) PAS stain and (**c**) Gomori SM stain showing fungal septate hyphae at acute angles of around 45°

CT scan is the initial investigation of choice as it shows typical findings in AFRS consisting of multiple sinus opacifications with central hyper-attenuation (central serpiginous or starry sky appearance), sinus mucocele, skull base erosions (56% of AFRS patients versus 5% of non-AFRS patients) and remodeling with a "pushing border" at skull base (Fig. 12.9c) [22, 23]. Intracranial and skull base aspergillomas are also better delineated on CT brain and skull base (Fig. 12.10) [24].

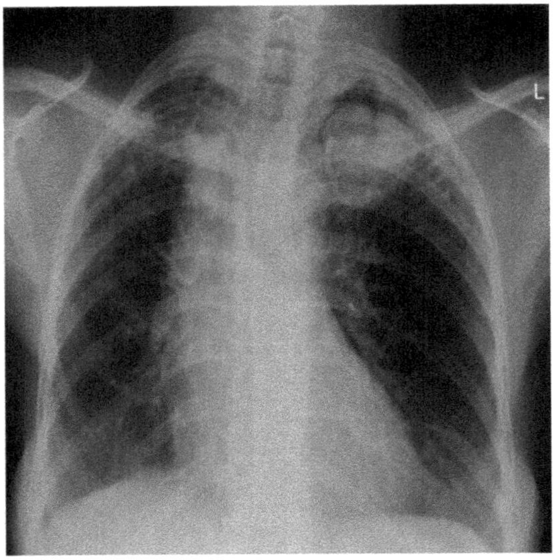

Fig. 12.7 Chest X-ray (CXR) demonstrating a left upper lobe aspergilloma in a patient with sarcoidosis [21]

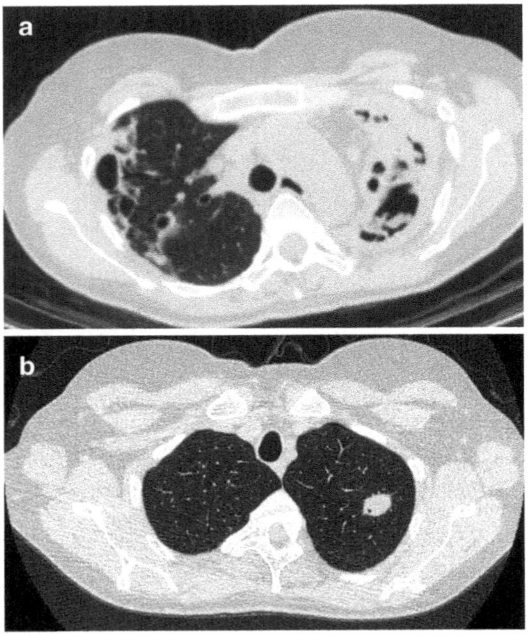

Fig. 12.8 (**a**) Chronic cavitatory pulmonary aspergillosis with involvement of the left upper lobe [21]. (**b**) Aspergillus nodule—CT scan from a patient with an isolated pulmonary nodule attributable to Aspergillus spp., unusually this lesion is showing signs of early cavitation [21]

MRI scan—In sinus and cerebral aspergillosis, CT along with gadolinium-enhanced MRI scan is crucial. It may show nodular or annular lesions having T1 W hypointense signal and T2 W hyperintense signal. Rarely mycotic aneurysms due to Aspergillus may occur [25, 26].

The characteristic features of AFRS include central low T1 and T2 void in sinuses which is due to the presence of eosinophilic mucin (>28% protein concentration) surrounded by low T1 and high T2 signal intensity of inflamed mucosa enhanced by intravenous gadolinium contrast Occasionally, iso-intense or hypo-intense T1/T2 signal may be visible, which is caused by ferromagnetic elements. High protein content of allergic mucin typically shows hyper attenuated signals in inspissated secretions [25] (Figs. 12.11 and 12.12).

12.6.5 Serology

- Type I hypersensitivity to fungi is demonstrated by either ImmunoCAP or skin prick test, the former being more specific and having a higher negative predictive value. It is observed that AFRS patients possess high levels of specific IgE to multiple fungi, which may aid in differentiating them from other CRS cases. Total IgE in these patients is often more than 1000 IU/mL [27].
- Surface-enhanced laser desorption/ionization time-of-flight mass spectrometry (SELDI-TOF MS): It allows protein profiling of serum and identifies AFRS patients with a sensitivity of 84% and specificity of 90%.
- Galactomannan (GM) has been the antigen of choice for the diagnosis of IPA since its discovery in the early 1970s. This has been due to the exquisite immunogenicity of the galactofuran side chain of the galactomannan, which has allowed the selection of monoclonal antibodies (MAbs) with high affinity and avidity. The method currently used is a sandwich ELISA based on a very efficient EB-A2 rat monoclonal antibody able to detect 05 to 1 ng of the galactofuran epitope. Sensitivity rates are ranging from 67% to 100%, and specificity rates, ranging from 86% to 99% [28].
- The (1,3)β-D-glucan assay is an amebocyte lysis assay with a sensitivity of 75–100% and

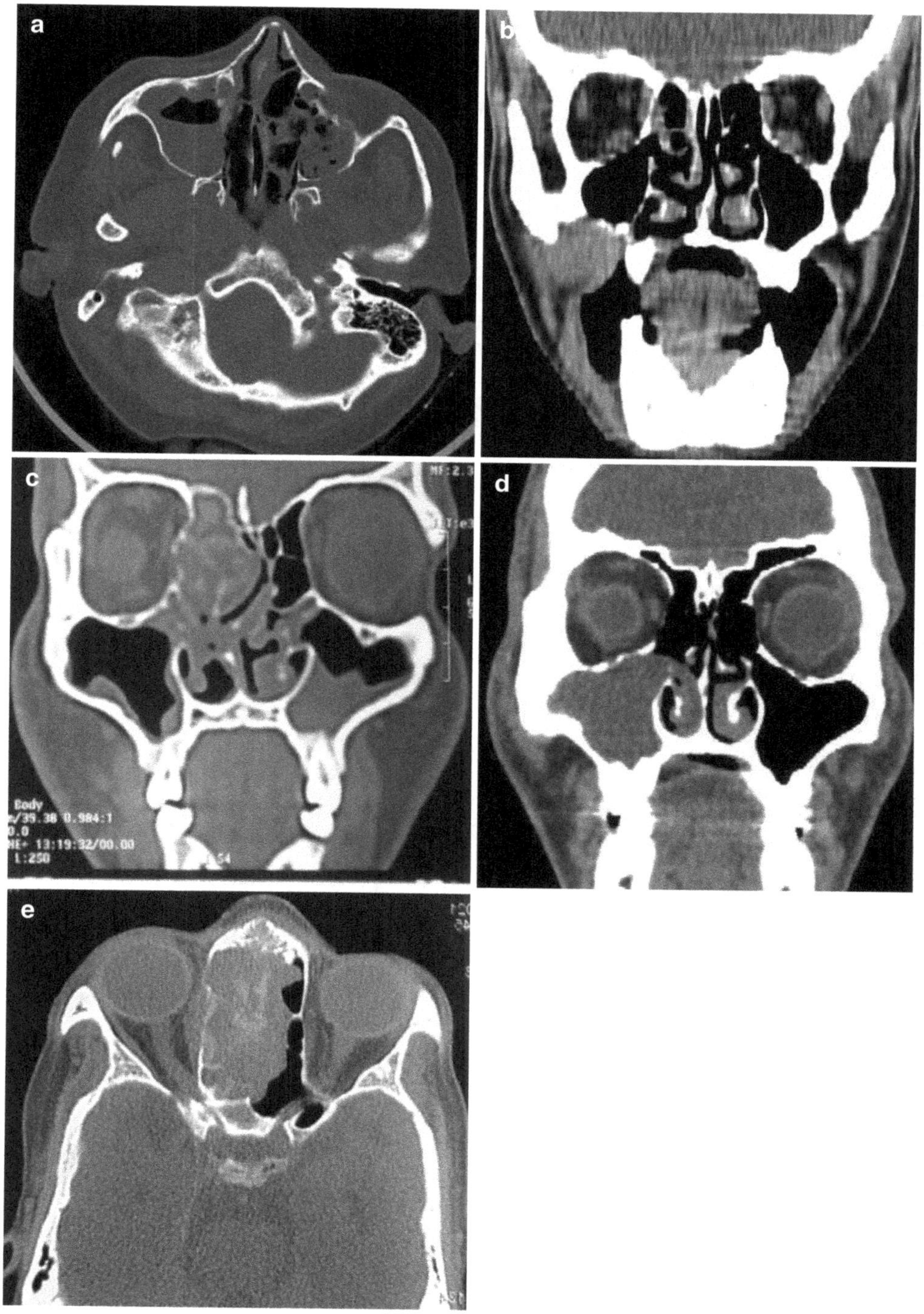

Fig. 12.9 (**a**) CT PNS axial view showing the destruction of nasal septum and medial walls of maxillary sinuses due to invasive aspergillosis. (**b**) CT PNS coronal view showing invasive fungal granuloma of right buccal space. (**c**) CT PNS coronal view of AFRS patient showing remodeling, "pushing border" of right skull base and lamina papyracea [22]. (**d**) CT PNS coronal view shows hyperattenuated focus with complete opacification of the right maxillary sinus. (**e**) CT PNS axial view of invasive aspergillosis patient showing opacification of right ethmoid sinuses with the destruction of medial orbital wall and the septum

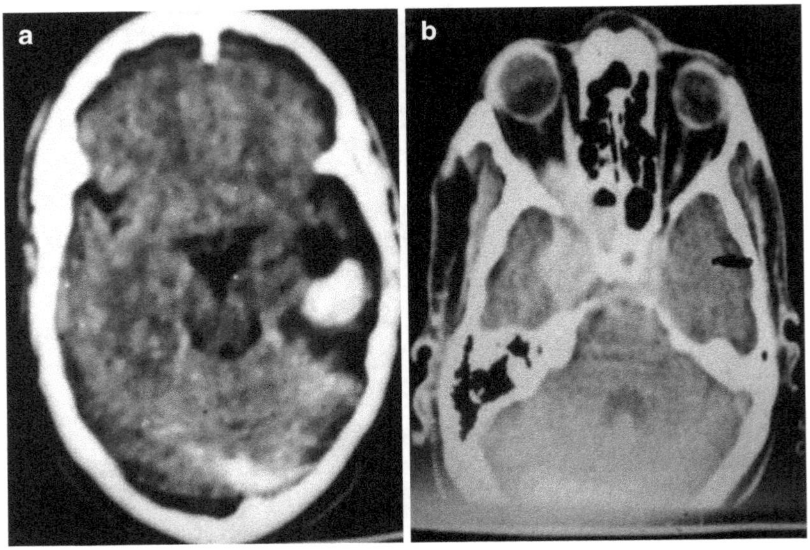

Fig. 12.10 Contrast CT scans showing densely enhancing left temporal intraparenchymal Aspergillus granuloma (**a**) and enhancing mass lesion in the ethmoid sinuses, right orbital apex, right extraparenchymal temporal fossa and left cavernous sinus skull base Aspergillus granuloma (**b**) [24]

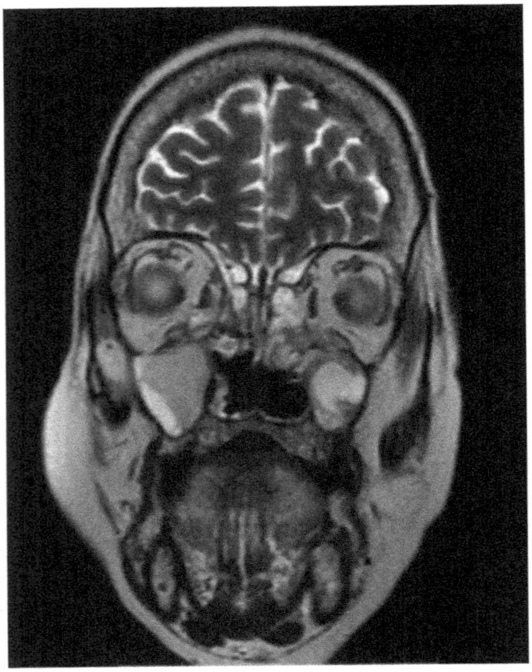

Fig. 12.11 Acute invasive fungal rhinosinusitis. T1-weighted MRI scan showing hyperintensity in bilateral maxillary and ethmoid sinuses with characteristic hyper attenuated thick inspissated secretions in maxillary sinuses

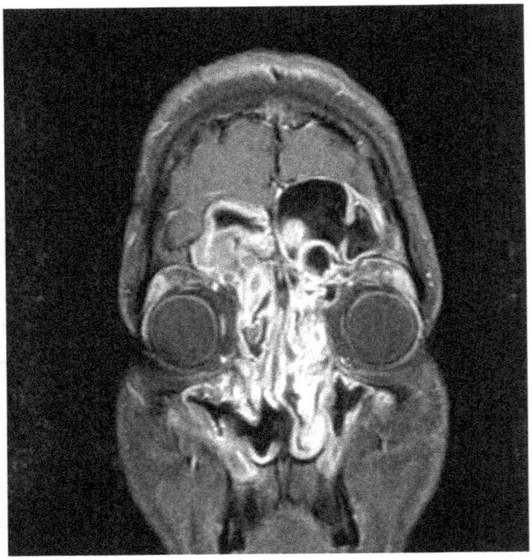

Fig. 12.12 Fungal rhinosinusitis. T1-weighted MRI with contrast shows enhancing mucosa characteristic of polyps in the ethmoid, frontal, and maxillary sinuses [26]

a specificity of 88–100%. It is a broad-spectrum assay that detects Aspergillus, Candida, Fusarium, Acremonium, and Saccharomyces species β-D-glucan is a cell wall component in a wide variety of fungi and can be detected based on its ability to activate factor G of the horseshoe crab coagulation cascade. The Fungitell assay may be used in the evaluation of invasive fungal infections caused by the fungi mentioned above [29].

- Aspergillus fumigatus-specific IgG: The precipitating IgG antibodies against *A. fumigatus* were the earliest immunological test used in the diagnosis of ABPA. Unfortunately, *A. fumigatus*-specific IgG detected using double gel diffusion technique has a sensitivity of only 27% in the diagnosis of ABPA [30].

12.6.6 Molecular Assay

It has demonstrated sensitivity of 100%, confirming its superiority over culture and also allows accurate identification by sequencing [31].

- PCR amplification targets either 28S RNA, the ITS1-5.8S region, or mitochondrial DNA. The DNA extraction protocol has been shown to be essential and is either manual or automated. Sources of the PCR samples are EDTA, blood, serum, or plasma [31].
- Meta-analyses have shown that the specificity of both GM and β1,3 glucan tests was significantly higher than that of PCR in serum samples. Recently, a combination of PCR/GM-EIA has been shown to be the most efficient diagnostic strategy, has reduced unnecessary antifungal therapy, and has improved fungal-free survival rates [31].

12.6.7 Other Tests

- Skin test—It helps in the diagnosis of allergic aspergillosis. For the skin test, a small amount of aspergillus antigen is injected into the forearm skin. Allergic skin reactions in the form of a red indurated patch can develop at the injection site, in the presence of fungal antibodies.
- Serum Total IgE Levels: Measurement of the serum total IgE is a useful test in the diagnosis and follow-up of patients with ABPA. A normal serum total IgE nearly excludes active ABPA as the cause of patient's symptoms. Although the sensitivity of serum total IgE (cut-off 500 IU/ml) in screening asthmatic patients for ABPA is good (96%), the specificity is poor (24%).
- Peripheral Blood Eosinophil Count: Total eosinophil count >1000 cells/μl is considered as an important criterion for the diagnosis of ABPA [30].
- Pulmonary Function Tests: These are essential in classifying the severity of lung disease. Bronchoprovocation testing with Aspergillus antigens has been used in the past; however, it can precipitate acute bronchospasm. The pulmonary function tests usually reveal obstructive defects with a reduction in diffusion capacity.[30].

12.7 Treatment

12.7.1 Invasive Aspergillosis (IA)

It is tretaed with IV antifungal medications (Voriconazole or liposomal Amphotericin B) in combination with surgical debridement [32–34].

- Voriconazole—6 mg/kg every 12 hrly on day 1 followed by 4 mg/kg every 12 hrly
- Liposomal Amphoterecin B—3–5 mg/kg/day

Since the pivotal trial by Herbrecht et al. demonstrated the superiority of voriconazole over amphotericin B deoxycholate, voriconazole has been the recommended first line antifungal agent for IA. This triazole antifungal agent is active against both *A. fumigatus* and *A. nidulans*, the most frequent fungal pathogens observed in IA, and has good central nervous system (CNS) penetration making it the first line of treatment as well in CNS aspergillosis. However, voriconazole is not without limitations; in keeping with other azoles, the pharmacokinetics are unpredictable and non-linear, necessitating therapeutic drug monitoring (TDM); short-and long-term side effects including visual disturbances; significant drug interactions; solar hypersensitivity and the risk of skin malignancy [34].

Another promising azole antifungal, isavuconazole, has recently been shown to be non-inferior to voriconazole in the invasive mold infections in adult allogeneic hematopoietic stem cell transplantation (HSCT) patients and adult patients with hematological malignancies [35].

12.7.2 Noninvasive Aspergillosis

For Allergic aspergillosis, the use of oral steroids for a prolonged period of time, preferably for 6–9 months, is preferred. Itraconazole is given with the steroids, as it is considered to have a "steroid-sparing" effect, causing the steroids to be more effective, allowing a lower dose [33, 34]. *A. fumigatus*, the most commonly infecting species, is intrinsically resistant to fluconazole [34].

12.7.3 Glucocorticoids

- Prednisolone: 0.5 mg/kg for 4 weak, 0.25 mg/kg for 4 weak, 0.125 mg/kg for 4 weak, then tapered by 5 mg every weak to continue for a total duration of at least 4 months.
- Inhaled Glucocorticoids (ICSs): Inhaled glucocorticoids (ICSs) achieve suitable concentrations in the airways, are associated with significantly fewer side effects and are the first-line therapy of bronchial asthma. These have also been used as anti-inflammatory agents in Allergic aspergillosis. (formoterol/budesonide, 24/1600 μg/day) [30].
- Intravenous Pulse Doses of Glucocorticoids: Pulse doses of glucocorticoids (intravenous infusion of 15 mg/kg of methylprednisolone for 3 consecutive days) have been used in children with ABPA as an alternative to daily glucocorticoid therapy [30].

12.7.4 Antifungal Drugs

- Oral azoles—Itraconazole (200 mg 12 hrly), Posaconazole (400 mg 12 hrly) and Voriconazole (200 mg 12 hrly), are preferred antifungal drugs.
- Nebulized amphotericin B—Inhaled amphotericin achieves high concentrations in the airways well above the minimal inhibitory concentration of *A. fumigatus* (0.5 mg/l), with negligible serum concentrations. Thus, there is clinical efficacy with minimal side effects.
- Topical antifungal drugs—in otomycosis, topical 1 % clotrimazole and in keratitis, topical Natamycin 5% is preferred.

12.7.5 Anti-IgE Therapy

While omalizumab, a monoclonal antibody, is indicated in patients with severe allergic asthma, it has also been evaluated in ABPA. The aim of therapy with omalizumab is to decrease the serum total IgE to <21 IU/ml, and the dose required to achieve this is 0.016 mg/kg/IU (IgE/ml). An upper limit of IgE of 1500 IU/ml and a maximum dose of omalizumab 1200 mg monthly have been specified by the manufacturer. In ABPA, the serum total IgE is highly elevated, and the dose required is very high [30].

12.7.6 Anti-Th2 Therapies

ABPA is characterized by an intense Th2 inflammation associated with excessive production of Th2 cytokines IL-4 and IL-5, which suggests a role for anti-IL-5 therapies [30].

12.7.7 Surgical Management

Because antifungal medications do not penetrate aspergillomas very well, surgery to remove the fungal mass is the first-choice treatment. Endoscopic excision of sinonasal fungal ball/granuloma is necessary for better penetration of antifungal medication. Functional endoscopic sinus surgery (FESS) has surpassed it as the surgery of choice. The main goal of surgical therapy is to remove the antigenic stimulus from the sinuses, relieve the obstruction by nasal polypectomy, removing mucin, debris, and fungal elements to improve ventilation, restore mucociliary function and provide easy access for further debridement or local therapy [36, 37].

12.8 Essential Features

- Aspergillosis refers to the diseases caused by infection by fungi of the genus Aspergillus.
- Out of 50 species, the five most clinically relevant that cause disease in humans include Aspergillus fumigates, *A. flavus*, *A. niger*, A. terreus, and *A. nidulans*, in order of frequency.
- Depending on the underlying immune status of the host, Aspergillus diseases can be roughly classified into three groups—saprophytic, allergic, and invasive aspergillosis.
- Saprophytic aspergillosis is commonly seen in immunocompetent individuals and includes aspergilloma (saprophytic colonization in a cavity) and chronic pulmonary aspergillosis.
- Allergic aspergillosis includes allergic bronchopulmonary aspergillosis, allergic rhinosinusitis and bronchocentric granulomatosis. It is observed in patients with atopy, asthma, or cystic fibrosis. It is commonly seen in immunocompetant hosts.
- Invasive form usually occurs in immunocompromised individuals and includes pulmonary invasive aspergillosis, acute necrotizing rhinosinusitis, chronic invasive rhinosinusitis, granulomatous invasive aspergillosis and cutaneous aspergillosis.
- Primary cutaneous form of aspergillosis includes otomycosis (ear infection), onychomycosis (nail bed infection), keratitis (eye infection) and Madura foot which follows traumatic inoculation of the spores directly into the affected tissues. These are less severe and respond well to local and oral antifungal medications.
- Secondary cutaneous aspergillosis has the potential to progress to systemic infection (disease dissemination) and is frequently lethal.
- Microscopy, culture, and histopathology form the mainstay of diagnosis, demonstrating septate branching hyphae at an acute angle of 45°. Special stains such as PAS and Gomori SM stain highlights the fungal sepatate branching hyphae.
- Imaging usually reveals fungal mass (aspergilloma), as well as characteristic signs of invasive and allergic bronchopulmonary aspergillosis.
- Galactomannan (GM) antigen testing with sandwich ELISA is the serological test of choice for the diagnosis of IPA.
- PCR amplification assay targets either 28S RNA, the ITS1-5.8S region, or mitochondrial DNA and has demonstrated sensitivity of 100%, confirming its superiority over culture and also allows accurate identification by sequencing.
- Total eosinophil count >1000 cells/μl and measurement of the serum total IgE is a useful test in the diagnosis and follow-up of patients with ABPA.
- The current medical treatments for aggressive invasive aspergillosis include voriconazole and liposomal amphotericin B in combination with surgical debridement. For the less aggressive allergic bronchopulmonary aspergillosis, findings use of oral steroids for 6–9 months is preferred. Itraconazole is given with steroids, as it is considered to have a "steroid-sparing" effect.
- Functional endoscopic sinus surgery (FESS) is the surgery of choice in sinonasal disease. The main goal of surgical therapy is to remove the antigenic stimulus from the sinuses, relieve the obstruction by nasal polypectomy, removing mucin, debris, and fungal elements to improve ventilation, restore mucociliary function, and provide easy access for further debridement or local therapy.

References

1. Smith N, Denning DW. Underlying conditions in chronic pulmonary aspergillosis including simple aspergilloma. Eur Respir J. 2011, April 1;37(4):865–72.
2. Alastruey-Izquierdo A, et al. Treatment of chronic pulmonary aspergillosis: current standards and future perspectives. Respiration. 2018;96:159–70. https://doi.org/10.1159/000489474.
3. Guinea J, et al. Pulmonary aspergillosis in patients with chronic obstructive pulmonary disease: inci-

dence, risk factors, and outcome. Clin Microbiol Infect. 2010;16(7):870–7.
4. Bongomin F et al. Chronic pulmonary aspergillosis: notes for a clinician in a resource-limited setting where there is no mycologist. J Fungi (Basel). 2020 Jun; 6(2):75. Published online 2020 Jun 2. https://doi.org/10.3390/jof6020075.
5. Chen J, et al. Risk factors for invasive pulmonary aspergillosis and hospital mortality in acute-on-chronic liver failure patients: a retrospective cohort study. Int J Med Sci. 2013;10(12):1625–31.
6. Garcia-Vidal C, et al. Epidemiology of invasive mold infections in allogeneic s tem cell transplant recipients: Biological risk factors for infection according to time after transplantation. Clin Infect Dis. 2008;47(8):1041–50.
7. Richard C. Barton. laboratory diagnosis of invasive aspergillosis: from diagnosis to prediction of outcome. Scientifica (Cairo) 2013; 2013:459405. Published online 2013 Jan 14. https://doi.org/10.1155/2013/459405.
8. Veress B, et al. Further observations on the primary paranasal aspergillus granuloma in the Sudan: a morphological study of 46 cases. Am J Trop Med Hyg. 1973;22:765–72.
9. Arunaloke Chakrabarti and Harsimran Kaur. Allergic aspergillus rhinosinusitis. J Fungi (Basel). 2016 Dec; 2(4):32. Published online 2016 Dec 8. https://doi.org/10.3390/jof2040032.
10. Muldoon EG, et al. Allergic and noninvasive infectious Pulmonary Aspergillosis syndromes. Clin Chest Med. 2017;38:521–34. https://doi.org/10.1016/j.ccm.2017.04.012.
11. Alastruey-Izquierdo A, et al. Treatment of chronic pulmonary aspergillosis: current standards and future perspectives. Respiration. 2018;96:159–70. https://doi.org/10.1159/000489474.
12. Denning DW, et al. Chronic pulmonary aspergillosis: rationale and clinical guidelines for diagnosis and management. Eur Respir J. 2016;47:45–68. https://doi.org/10.1183/13993003.00583-2015.
13. Kosmidis C, Denning DW. The clinical spectrum of pulmonary aspergillosis. Thorax. 2015;70:270–7. https://doi.org/10.1136/thoraxjnl-2014-206291.
14. Agarwal R, et al. Developments in the diagnosis and treatment of allergic bronchopulmonary aspergillosis. Expert Rev Respir Med. 2016;10:1317–34. https://doi.org/10.1080/17476348.2016.1249853.
15. Knutsen AP, Slavin RG. Allergic bronchopulmonary aspergillosis in asthma and cystic fibrosis. Clin Dev Immunol. 2011;2011:843763.
16. DeShazo RD, et al. A new classification and diagnostic criteria for invasive fungal sinusitis. Arch Otolaryngol Head Neck Surg. 1997;123:1181–8. https://doi.org/10.1001/archotol.1997.01900110031005.
17. van Burik J-AH, et al. Cutaneous Aspergillosis J Clin Microbiol 1998 Nov; 36(11): 3115–3121.
18. Hoffman JJ. Mycotic keratitis—a global threat from the filamentous fungi. J Fungi (Basel). 2021 Apr; 7(4):273. Published online 2021 Apr 3. https://doi.org/10.3390/jof7040273
19. Bauters TGM, Nelis HJ. Rapid and sensitive plate method for detection of Aspergillus fumigatus. J Clin Microbiol. 2000;38(10):3796–9.
20. Guarner J, Brandt ME. Histopathologic diagnos is of fungal infections in 21st century. Clin Microbiol Rev. 2011;24:247–80.
21. Gemma E, et al. Chronic pulmonary aspergillosis—where are we? and where are we going? J Fungi (Basel). 2016 Jun; 2(2):18. Published online 2016 Jun 7. https://doi.org/10.3390/jof2020018.
22. Chakrabarti A, Kaur H. Allergic aspergillus rhinosinusitis. J Fungi (Basel). 2016 Dec; 2(4):32. Published online 2016 Dec 8. https://doi.org/10.3390/jof2040032.
23. Manning SC, et al. Computed tomog raphy and magnetic resonance diagnosis of allergic fungal sinusitis. Laryngoscope. 1997;107:170–6. https://doi.org/10.1097/00005537-199702000-00007.
24. Sundaram C, Murthy JMK. Intracranial aspergillus granuloma. Pathol Res Int. 2011, 2011:5. https://doi.org/10.4061/2011/157320. Article ID 157320
25. Aribandi M, et al. Imaging features of invasive and noninvasive fungal sinusitis: a review. Radiographics. 2007;27:1283–96. https://doi.org/10.1148/rg.275065189.
26. Soler ZM, Schlosser RJ. The role of fungi in diseases of the nose and sinuses. Am J Rhinol Allergy. 2012 Sep–Oct;26(5):351–8. https://doi.org/10.2500/ajra.2012.26.3807.
27. Calabria CW, et al. Comparison of serum-specific IgE (ImmunoCAP) and skin-prick test results for 53 inhalant allergens in patients with chronic rhinitis. Allergy Asthma Proc. 2009;30:386–96. https://doi.org/10.2500/aap.2009.30.3258.
28. Stynen D, Sarfati J, et al. Rat monoclonal antibodies against Aspergillus galactomannan. Infect Immun. 1992;60:2237–45.
29. Lamoth F. Galactomannan and 1,3-β-d-glucan testing for the diagnosis of invasive aspergillosis. J Fungi. 2016;2:22. https://doi.org/10.3390/jof2030022.
30. Agarwal R, et al. Allergic bronchopulmonary aspergillosis. Indian J Med Res. 2020 Jun;151(6):529–49. https://doi.org/10.4103/ijmr.IJMR_1187_19.
31. Reinwald M, Spiess B, et al. Diagnosing pulmonary aspergillosis in patients with hematological malignancies: a multicenter prospective evaluation of an Aspergillus PCR assay and a galactomannan ELISA in bronchoalveolar lavage samples. Eur J Haematol. 2012;89:120–7. https://doi.org/10.1111/j.1600-0609.2012.01806.x.
32. Cornely OA, et al. Posaconazole vs. fluconazole or itraconazole prophylaxis in patients with neutropenia. N Engl J Med. 2007;356(4):348–59.
33. Walsh TJ, et al. Treatment of aspergillosis: clinical practice guidelines of the infectious diseases society of America. Clin Infect Dis. 2008;46(3):327–60.
34. Herbrecht R, et al. Voriconazole vs. amphotericin b for primary therapy of invasive aspergillosis. N Engl

J Med. 2002;347:408–15. https://doi.org/10.1056/NEJMoa020191.
35. King J et al. Aspergillosis in chronic granulomatous disease. J Fungi (Basel). 2016 Jun; 2(2):15. Published online 2016 May 26. https://doi.org/10.3390/jof2020015.
36. Herbrecht R, et al. Invasive fungal infections Group of the European Organisation for research and treatment of Cancer and the global Aspergillus study group. "Voriconazole versus amphotericin B for primary therapy of invasive aspergillosis". N Engl J Med. 2002;347(6):408–15.
37. Gan EC, et al. Medical management of allergic fungal rhinosinusitis following endoscopic sinus surgery: an evidence-based review and recommendations. Int Forum Allergy Rhinol. 2014;4:702–15. https://doi.org/10.1002/alr.21352.

Mucormycosis

13

Abstract

Mucormycosis is an angioinvasive fungal infection, due to fungi of the order Mucorales. It is an opportunistic infection especially associated with diabetes. In developed countries, the most common underlying diseases are hematological malignancies and transplantation. Depending on the clinical presentation it is classified as rhinocerebral (commonest presentation), pulmonary, cutaneous, gastrointestinal, and disseminated. Diagnosis of mucormycosis remains challenging. The clinical approach to diagnosis has a low sensitivity and specificity; it helps however in raising suspicion and prompting the initiation of laboratory testing. Histopathology, direct examination, and culture remain essential tools, although the molecular methods are improving. First-Line Monotherapy is with liposomal Amphoterecin-B (AmB). For patients refractory to AmB, salvage Therapy with Posaconazole or Isavuconazole is preferred. Surgical debridement improves the penetration of antifungal drugs in the soft tissue and helps in the complete clearance of disease. Rhinocerebral mucormycosis is one of the most common life-threatening opportunistic fungal infections associated with moderate to severe Coronavirus disease 2019 (COVID-19). Uncontrolled diabetes mellitus and the use of corticosteroids increase the risk of invasive fungal infection with mucormycosis which can develop during the course of the illness or as a sequelae. A high index of suspicion, early diagnosis, and appropriate management can improve survival.

Synonyms
Zygomycosis; Phycomycosis [1, 2].

13.1 Background

Mucormycosis is a fungal infection caused by fungi in the order Mucorales and class zygomycetes. The disease was first described in 1876 when Furbinger described in Germany a patient who died of cancer and in whom the right lung showed a hemorrhagic infarct with fungal hyphae and a few sporangia. In 1885, Arnold Paltauf published the first case of disseminated mucormycosis, which he named "Mycosis mucorina" [2]. Currently, Mucorales fungi are the next most common mold pathogens after Aspergillus, leading to invasive fungal disease in patients with malignancies or transplantation. The incidence of mucormycosis has also increased significantly in patients with diabetes, which is the commonest underlying risk factor globally. Usually, the Mucor, Rhizopus, Absidia, and Cunninghamella species are most often implicated. The disease is characterized by hyphae growing in and around blood vessels and can be potentially life-

S. V. Nemade, K. J. Shinde, *Granulomatous diseases in Otorhinolaryngology, Head and Neck*,
https://doi.org/10.1007/978-981-16-4047-6_13

threatening in diabetic or severely immunocompromised individuals. It presents in the four clinical forms: rhinocerebral, gastrointestinal, pulmonary, and disseminated, in the decreasing frequency of occurrence [1–3].

13.2 Epidemiology

Mucormycosis is a very rare angioinvasive fungal infection. Therefore, the ability to determine the burden of disease is limited [4] during the past 2 decades, mucormycosis has emerged as an important fungal infection with high associated mortality rates. Global population-based incidence estimates to vary between 0.5 and 4 cases per 1 million population with a mortality rate of 54% [5]. Globally, mucormycosis is found in 1% of patients with acute leukemia patients [4, 6].

In India, the prevalence of mucormycosis is approximately 0.14 cases per 1000 population, which is about 80 times the prevalence of mucormycosis in developed countries [6].

13.3 Etiopathogenesis

Mucormycosis is a ubiquitous fungus, usually avirulent, causing opportunistic infections in immunocompromised individuals.

13.4 Classification

- Class: Phycomycetes/zygomycetes
- Order: Mucorales
- Family: Mucoraceae.
- Genera: Rhizopus, Mucor, Lichtheimia and Cunninghamella.
- It is a basophilic branched, non-septate fungus with rounded pigmented multicellular sporangia with multiple sporangiophores.
- The order Mucorales comprises 261 species in 55 genera, 38 of which have been associated with human infections. The most common species all over the world is Rhizopus arrhizus (formerly Rhizopus oryzae). Other isolated fungi belong to the genera Lichtheimia, Mucor, Rhizomucor, Cunninghamella, Saksenaea, Apophysomyces, Cokeromyces, Actinomucor and Syncephalastrum. In the global review by Jeong et al., Rhizopus spp., Lichtheimia spp., and Mucor spp. accounted for 75% of all cases [2, 6].

13.4.1 Predisposing Factors

- Diabetes Mellitus
- Hematological malignancy
- Organ transplants
- Immunosuppressants
- Uremia
- Burns
- Severe malnutrition and diarrhoeal disease

The fungus is present in air, dust, plants, and decaying matter. It adheres to dust particles and is inhaled and deposited in the nose and paranasal sinus mucosa. The warm moist environment with decreased immunity of the host enhances the fungal growth. It invades blood vessels and causes plugging by fungal mycelia. This leads to thrombosis and ischemic necrosis. This necrotic tissue is the nidus for organism growth, and it thrives there and subsequently invades the surrounding tissue through blood vessels. It also induces IgE hypersensitivity, which is enhanced in a hypoxic environment.

13.5 Clinical Features

Constitutional symptoms such as fever, malaise, lethargy are common in all types of clinical presentations.

Rhinocerebral disease: This is the most common presentation. Nasal obstruction, rhinorrhoea, epistaxis, nasal hypoesthesia, facial pain, facial numbness, and headache are the most common complaints. Typical black colored fungal debris is found in the nasal cavity and sinuses (Fig. 13.1a, b). The most common site involved is middle turbinate, followed by middle meatus and septum. In undiagnosed and untreated cases, it is associated with extensive destruction of nasal

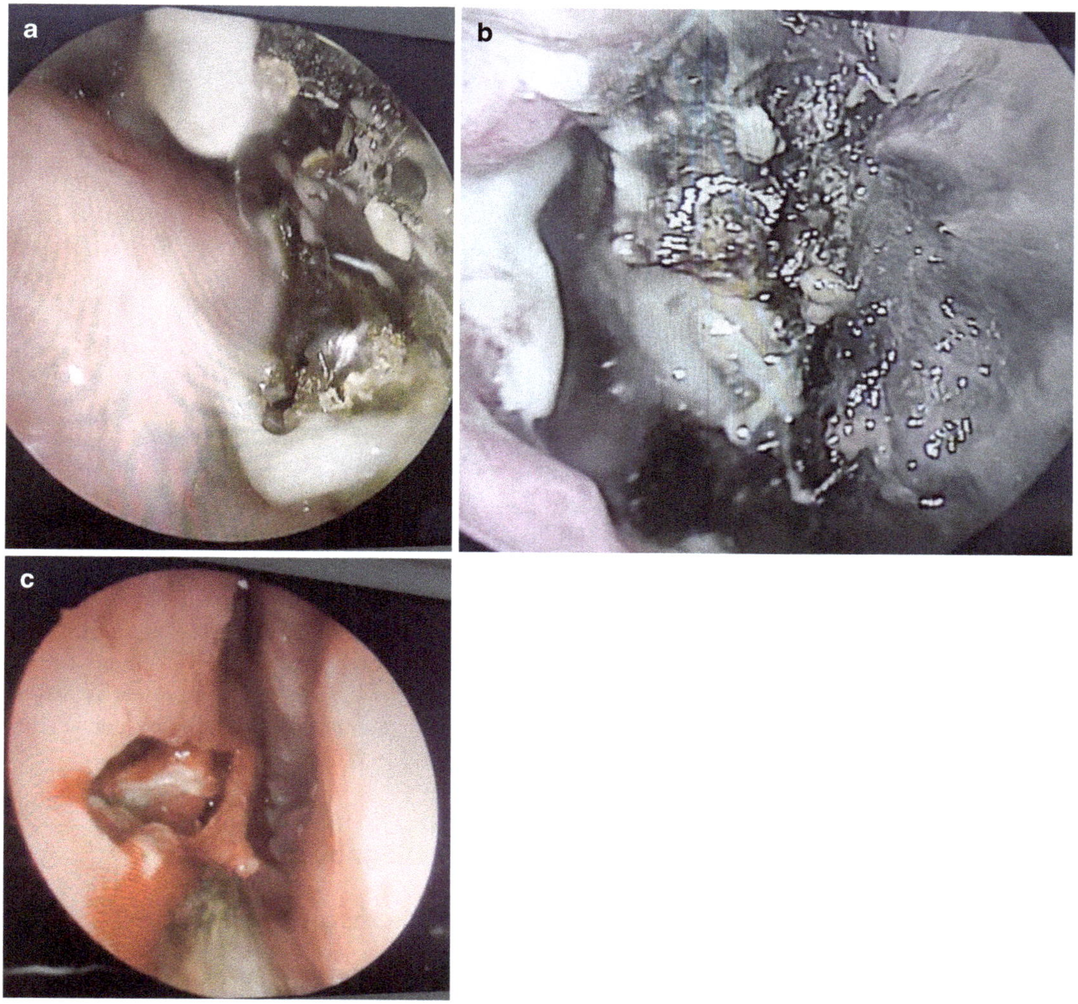

Fig. 13.1 (**a**, **b**) Nasal endoscopy showing black colored fungal debris with purulent secretions. (**c**) Septal perforation with bony sequestrum

septum, bony walls of sinuses with the extension of disease in the oral cavity, orbit or cranial cavity through the involvement of sphenopalatine and internal maxillary arteries. Nasal/facial/palatal necrosis and bony sequestration are the typical features (Figs. 13.1c, 13.2, 13.3, and 13.4). Intraorbital disease leads to orbital cellulitis and/or loss of vision (Fig.13.5). Common eye complaints are retro-orbital or periorbital pain, diplopia, chemosis, and blurring of vision. The involvement of internal carotid artery and cavernous sinus thrombosis is common only in long-standing cases. Intracranial extension manifests as disorientation, comatose state, convulsions, and cranial nerve palsies [6–8].

Gastrointestinal disease: It is usually secondary to hematological spread of disease secondary to fulminant rhinocerebral disease. Abdominal cramps, hematemesis, diarrhea with blood-stained stools, dehydration are the features [6].

Pulmonary disease: Isolated pulmonary involvement without nasal disease is rare. It presents with cough, hemoptysis, dyspnoea, and pleural effusion.

Disseminated disease: Hematological spread may lead to multisystem failure due to ischemic

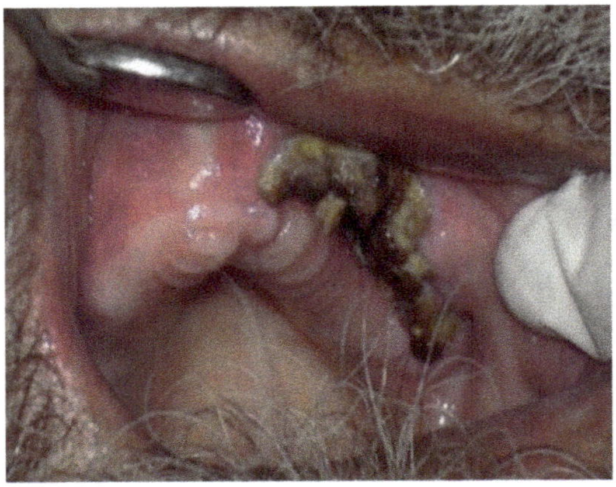

Fig. 13.2 Intra-oral photograph showing necrosis of mucosa and underlying bone in relation to canine to tuberosity area of left vestibular region of maxilla along with abnormal communication between vestibule and palate [7]

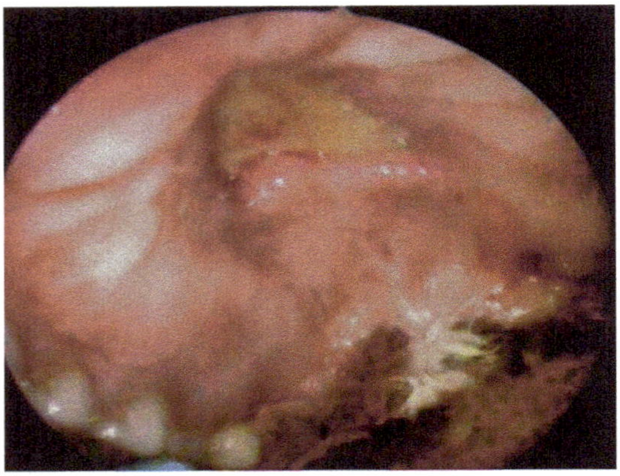

Fig. 13.3 Palatal perforation covered with slough

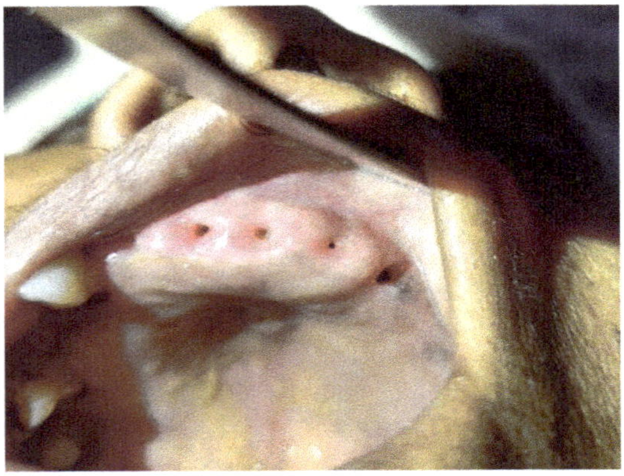

Fig. 13.4 Multiple oro-antral fistulas with palatal destruction

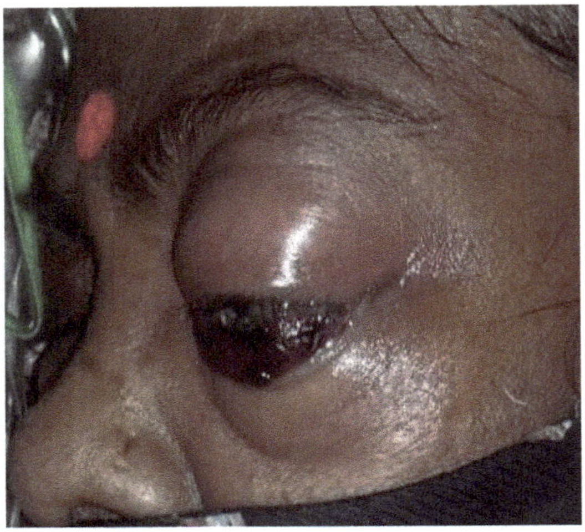

Fig. 13.5 Orbital mucormycosis

necrosis and is often fatal. Cutaneous involvement is commonly seen (Fig. 13.6). Ear involvement is extremely rare [7, 9]. The cholesteatoma with mucormycosis of the middle ear is associated with perineural involvement and causes facial palsy [9, 10].

13.6 Diagnosis

13.6.1 Microscopy and Culture

For a rapid presumptive diagnosis of mucormycosis direct microscopy of KOH wet mounts can be used. It can be applied to all materials (secretions or tissue specimens) sent to the clinical laboratory, preferably using fluorescent brighteners such as Blankophor and Calcofluor White together with KOH, which enhance the visualization of the characteristic non-pigmented thin-walled, ribbon-like pauciseptate fungal hyphae. The use of fluorescent brighteners requires a fluorescent microscope [11, 12].

13.6.2 Culture

Fungal culture of nasal secretions, sputum, GI secretions or tissue specimen is essential for the diagnosis of mucormycosis since it allows identification to the genus and species level, and even-

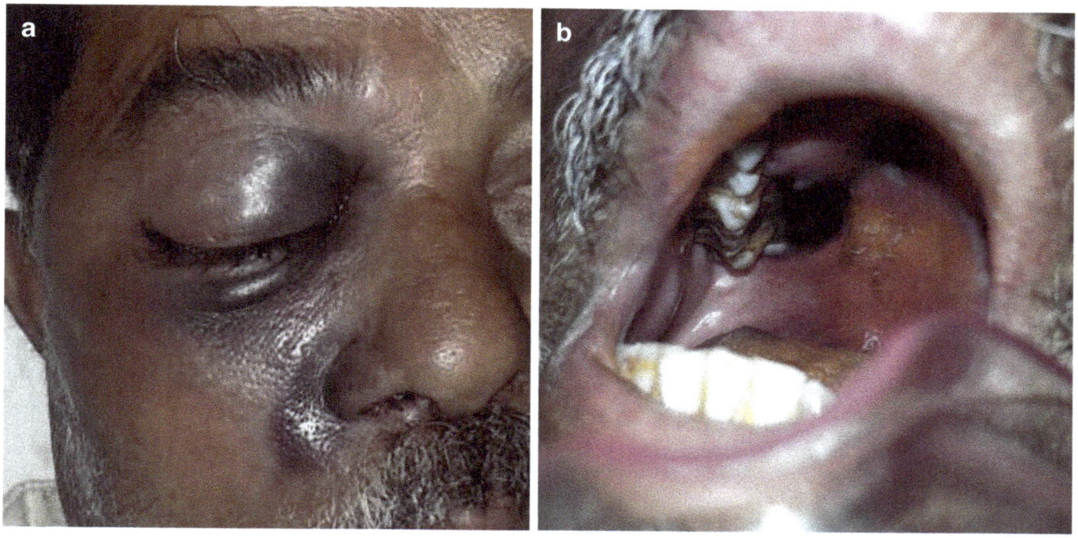

Fig. 13.6 Local as well as disseminated sinonasal mucormycosis involving (**a**) right orbit, skin, and (**b**) palate

tually antifungal susceptibility testing. Most of the Mucorales are thermotolerant and are able to grow rapidly at temperatures of 37 °C. They grow on virtually any carbohydrate substrate, colonies appearing usually within 24–48 h and identification is based on colonial and microscopic morphology and growth temperature. Characteristic non-pigmented, wide (5–20 μm), thin-walled, ribbon-like fungal hyphae with no or few septations (pauciseptate) and right-angle branching confirms the diagnosis [11, 12].

A positive culture from a sterile site confirms the diagnosis, while a positive culture from a non-sterile site could be due to a contaminant and must be combined with clinical and radiological data to establish a probable diagnosis. Hence, there is a caveat for falsely positive results, especially when histopathology is not available [5]. The major concern about culture, however, is its low sensitivity, as it can be falsely negative in up to 50% of mucormycosis cases [5, 13, 14].

13.6.3 Histopathology

A definitive diagnosis is based on the demonstration of fungal hyphae typical for mucormycetes in biopsies of affected tissues. Histopathology is a very important diagnostic tool since it distinguishes the presence of the fungus as a pathogen in the specimen from a culture contaminant and is indispensable to define whether there is blood vessel invasion. It can furthermore reveal coinfections with other molds. Mucorales genera produce typically non-pigmented, wide (5–20 μm), thin-walled, ribbon-like hyphae with no or few septations (pauciseptate) and right-angle branching, in contrast to those of the Aspergillus species or other hyaline molds, which are typically 3–5 μm wide, septate and form acute-angle branching (Fig. 13.7). Routine hematoxylin and eosin (H&E) stains may show only the cell wall with no structures inside and very degenerate hyphae (Fig. 13.8). Stains that can help highlight the fungal wall include Grocott methenamine-silver (GMS) (Fig. 13.9a) and periodic acid-Schiff PAS stains (Fig. 13.9b), although PAS gives a better visualization of the surrounding tissue compared to GMS [8, 15].

13.6.4 Serology

Serological tests for diagnosis of zygomycosis are detection of antigen and/or antibody. Antibodies to Zygomycetes can be detected by enzyme-linked immunosorbent assays (ELISAs) and double diffusion. Immunoblot analyses have also been used to detect Rhizopus antigens [16].

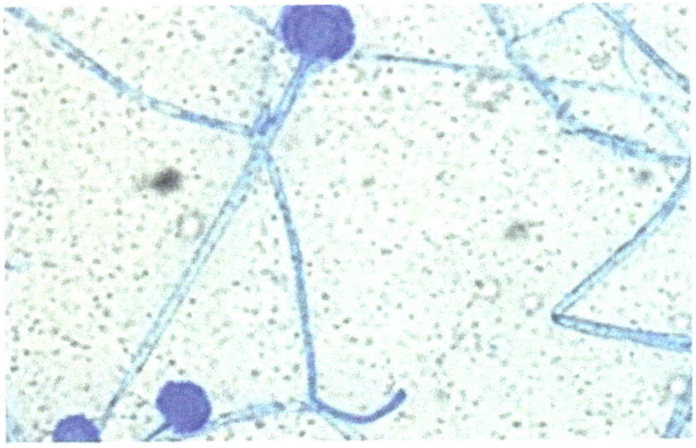

Fig. 13.7 Direct examination of culture specimen of Cunninghamella spp. after 48 h of incubation on Sabouraud agar [12]

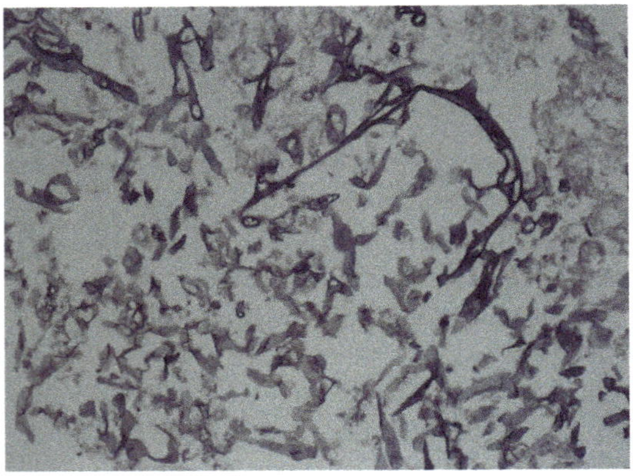

Fig. 13.8 Hematoxylin and eosin (H&E) stain demonstrating fungal hyphae

13.6.5 Molecular Assay

- Polymerase chain reaction (PCR) assay of tissue specimens—It has been found to be more sensitive for early detection of mucor infection [14].
- A multiplex real-time quantitative PCR (qPCR) targeting ITS1/ITS2 region with specific probes for *R. oryzae*, *R. microsporus*, and Mucor spp. [17].
- A real-time qPCR with specific primers that are designed to amplify a part of the cytochrome b gene, a specific qPCR targeting the 28S rDNA [17].
- Two independent mucorales specific real-time qPCR assays (targeting two different regions of the multicopy ribosomal operon-18S and 28S) that are able to detect DNA from a broad range of clinically relevant mucorales species are useful for the diagnosis of mucor infection [17]. The Mucorales qPCR performed on serum or plasma is a non-invasive technique that can be performed in all patients, with an acceptable time frame and a reasonable cost [17].

13.6.6 Imaging

CT and MRI scans show a spectrum of findings in all types of mucormycosis [6, 10].

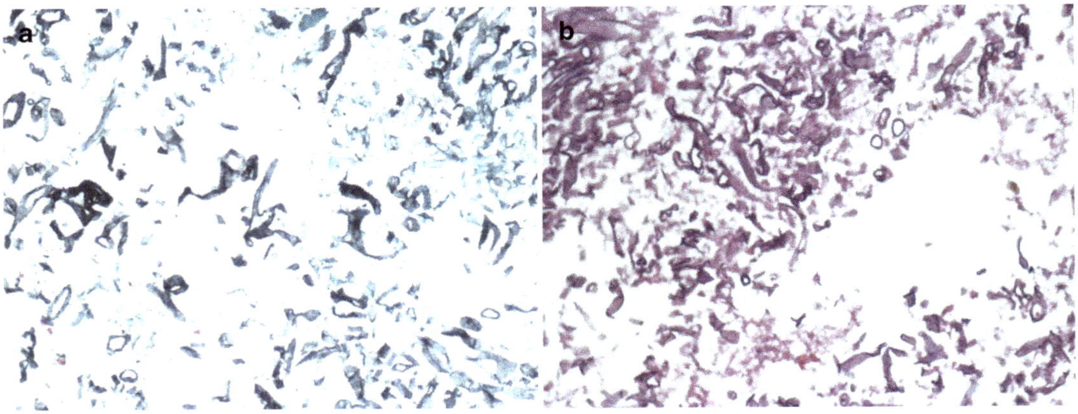

Fig. 13.9 (**a**) Gomori methenamine silver (GMS) stain highlighting the fungal wall and the pathognomonic pauci-septate right-angle branching hyphae. (**b**) High-power PAS stain demonstrating hyphae and inflammatory cells with brisk neutrophilic infiltrate and limited blood elements

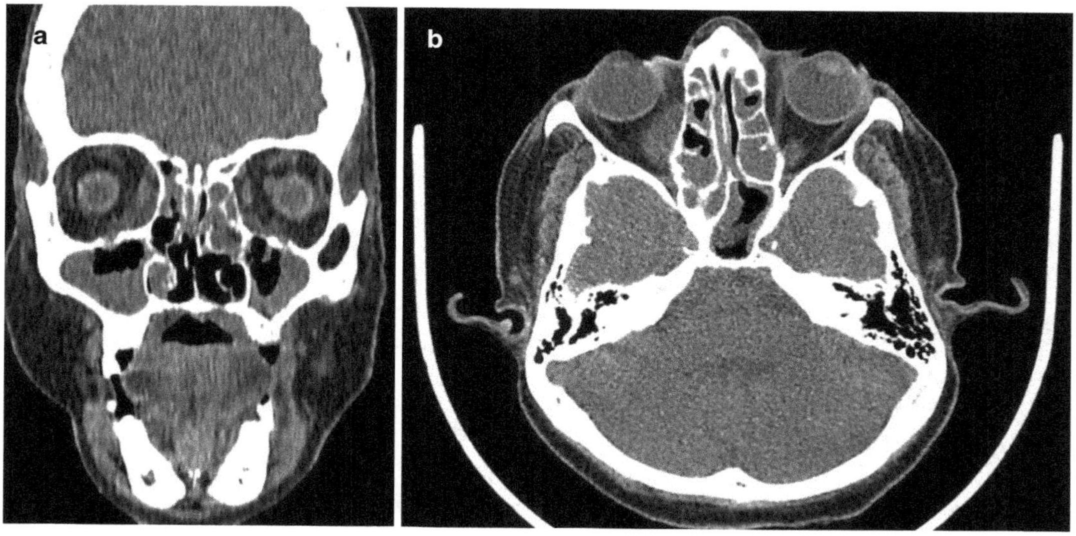

Fig. 13.10 (**a**) CT PNS coronal section demonstrating the involvement of bilateral maxillary and ethmoidal sinuses. (**b**) CT PNS axial section demonstrating the involvement of bilateral ethmoidal sinuses

- Rinocerebral disease—CT shows minimally enhancing hypodense soft tissue thickening as the predominant finding in the involved areas, while MRI shows T2 isointense to mildly hypointense soft tissue thickening and heterogenous post-contrast enhancement as the main finding. CT may reveal bone erosions in advanced disease (Figs. 13.10, 13.11 and 13.12)
- Pulmonary disease—CT shows consolidation with surrounding ground-glass opacity (Halo sign). In the advanced disease, it may progress to "reverse halo sign" (central ground-glass opacity with the surrounding irregular rim of consolidation). Pleural thickening may be the additional finding.

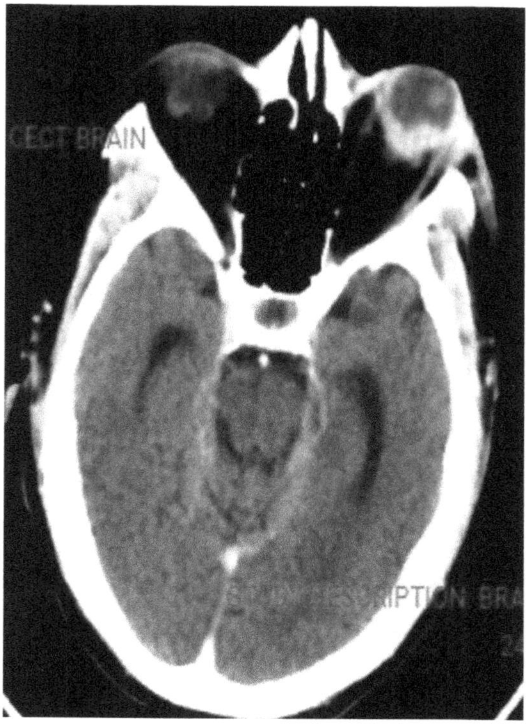

Fig. 13.11 CT axial section showing isolated involvement of left orbit with normal sinuses

13.7 Treatment

The successful treatment of mucormycosis requires four steps: (1) early diagnosis; (2) reversal of underlying predisposing risk factors, if possible; (3) prompt antifungal therapy; and (4) surgical debridement where applicable.

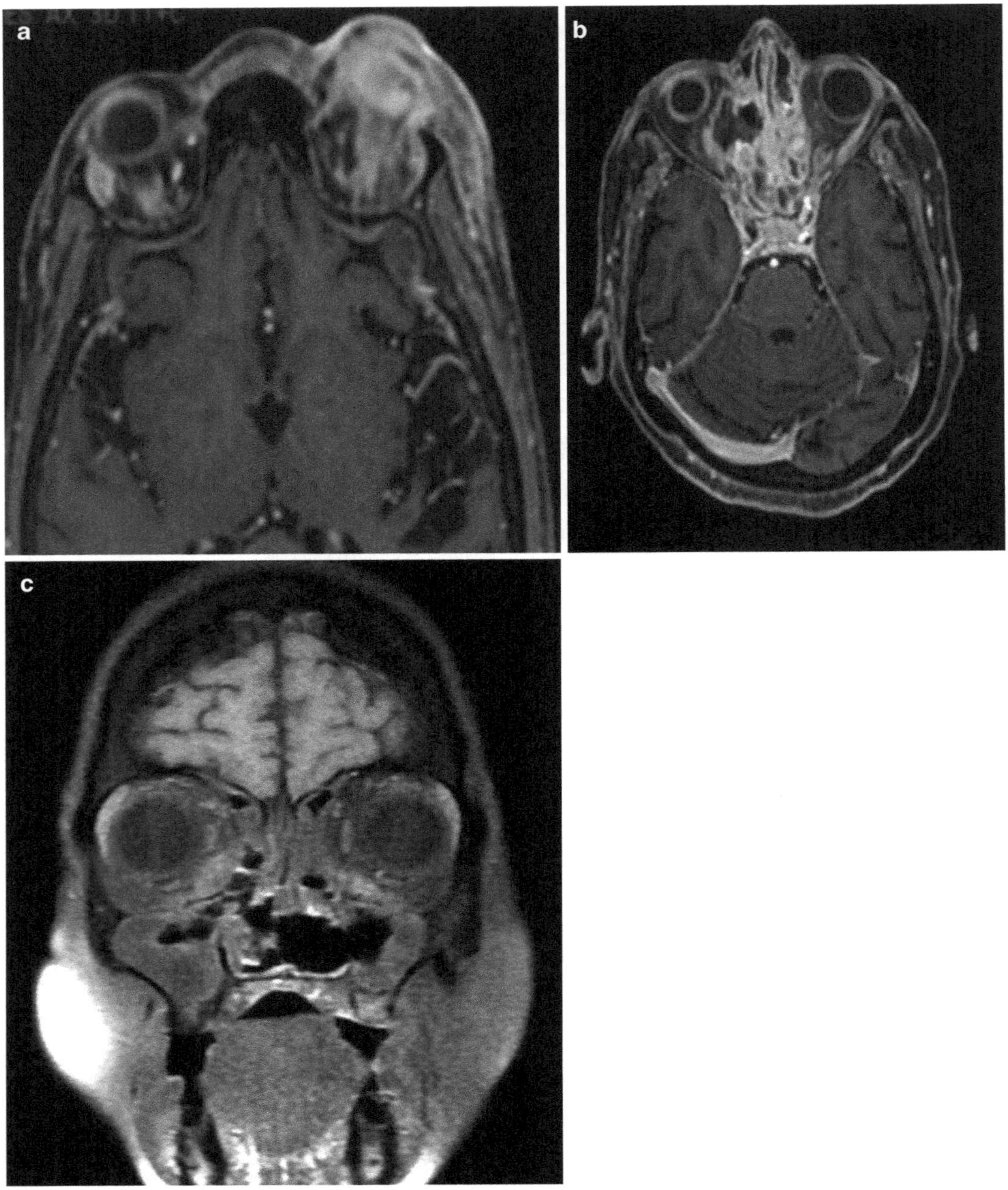

Fig. 13.12 (**a**) MRI PNS axial section showing isolated involvement of left orbit with normal sinuses. (**b**) MRI PNS axial section demonstrating the involvement of bilateral ethmoid sinuses with intraorbital extension on the right side. (**c**) MRI PNS coronal section showing involvement of maxillary and ethmoid sinuses with the destruction of medial wall of maxilla and nasal septum

1. Establishing an early diagnosis of mucormycosis is critical to enable the early initiation of active antifungal therapy and to improve the survival rate.
2. Reversal of Underlying Disease

   It is critical to reverse/prevent underlying defects in host defense when treating patients with mucormycosis. Immunosuppressive

medications, particularly corticosteroids, should be dose reduced or stopped if possible. Aggressive management to rapidly restore euglycemia and normal acid-base status is critical in diabetic patients in ketoacidosis.
3. Prompt antifungal therapy

13.7.1 First-Line Monotherapy

In general, primary antifungal therapy for mucormycosis should be based on a polyene, if possible. Although amphotericin B deoxycholate (AmB) was the cornerstone of mucormycosis therapy for decades, lipid formulations of Amphoterecin are significantly less nephrotoxic and can be safely administered at higher doses for a longer period of time than AmB deoxycholate.

13.7.2 Dose of AmB (amphotericin B deoxycholate)

- First day: 0.25 mg/kg of body weight IV over 45–60 min.
- Second day: 0.5 mg/kg; Third day: 0.75 mg/kg. Then alternate day 0.75 mg/kg. Liver function and kidney function should be monitored weekly till the completion of antifungal therapy.
- Dose of Liposomal formulation (AmBisome)—It is the drug of choice based on efficacy and safety data. Lipid preparations of amphotericin B are used at 5 mg/kg/d [1]. Some have used doses of up to 7.5–10 mg/kg/d to treat mucormycosis, especially CNS disease [18, 19].

13.7.3 Salvage Therapy

- Posaconazole or deferasirox are reasonable salvage options for patients with mucormycosis refractory to or intolerant of polyene therapy. Oral Posaconazole (400 mg twice a day) has been recently approved by FDA to treat invasive mucormycosis. Posaconazole appears to be quite safe despite months to years of administration [11, 12, 20].
- Isavuconazole (Cresemba) is a novel triazole antifungal agent that was approved for the treatment of mucormycosis in March 2015. Isavuconazole offers several advantages over other triazoles (i.e., posaconazole, voriconazole), apart from its wider spectrum of antifungal activity. The drug has excellent oral bioavailability not reliant on food intake or gastric pH and is also available in an intravenous formulation [21].
- Deferasirox and deferiprone are iron-chelating agents which do not act as a siderophore to the fungus. Unsaturated serum transferrin acts as a fungistatic agent by suppressing fungal growth. Iron chelators modify the fungistatic activity of transferrin and also inhibit the iron-catalyzed peroxidase-dependent production of free radicals, which kills fungi. The DEFEAT mucor (Deferasirox-AmBisome Therapy) for Mucormycosis randomized trial showed increased mortality in patients who received a combination of amphotericin and deferasirox than those who received amphotericin alone [22].
- The role of hyperbaric oxygen therapy is yet to be established, though hyperbaric oxygen is expected to alleviate severe hypoxia and acidosis, thereby inhibiting fungal multiplication. Also, the higher oxygen pressure increases the ability of neutrophils to kill the organism [12, 23].

13.7.4 Surgical Management

Blood vessel thrombosis and resulting tissue necrosis during mucormycosis can result in poor penetration of antifungal agents to the site of infection. Therefore, debridement of necrotic tissues may be critical for the complete eradication of mucormycosis. Surgical debridement includes extensive resection of infected and necrotic tissues as a part of source control and reduction of fungal load (Fig. 13.13a, b). Debridement also provides adequate tissue biopsy specimens for

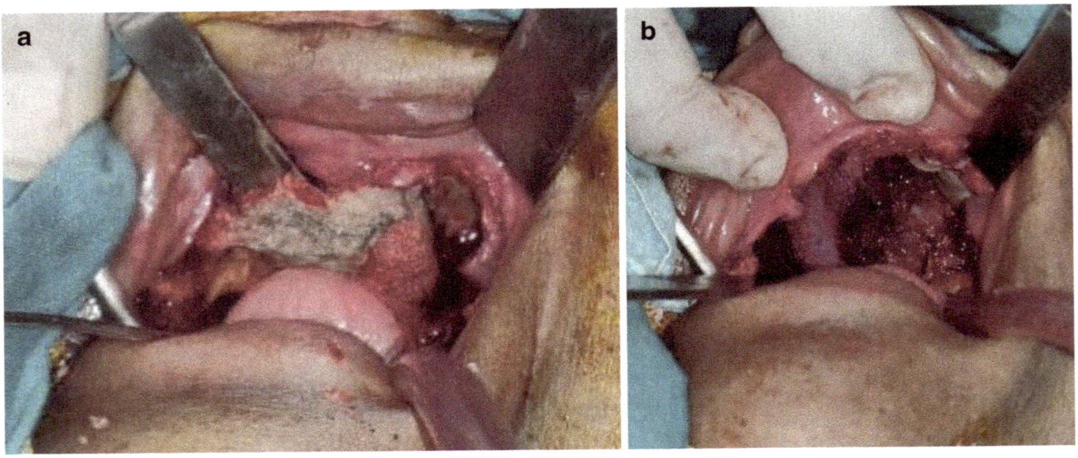

Fig. 13.13 (**a**) Extensive necrosis of palate with mucormycosis. (**b**) Intraoperative photograph after excision of the palate

definite histopathologic confirmation. Dissection is usually continued until normal, well-perfused bleeding tissue is reached since mucormycotic tissues are less likely to bleed due to extensive thrombosis of vessels. Removal of the palate, nose cartilage, and orbit would cause significant disfigurement. The orbital involvement may need orbital decompression or exenteration [24].

The prognosis of mucormycosis is poor and has varied mortality rates depending on its form and severity. In the rhinocerebral form, the mortality rate is between 30% and 70%, whereas in disseminated mucormycosis presents mortality rate is up to 90% [9]. Patients with AIDS have a mortality rate of almost 100% [2, 11]

13.7.5 Post Covid-19 Mucormycosis (From Frying Pan to Fire)

COVID-19 pandemic has resulted in widespread mortality, morbidity, social and economic upheavals of an unprecedented magnitude. Post COVID-19 sepsis is what occurs after SARS-CoV-2 infection has had a rampage in the human body. It leads to a dysregulated innate immune response, ciliary dysfunction, cytokine storm, thrombo-inflammation, microvascular coagulation, and eventual immune exhaustion. This cascade of events facilitates secondary bacterial and fungal infections especially in critically ill patients subjected to emergency invasive procedures, mechanical ventilation, prolonged hospital stays, and breaches in asepsis. Further, the use of corticosteroid treatment and anti-IL-6-directed strategies in these highly susceptible hosts along with high fungal spore counts in the environment creates the perfect setting for mold infections [25, 26].

The most common form of mucormycosis in post-Covid 19 infection is Rhino-orbital cerebral mucormycosis. It is associated with angioinvasion and with high morbidity and mortality despite treatment. Suspicion or diagnosis of rhino-orbital cerebral mucormycosis is a medical as well as surgical emergency. Song et al. noted that fungal infections are more likely to develop during the middle and later stages of COVID-19 infection [27]. The mortality rate is also higher (53% with vs. 31% without invasive fungal infection) amongst the patients of COVID-19 with secondary fungal infection [28]. A high index of suspicion among caregivers, a rapid workup, early initiation of amphotericin, and surgical debridement in all suspected cases are a must for improved outcomes. Surgical debridement reduces the fungal load as well as enables tissue diagnosis. Significant disfigurement is common after debridement. An interprofessional team approach with close interaction and coordination among various medical and surgical specialties indisputably ensures a better outcome [25, 26].

13.8 Essential Features

- Also known as zygomycosis or mucormycosis caused by ubiquitous fungi of class Zygomycetes.
- Opportunistic infection is especially associated with diabetes; other predisposing factors are neutropenia, corticosteroid therapy, iron overload, and mucocutaneous trauma.
- Rhinocerebral disease is the most common presentation. Manifests with nasal obstruction, epistaxis, headache, disorientation, cranial nerve palsies, cavernous sinus thrombosis, orbital cellulitis, nasal/facial/palatal necrosis, and bony sequestration.
- Pulmonary disease and GI involvement are usually secondary to rhinocerebral mucormycosis.
- Disseminated disease: Hematological spread may lead to multisystem failure due to ischemic necrosis and is often fatal.
- Microscopy and culture of nasal secretions, sputum, or GI secretions: Characteristic non-pigmented, wide (5–20 μm), thin-walled, ribbon-like fungal hyphae with no or few septations (pauciseptate) and right-angle branching confirms the diagnosis.
- Histopathology with special stains that can help highlight the fungal wall includes Grocott methenamine-silver (GMS) and periodic acid-Schiff PAS.
- Polymerase chain reaction (PCR) assay of tissue specimens has been found to be more sensitive for early detection of mucor infection.
- CT and MRI help to delineate the integrity, extent of disease along with destruction and angioinvasion.
- Euglycemia and normal acid-base status maintenance, correction of underlying immunocompromised situation are important.
- First-Line Monotherapy is with liposomal Amphoterecin-B (AmB).
- For patients refractory to AmB, salvage Therapy with Posaconazole or Isavuconazole is preferred.
- Hyperbaric oxygen therapy is used along with pharmacotherapy, thereby inhibiting fungal multiplication.
- Surgical debridement improves the penetration of antifungal drugs in the soft tissue and helps in the complete clearance of disease.
- Mucormycosis is frequently encountered in Post COVID-19 sepsis and warrants a high index of suspicion, rapid workup, early initiation of amphotericin, and surgical debridement for a better outcome.

References

1. James WD, Berger TG. Andrews diseases of the skin: clinical dermatology. London: Saunders Elsevier; 2006. isbn 0-7216-2921-0
2. Skiada A, et al. Epidemiology and diagnosis of mucormycosis: an update. J Fungi (Basel). 2020 Dec; 6(4):265. Published online 2020 Nov 2. https://doi.org/10.3390/jof6040265.
3. Lee FY, et al. Pulmonary mucormycosis: the last 30 years. Arch Intern Med. 1999;159(12):1301–9.
4. Ibrahim AS, et al. Pathogenesis of mucormycosis. Clin Infect Dis. 2012;54(Suppl 1):S16–22.
5. Cornely OA, et al. Global guideline for the diagnosis and management of mucormycosis: an initiative of the European Confederation of Medical Mycology in cooperation with the mycoses study group education and research consortium. Lancet Infect Dis. 2019;19:e405–21. https://doi.org/10.1016/S1473-3099(19)30312-3.
6. Chander J, et al. Saksenaea erythrospora, an emerging mucoralean fungus causing severe necrotizing skin and soft tissue infections —a study from a tertiary care hospital in North India. Infect Dis. 2017;49:170–7. https://doi.org/10.1080/23744235.2016.1239027.
7. Sahota R, et al. Rhinocerebral Mucormycosis: report of a rare case. Ethiop J Health Sci. 2017 Jan;27(1):85–90. https://doi.org/10.4314/ejhs.v27i1.11.
8. Walsh TJ, et al. Development of new strategies for early diagnosis of mucormycosis from bench to bedside. Mycoses. 2014;57(Suppl 3):2–7.
9. Hazarika P, et al. Mucormycosis of the middle ear: a case report with review of literature. Indian J Otolaryngol Head Neck Surg. 2012;64:90–4.
10. Mohamed MS, et al. Management of rhino-orbital mucormycosis. Saudi Med J. 2015;36:865–8.
11. Walsh TJ, et al. Early clinical and laboratory diagnosis of invasive pulmonary, Extrapulmonary, and disseminated Mucormycosis (Zygomycosis) Clin. Infect Dis. 2012;54:S55–60. https://doi.org/10.1093/cid/cir868.
12. Mascarella MA, et al. The infectious thyroid nodule: a case report of mucormycosis associated with ibrutinib therapy. J Otolaryngol Head Neck Surg. 2019; 48:49. Published online 2019 Oct 16. https://doi.org/10.1186/s40463-019-0376-1

13. Kermani W, et al. ENT mucormycosis. Report of 4 cases. Eur Ann Otorhinolaryngol Head Neck Dis. 2016;133:83–6.
14. Lackner M, et al. Laboratory diagnosis of mucormycosis: current status and future perspectives. Future Microbiol. 2014;9:683–95. https://doi.org/10.2217/fmb.14.23.
15. Skiada A, et al. Epidemiology and diagnosis of mucormycosis: an update. J Fungi (Basel). 2020 Dec; 6(4):265. Published online 2020 Nov 2. https://doi.org/10.3390/jof6040265.
16. Wysong D, Waldorf AR. Electrophoretic and immunoblot analyses ofRhizopus arrhizusantigens. J Clin Microbiol. 1987;25:358–63.
17. Millon L, et al. Molecular Strategies to Diagnose Mucormycosis. J Fungi (Basel). 2019 Mar; 5(1): 24. Published online 2019 Mar 20. https://doi.org/10.3390/jof5010024.
18. Spellberg B, et al. Recent advances in the management of mucormycosis: from bench to bedside. Clin Infect Dis. 2009 Jun 15;48(12):1743–51.
19. Roden MM, et al. Epidemiology and outome of zygomycosis: a review of 929 reported cases. Clin Infect Dis. 2005 Sep 1;41(5):634–53.
20. Spellberg B, Ibrahim AS. Recent advances in the treatment of Mucormycosis. Curr Infect Dis Rep. 2010; 12(6): 423–429. Published online 2010 Aug 10. https://doi.org/10.1007/s11908-010-0129-9.
21. Marty FM, et al. Isavuconazole treatment for mucormycosis: a single-arm open-label trial and case-control analysis. Lancet Infect Dis. 2016 Jul.;16(7):828–37.
22. Spellberg B, et al. The Deferasirox-AmBisome therapy for Mucormycosis (DEFEAT Mucor) study: a randomized, double-blinded, placebo-controlled trial. J Antimicrob Chemother 2012 Mar.
23. Yohai RA, et al. Survival factors in rhino-orbital-cerebral mucormycosis. Surv Ophthalmol 1994 Jul–Aug.
24. Chander J, et al. Mucormycosis: battle with the deadly enemy over a five-year period in India. Journal of fungi (Basel, Switzerland). 2018 Apr 6.
25. Prakash H, Chakrabarti A. Global epidemiology of Mucormycosis. J Fungi (Basel). 2019;5:26.
26. Chakrabarti A, et al. Epidemiology and clinical outcomes of invasive mould infections in Indian intensive care units (FISF study). J Crit Care. 2019;51:64–70.
27. Song G, et al. Fungal co-infections associated with global COVID-19 pandemic: a clinical and diagnostic perspective from China. Mycopathologia. 2020:1–8. https://doi.org/10.1007/s11046-020-00462-9.
28. Mehta S, Pandey A. Rhino-orbital mucormycosis associated with COVID-19? Cureus. 2020;12::e10726. https://doi.org/10.7759/cureus.10726.

Rhinosporidiosis

14

Abstract

Rhinosporidiosis is a chronic granulomatous infective disorder commonly affecting the mucous membranes of the nose, nasopharynx, and less commonly other sites. Infection of nose and nasopharynx is involved in 70% of cases and infection of palpebral conjunctiva is seen in 15% of cases. Other structures such as the mouth, larynx, tracheobronchial tree, and lacrimal sac may be sites of disease. In these cases, it is usually secondary to nasal rhinosporidiosis with inoculation of spores in the adjacent mucosa (auto-inoculation). Other (atypical) sites of rhinosporidiosis are scalp, skin, penis, urethra, vulva, and bone. This organism was previously considered to be a fungus, and rhinosporidiosis is classified as a fungal disease under ICD-10. It is now considered to be a protist classified under Mesomycetozoea. Its causative agent is *Rhinosporidium seeberi*. The disease is more prevalent in the Indian subcontinent. Clinically nasal rhinosporidiosis is characterized by the development of a single pedunculated polyp, multiple sessile polypoid tumors, or a combination of both. Histopathological examination showing submucosal globular sporangia in different stages of development is pathognomonic of rhinosporidiosis. Surgical excision remains the mainstay of treatment for rhinosporidiosis lesions. Wide, complete, and meticulous excision of the polyp followed by thorough electro-cautery of the lesion's base is recommended.

14.1 Background

Rhinosporidiosis is a chronic granulomatous infective disorder that is caused by *Rhinosporidium seeberi*. It usually presents as a soft polypoidal, pedunculated, or sessile mass arising from the nasal mucosa. Common sites of occurrence of rhinosporidiosis are nasal cavity and nasopharynx; it can also be found in conjunctiva, larynx, and maxillary sinuses [1–3].

The first case was described by Guillermo Seeber from Buenos Aires in 1900 [4, 5]. The etiologic agent, *Rhinosporidium seeberi*, has never been successfully propagated in vitro. Initially thought to be a parasite, for more than 50 years *R. seeberi* had been considered to be a water mold [6, 7]. Molecular biological techniques have more recently demonstrated this organism to be an aquatic protistan parasite, and it has been placed into a new class, the Mesomycetozoea, along with organisms that cause similar infections in amphibians and fish [3–5].

S. V. Nemade, K. J. Shinde, *Granulomatous diseases in Otorhinolaryngology, Head and Neck*,
https://doi.org/10.1007/978-981-16-4047-6_14

14.2 Epidemiology

Rhinosporidiosis has been found to occur in roughly 70 countries around the world and thrives in warm, tropical climates. The fact that sporangia are induced to extrude their endospores by watery substances helps explain the pervasiveness of the disease in areas with wet environments.

It is endemic in India, Sri Lanka, South America, and Africa. Cases from the United States and Southeast Asia, as well as scattered occurrences throughout the world, have also been reported. Most cases of rhinosporidiosis occur in persons from or residing in the Indian subcontinent or Sri Lanka [3]. Rhinosporidiosis has no known racial predilection. Men are affected more commonly than women, with a male-to-female ratio of 4:1. It most commonly occurs in children and in individuals aged 15–40 years. It has been associated with rural residence, occupation in farming or agriculture, and bathing in ponds or rivers [8].

14.3 Etiopathogenesis

The causative organism was initially considered a fungus, and Ashworth in 1923 described its life cycle establishing the nomenclature *Rhinosporidium seeberi* [3, 5]. It is presumed to be transmitted by exposure to the pathogen when taking a bath in stagnant water pools where animals also bathe [3, 5]. The mode of infection from the natural aquatic habitat of *R. seeberi* is through the traumatized epithelium ("transepithelial infection"), most commonly in nasal sites. It affects the mucous membrane of the nasopharynx, oropharynx, conjunctiva, rectum, and external genitalia [1].

- Infection of nose and nasopharynx—70%
- Infection of palpebral conjunctiva—15%

Other structures such as the mouth, larynx, tracheobronchial tree, and lacrimal sac may be sites of disease. In these cases, it is usually secondary to nasal rhinosporidiosis with inoculation of spores in the adjacent mucosa. This is known to be auto-inoculation.

Autoinoculation—Spillage of endospores from polyps after trauma or surgery is thought to be followed by "autoinoculation" through the adjacent epithelium. Laryngeal rhinosporidiosis may be due to inoculation from the nose during endotracheal intubation. After inoculation, the organism replicates locally, resulting in hyperplasia of host tissue and localized immune response.

Disease of the skin, ear, genitals, and rectum has also been described. Genital rhinosporidiosis has been described in the vagina, penile urethra or meatus, and scrotum [8]. Trauma from *R. seeberi* contaminated stones used for mopping-up residual drops of urine is claimed to be responsible for anterior urethral rhinosporidiosis in the males.

Hematogenous dissemination with the cutaneous and multisite disease is also reported, but this is much less common. The development of subcutaneous granulomata in the limbs, without breach of the overlying skin, could be attributed to such hematogenous dissemination. Isolated cases of dissemination involving deep organs have been rarely reported [8, 9].

Rhinosporidiosis is an infective disease in the sense that the tissue lesions are always associated with the presence of the pathogen. No evidence has been adduced that it is also an infectious disease, as no transmission has ever been documented of cross-infection between members of the same family or between animals and humans.

14.4 Clinical Features

Rhinosporidiosis involving nose and nasopharynx is the commonest presentation (70%).

14.4.1 Symptoms

- Unilateral nasal obstruction
- Epistaxis
- Local pruritus
- Rhinorrhea
- Rhinitis with sneezing

- Postnasal discharge with cough
- Foreign body sensation
- History of exposure to contaminated water [8, 10].

14.4.2 Signs of Nasal Rhinospridiosis Mass

- Pink to deep red nasal mass which is granular, polypoidal sessile, or pedunculated (Fig. 14.1) [12].
- Strawberry-like appearance. This appearance results from sporangia, which are visible as gray or yellow pinhead dots on the vascular mass [10].
- Friable mass that bleeds easily upon manipulation.

Extra-nasal (atypical) sites of rhinosporidiosis are orbital region, lip, palate, uvula, larynx, trachea, buccal cavity, lacrimal sac, scalp, skin, penis, urethra, vulva, and bone. Presumptive diagnosis of primary rhinosporidiosis at the extra-nasal site is often difficult. Some cases of extra-nasal rhinosporidiosis are associated with nasal involvement also [13].

Epiphora and photo-phobia are common symptoms in infection of the palpebral conjunctiva. There are several clinical pointers that raise suspicion of lacrimal sac rhinosporidiosis during clinical evaluation—a boggy lacrimal sac swelling with a "bag of worms" feel, presence of bloody tears, history of bathing in stagnant pond water, and residence in or recent travel to an endemic area [14].

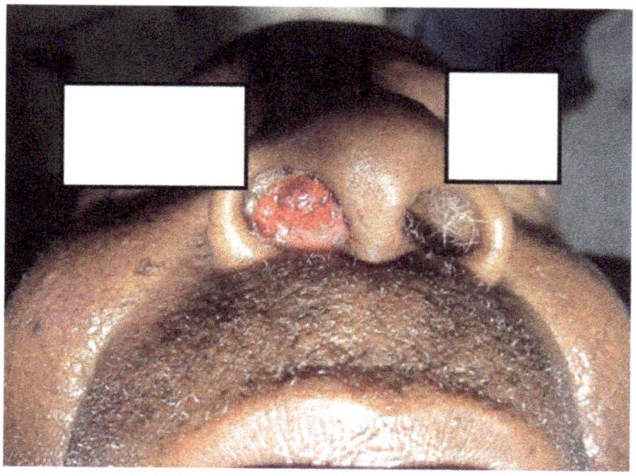

Fig. 14.1 Polypoidal mass of rhinosporidiosis in the right nasal cavity [11]

Few cases of disseminated rhinosporidiosis have also been reported. Extra-nasal rhinosporidiosis often presents with cutaneous or subcutaneous nodular swelling or sometimes with a reddish polypoid mass lesion. Rhinosporidial granulomas in disseminated cases occur as subcutaneous lumps with unbroken skin. These sometimes present clinically as ulcerated growths which could mimic malignant lesions such as sarcomas and carcinomas [13, 14]

14.5 Diagnosis

Nasal rhinosporidiosis is easier to diagnose clinically because of its typical polypoid presentation with a granular red surface with pinheaded spots. In contrast, diagnosis of extra-nasal rhinosporidiosis is difficult on the basis of clinical presentation because it may be confused with benign cystic lesions, soft tissue tumors, and papillomas. Hence, aspiration cytology is helpful in preoperative diagnosis of these atypical presentations of rhinosporidiosis and for exclusion of differential diagnoses.

14.5.1 Cytology and Histopathology

Cytological diagnosis depends on the demonstration of sporangia in different stages of maturation and endospores admixed with mixed inflammatory cells. Sporules may be present as well-circumscribed round structures with several endospores inside. Sometimes epithelial cells may be confused with endospores especially in respiratory secretions, in which the residual cytoplasm and large nuclei might simulate the residual mucoid sporangial material around the endospores (referred to as "comet" forms by Beattie) [8, 10]. The Periodic acid-Schiff stain help to discriminate between these, as the endospores stain markedly magenta while the epithelial cells are PAS-negative. The presence of electron-dense bodies in the endospores is useful in the confirmation of rhinosporidial identity. The organism can be observed with typical fungal stains (Gomori methenamine silver [GMS], periodic acid-Schiff [PAS]), as well as with standard Hematoxylin and Eosin (H&E) staining. Smears can also be assessed with10% potassium hydroxide (KOH) preparation [10].

In most histological sections, the organism is present in all stages of its development. They are associated with immune cells, including neutrophils, lymphocytes, plasma cells, and multinucleated giant cells, often in scattered granuloma. Papillomatous hyperplasia and hypervascularity are also common [15, 16]. Several round or oval large (100–450 microns), thick-walled sporangia with 1000+ endospores, each 6–10 microns, and spores which may be seen bursting through its chitinous wall is characteristic appearance (Figs. 14.2 and 14.3) [12, 17]. The sporangiaof *R. seeberi* are observed under the normal epithelium.

14.5.2 Serology

Serological identification of antirhinosporidial antibody by Immunoblot- Enzyme-linked immunosorbent assay [ELISA] has been developed and used for epidemiologic studies in endemic areas, but this test is not routinely available [10, 17].

14.5.3 Imaging

Computed tomography (CT) imaging helps to delineate the site and extent of the disease. Moderate-to-intense enhancement on CT is the characteristic feature [17].

On CT, rhinosporidiosis mass looks like irregular or lobulated lesions of soft tissue density showing moderate-to-intense postcontrast enhancement. Small foci of calcification and air can be seen within the lesions. Multiple dilated vessels can be also seen arising from nasopharyngeal mucosa which can be seen supplying the lesion. Lesions arising from oropharynx or tra-

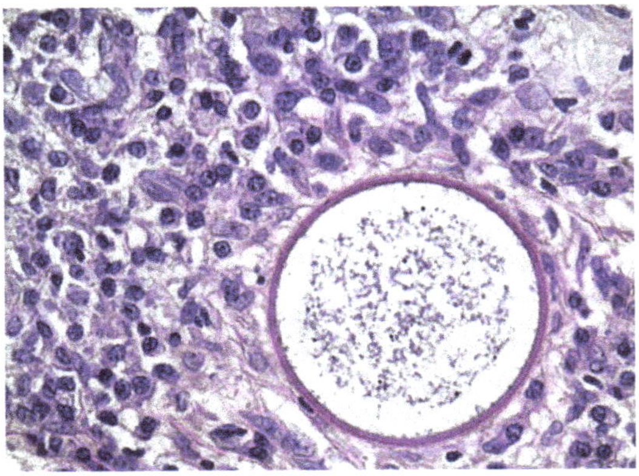

Fig. 14.3 Sporangium at higher magnification filled with endospores and surrounded by plasma cells and lymphocytes (H&E × 40) [16]

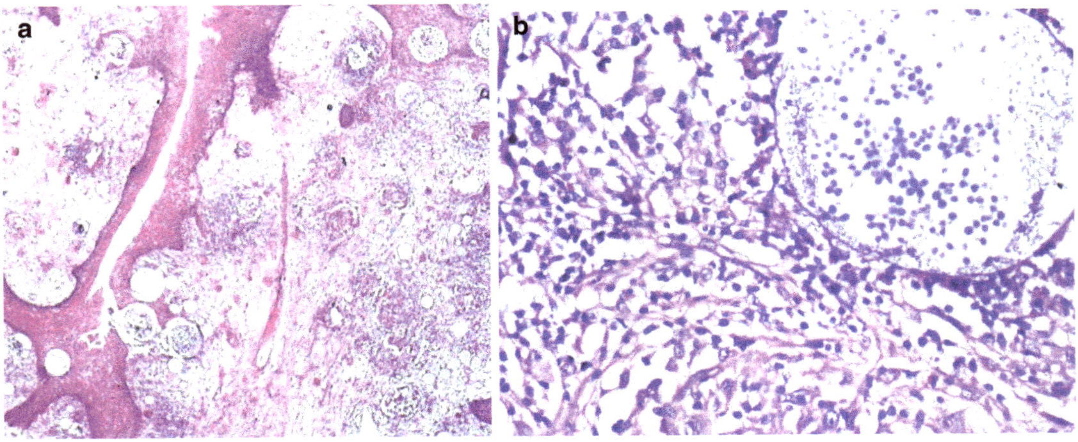

Fig. 14.2 (**a**) H&E stain showing multiple sporangia with inflammatory infiltrate. (**b**) High magnification view showing sporangia filled with endospores and surrounded by inflammatory cells

chea can be relatively hypoenhancing compared to the lesions at other sites. Bony involvement may appear as thinning of wall, rarefaction, or complete erosion [18, 19].

MRI shows heterogeneously mixed density mass lesion with prominent flow voids on T2-weighted imaging. Postcontrast imaging shows intense enhancement of the mass. Multilobulated appearance may give rise to cerebriform appearance as described for inverted papilloma in the literature. The main imaging differentials are inverted papilloma, juvenile angiofibroma, lobular capillary hemangioma, angiomatous polyp, and sinonasal malignancy [25, 26] (Fig. 14.4).

14.6 Treatment

Although cases of spontaneous regression have been recorded, they are rare, and surgical excision remains the mainstay of treatment for rhinosporidiosis lesions. Wide, complete, and meticulous excision of the polyp followed by thorough electro-cautery of the lesion's base is recommended. It is hypothesized that cauterization of the lesion's base may abate recurrence resulting from spillage of endospores on the adjacent mucosa [20, 21]. Diathermy excision is an acceptable treatment modality in cases of the nose and nasopharyngeal presentations. However, when there is the involvement of the tracheobronchial tree, a more radical approach may be considered. The choice of treatment may be cauterization with LASER through a bronchoscope [15, 22].

The lacrimal sac, being a relatively isolated organ compared to the other involved sites in the body, lends itself to complete removal more easily than most other tissues. The most commonly recommended treatment modality for lacrimal sac rhinosporidiosis is complete excision of the infected lacrimal sac or dacryocystectomy (DCT). This modality, though apparently safe and curative, also produces constant and debilitating postoperative epiphora in the patient that is

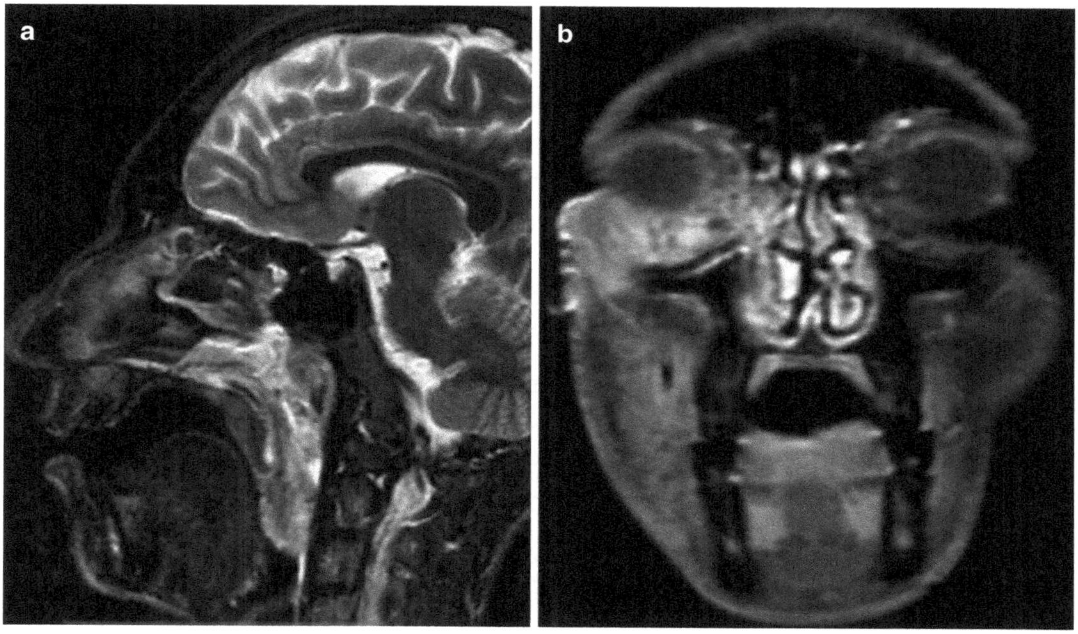

Fig. 14.4 (**a**) T2-weighted MRI sagittal section showing heterogeneously hyperintense multilobulated mass originating from nasal cavity and nasopharynx and extending into oropharynx. Lesion shows few flow voids within. (**b**) Postcontrast T1-weighted MRI coronal section showing enhancing mass lesion in inferior portion of right orbit. There are few nonenhancing areas within. Lesion is extending into the inferior turbinate via the nasolacrimal duct [19]

difficult to relieve. In contrast, a dacryocystorhinostomy (DCR) performed after excision of the sac granuloma with appropriate precautions is a suitable alternative that appears to have very good long-term outcomes [14, 22].

Medical treatment is not so effective but treatment with a year-long course of Dapsone (4, 4- diaminodiphenyl sulphone-2 mg/kg/day) is believed to be effective in tackling local subepithelial and subcutaneous spread and acts by causing maturation arrest of sporangia and accelerates their degeneration. These non-dividing sporangia are removed by an accentuated granulomatous response [22]. Other drugs like griseofulvin, amphotericin B have been tried especially in individuals with multisystem rhinosporidiosis. However, by far there has been no tangible success with medical therapy [14, 23].

14.7 Essential Features

- Caused by *Rhinosporidium seeberi*, traditionally thought to be a fungus but now considered to be an aquatic protistan parasite.
- Endemic in southern India, Sri Lanka, and emigrants from this region rare indigenous cases in the USA.
- Natural aquatic habitat, transmitted through traumatized epithelium, most commonly in nose and eye, also skin, ear, genitals, and rectum.
- Manifests predominantly in the nose (70–85% of the patients).
- Less commonly, the nasopharynx, other mucous membranes of the upper aerodigestive tract, the skin, and internal organs are affected. Dissemination of the disease is rare and mostly fatal.
- Presents as a hyperplastic, polypoid, red, granular mass commonly in the nasal cavity. Strawberry-like appearance of the mass is a characteristic feature. This appearance results from sporangia, which are visible as gray or yellow pinhead dots on the vascular mass.
- Common symptoms of nasal involvement are epistaxis, nasal obstruction, and rhinorrhea.
- In infection of the palpebral conjunctiva, epiphora and photo-phobia are common manifestations.
- Histopathology is characterized by large (100–450 microns), thick-walled sporangia with 1000+ endospores, each 6–10 microns, accompanied by a mixed inflammatory infiltrate.
- Treatment is surgical excision with electrocoagulation of the lesion base to prevent recurrence.
- No effective medical treatment alone. In cases of recurrences, steroid, dapsone, and amphotericin B are preferred.

References

1. Capoor MR, et al. Rhinosporidiosis in Delhi, North India: case series from a non-endemic area and mini-review. Mycopathologia. 2009 Aug.;168(2):89–94.
2. Gaines JJ Jr, et al. Rhinosporidiosis: three domestic cases. South Med J. 1996 Jan.;89(1):65–7.
3. Hospenthal DR. Uncommon Fungi and related species. In: Bennett JE, Dolin R, Blaser MJ, editors. Mandell, Douglas, and Bennett's principles and practice of infectious diseases. 8th ed. Philadelphia, PA: Elsevier Saunders; 2015. p. 3003–15.
4. Fredricks DN, et al. Rhinosporidium seeberi: a human pathogen from a novel group of aquatic protistan parasites. Emerg Infect Dis. 2000 May–Jun.;6(3):273–82.
5. Kwon-Chung KJ, Bennett JE. Rhinosporidiosis. Medical mycology. Philadelphia, PA: Lea & Febiger; 1992. p. 695–706.
6. Hospenthal DR. Entomophthoramycosis, Lobomycosis, Rhinosporidiosis, and Sporotrichosis. In: Guerrant RL, Walker DH, Weller PF, editors. Tropical infectious diseases. Principles, pathogens, & practice. 3rd ed. Philadelphia, PA: Saunders Elsevier; 2011. p. 603–7.
7. Ashworth JH. On Rhinosporidium seeberi (Wernicke 1903) with special reference to its sporulation and affinities. Trans R Soc Edinburgh. 1923;53:301–42.
8. Saha J, et al. Atypical presentations of rhinosporidiosis: a clinical dilemma? Indian J Otolaryngol Head Neck Surg. 2011;63:243–6.
9. Agrawal S, et al. Generalized rhinosporidiosis with visceral involvement; report of a case. AMA Arch Derm. 1959 Jul.;80(1):22–6.
10. Arseculeratne SN, et al. Patterns of rhinosporidiosis in Sri Lanka: comparison with international data. Southeast Asian J Trop Med Public Health. 2010 Jan.;41(1):175–91.
11. Uledi S, Fauzia A. Human nasal rhinosporidiosis: a case report from Malawi. Pan Afr Med J. 2011; 9:27.

Published online 2011 Jul 18. https://doi.org/10.4314/pamj.v9i1.71203
12. Sudasinghe T, et al. The regional sero-epidemiology of rhinosporidiosis in Sri Lankan humans and animals. Acta Trop. 2011 Oct–Nov.;120(1–2):72–81.
13. Pal S, et al. Cytodiagnosis of extra-nasal Rhinosporidiosis: a study of 16 cases from endemic area. J Lab Physicians. 2014 Jul–Dec;6(2):80–3. https://doi.org/10.4103/0974-2727.141501.
14. Bothra N, et al. External dacryocystorhinostomy for isolated lacrimal sac rhinosporidiosis - a suitable alternative to dacryocystectomy. Indian J Ophthalmol. 2019 May;67(5):665–8. https://doi.org/10.4103/ijo.IJO_1136_18.
15. Arseculeratne SN, et al. Patterns of rhinosporidiosis in Sri Lanka comparison with international data. Southeast Asian J Trop Med Public Health. 2010;41(1):175–91.
16. Gichuhi S, et al. Ocular rhinosporidiosis mimicking conjunctival squamous papilloma in Kenya – a case report. BMC Ophthalmol. 2014; 14:45. Published online 2014 Apr 8. https://doi.org/10.1186/1471-2415-14-45
17. Prabhu SM, et al. Imaging features of rhinosporidiosis on contrast CT. Indian J Radiol Imaging. 2013 July;23(3):212–8.
18. Prabhu SM, et al. Imaging features of rhinosporidiosis on contrast CT. Indian J Radiol Imaging. 2013;23(3):212–8. https://doi.org/10.4103/0971-3026.120267.
19. Dey AK, et al. Rhinosporidiosis: a rare cause of proptosis and an imaging dilemma for sinonasal masses. Case Rep Otolaryngol. 2016; 2016: 3573512. Published online 2016 Nov 30. doi: https://doi.org/10.1155/2016/3573512.
20. Job A, et al. Medical therapy of rhinosporidiosis with dapsone. J Laryngol Otol. 1993 Sep.;107(9):809–12.
21. Madke B, et al. Disseminated cutaneous with nasopharyngeal rhinosporidiosis: light microscopy changes following dapsone therapy. Australas J Dermatol. 2011 May;52(2):e4–6.
22. Kameswaran M, et al. KTP-532 laser in the management of rhinosporidiosis. Indian J Otolaryngol Head Neck Surg. 2005;57:298–300.
23. Nayak S, et al. Disseminated cutenous rhinosporidiosis. Indian J Dermatol venereol leprol. 2007;73:185–7.

15 Candidiasis

Abstract

Candidiasis is a fungal infection caused by yeasts from the genus Candida. *Candida albicans* is the predominant cause of the disease. Candida species produce a wide spectrum of diseases, ranging from cutaneous, mucocutaneous disease to invasive illness. Mucocutaneous candidiasis predominantly includes oropharyngeal, esophageal, respiratory, and genitourinary candidiasis. The systemic form includes candidemia and disseminated candidiasis with multisystem involvement. Primary oropharyngeal candidiasis includes Pseudomembranous, Erythematous, or Hyperplastic (nodular) types. Candid granuloma is a type of chronic mucocutaneous candidiasis and is often associated with systemic candidiasis. Exfoliative smear from oral, esophageal, or genital lesions shows candidal hyphae when stained with gram stain or PAS. Histopathology reveals inflammatory cell infiltration of the epithelium and lamina propria. Epithelial patterns may show hyperplasia, dysplasia, atrophy, or parakeratosis depending upon the clinical type of candidiasis. Serological tests such as Candida mannan assay, enolase assay, and (1,3)β-D-glucan assay carry high sensitivity, however not specific for *C. albicans*. Polymerase chain reaction (PCR) assay and DNA probes appear promising in the rapid diagnosis of Candida infections. The mainstay of treatment is topical antifungal agents, oral Fluconazole, improving oral hygiene, and treatment of the underlying immunocompromised condition. Surgical excision of the nodular/granulomatous lesions may be required in cases refractory to anti-fungal medications.

Synonyms

Candidosis, moniliasis, oidiomycosis [1].

15.1 Background

As mentioned by the famous Greek physician, Hippocrates in his findings, it commonly presents as superficial infections of the oral and vaginal mucosa. However, it was not until the mid-1800s that the documented research on the pathogenesis of candidiasis was instigated. The principal yeast pathogen, *Candida albicans*, itself, was identified in the nineteenth century [2]. *C. albicans* is a normal commensal of oral cavity, throat, intestines, vagina, and skin. It can become pathogenic in response to changes in the environment or certain triggers. Infections are frequently seen in immunocompromised patients. Candida species produce a wide spectrum of diseases, ranging from cutaneous, mucocutaneous disease to invasive illnesses. Mucocutaneous candidiasis predominantly includes oropharyngeal, oesophageal, respiratory, and genitourinary candidiasis.

S. V. Nemade, K. J. Shinde, *Granulomatous diseases in Otorhinolaryngology, Head and Neck*,
https://doi.org/10.1007/978-981-16-4047-6_15

The systemic form includes candidemia and disseminated candidiasis with multisystem involvement. Early therapeutic intervention whether surgical, or medical, or both significantly diminishes mortality [2].

15.2 Epidemiology

The incidence of nosocomial candidiasis has increased over the past few decades. Moreover, Candida bloodstream infection incidence is bimodal, with older people and premature babies having the highest risk. Invasive candidiasis is associated with unacceptably high mortality rates in the excess of 40% even with the introduction of newer antifungal agents. The total burden of invasive candidiasis is around 160,000 cases across 39 countries. The incidence is high in developing countries. This can be linked to compromised health care systems, deficiency in resources, poor infection control implementation, unavailability of diagnostic aids allowing excess empirical therapy, impaired knowledge about the fungal infections, or misuse of antibiotics.

15.2.1 Global Emergence of *Candida Auris*

Candida auris is an emerging multidrug-resistant type of Candida that presents a serious global health threat, including in the United States. It can cause severe infections and spreads easily in healthcare facilities. *C. auris* has caused bloodstream infections, wound infections, and ear infections. It also has been isolated from respiratory and urine specimens, but it is unclear if it causes infections in the lung or bladder.

15.2.2 3 Major Concerns About It Are

- It is often multidrug-resistant, meaning that it is resistant to multiple antifungal drugs commonly used to treat Candida infections.
- It is difficult to identify with standard laboratory methods, and it can be misidentified in labs without specific technology. Misidentification may lead to inappropriate management.
- It has caused outbreaks in healthcare settings [3, 4].

15.3 Etiopathogenesis

The causative organism is usually *Candida albicans* or less commonly other Candida species such as (in decreasing order of frequency) *Candida tropicalis, Candida glabrata, Candida parapsilosis*, Canida krusei, or other species (*Candida stellatoidea*, Candida pseudotropicalis, *Candida famata, Candida rugosa, Candida geotrichium, Candida dubliniensis*, and *Candida guilliermondii*). *C. albicans* accounts for about 50% of oral candidiasis cases, and together *C. albicans, C. tropicalis,* and *C. glabrata* account for over 80% of cases [4, 5].

Infections caused by Candida species occur very frequently in immunocompromised patients. Immunocompromised status can result from trauma, burns, cancer especially hematologic malignancies, cancer chemotherapy, irradiation, and immunosuppressive therapy [6]. Apart from predisposing factors such as the immunocompromised status of the host, the microorganism must possess specific factors or mechanisms of pathogenesis that enable them to cause infection.

15.3.1 Virulence Properties of Candida Species

- Cell surface hydrophobicity
- Adherence to host cells or surfaces
- Yeast receptors that bind a complement component
- Hydrolytic enzymes (Proteinases, phospholipases, lysophospholipases)
- Dimorphism and phenotypic switching [6, 7]

Adherence is the first step to establish colonization and infection. *C. albicans* is known to colonize humans more frequently than other fungi. Variations among strains of *C. albicans* to adhere to epithelial cells have been demonstrated, and in some studies, a close correlation was observed between the adherence ability of a strain and virulence [8, 9]. Relevant factors that enhance adherence include fungal cell surface hydrophobicity (CSH), environmental factors, the phenotype of the organism, pH, and temperature. CSH enhances candidal adherence to epithelial cells and the virulence increases due to the ability of hydrophobic cells to bind host tissue. Production of extracellular hydrolytic enzymes has been demonstrated in some strains of *C. albicans*. A few of them have been found associated with pathogenesis, including acid phospho-monoesterase, phospho-lipase, and acid protease. Isolates with greater in vitro enzyme activity are usually more virulent [10–12].

15.4 Clinical Features

1. Cutaneous and mucocutaneous candidiasis:

This type of candidiasis describes a group of Candida infections of the skin, hair, nails, and mucous membranes that tends to have a protracted and persistent course.

a. Oropharyngeal candidiasis

The patient usually has a history of HIV infection, wearing dentures, diabetes mellitus, or has been exposed to broad-spectrum antibiotics or inhaled steroids. Patients are frequently asymptomatic. Candidiasis in the mouth and throat is also called thrush or oropharyngeal candidiasis [2].Classification of oropharyngeal candidiasis [3, 13]:

- Primary candidiasis (group I)
  - Pseudomembranous (acute or chronic):
  - Erythematous (acute or chronic)
  - Hyperplastic: plaque-like, nodular
  - Candida-associated lesions: Denture related stomatitis, angular stomatitis, median rhomboid glossitis, linear gingival erythema
- Secondary candidiasis (group II)
  - Oral and throat manifestations of systemic mucocutaneous candidiasis (due to diseases such as thymic aplasia and candidiasis endocrinopathy syndrome)
- Candida-associated Lesions
  - Denture stomatitis
  - Angular cheilitis
  - Median rhomboid glossitis
  - Linear gingival erythema

15.4.1 Primary Candidiasis

Acute pseudomembranous candidiasis is a classic form of oral candidiasis, commonly known as thrush. It presents as individual patches of pseudomembranous white slough sometimes described as "curdled milk," or "cottage cheese" (Figs. 15.1 and 15.2). As the name suggests, the pseudomembrane can be easily wiped off to reveal a reddish patch that minimally bleeds. It can involve any part of the mouth, but usually, it appears on the tongue, buccal mucosae, or palate [15].

Erythematous (atrophic) candidiasis is when the condition appears as a red, raw-looking lesion (Fig. 15.3). Acute erythematous candidiasis usually occurs on the dorsum of the tongue in persons taking long-term corticosteroids or antibiotics, but occasionally it can occur after only a few days of using a topical antibiotic. This is usually termed "antibiotic sore mouth," "antibiotic sore tongue," or "antibiotic-induced stomatitis" because it is commonly painful as well as red. It may precede the pseudomembrane formation [16].

Chronic erythematous candidiasis is usually associated with denture wearing.

Hyperplastic/Nodular candidiasis: This variant is also sometimes termed "plaque-like candidiasis" or "nodular candidiasis" [17]. The most common appearance of hyperplastic candidiasis is a persistent white plaque that does not rub off (Fig. 15.4). The lesion may be rough or nodular in texture in severe cases, with deep invasion, it causes hyperplastic nodules [17, 19].

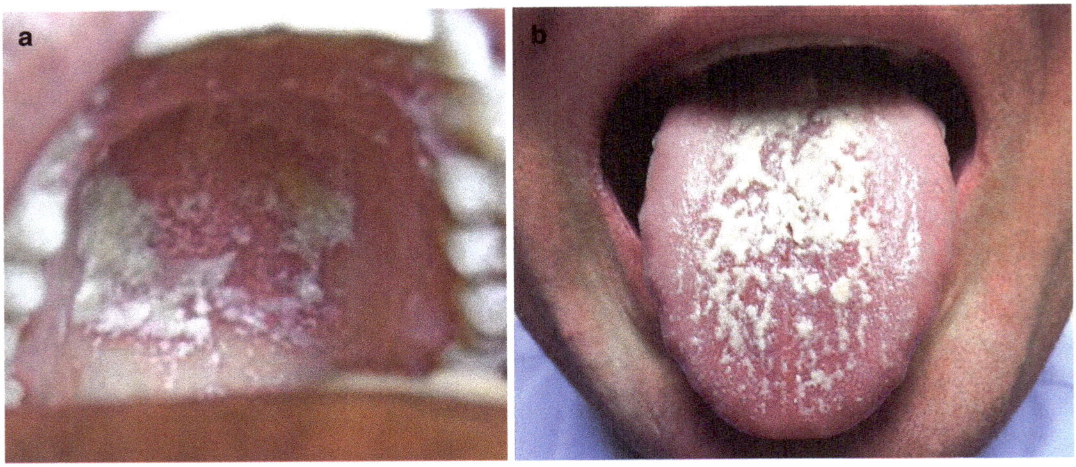

Fig. 15.1 Pseudomembranous candidiasis involving (**a**) hard palate and (**b**) tongue

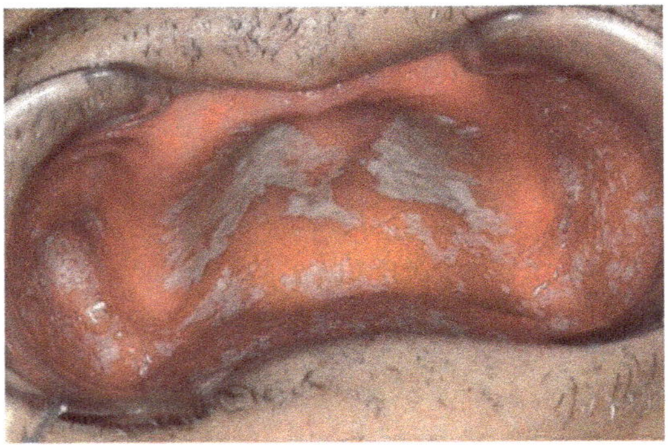

Fig. 15.2 Pseudomembranous candidiasis of alveolus and buccal mucosa [14]

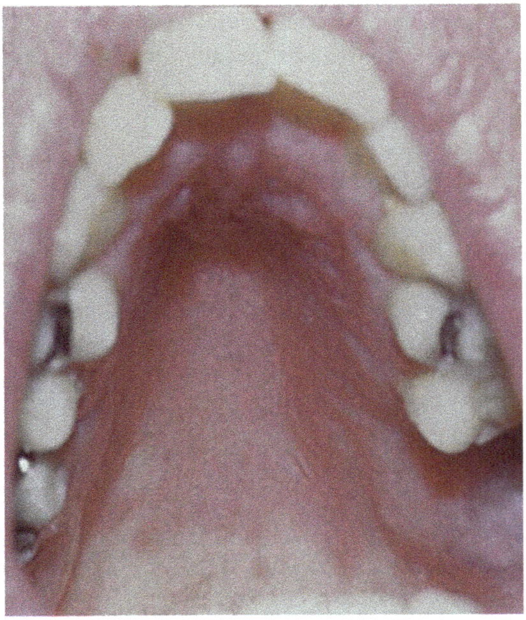

Fig. 15.3 Erythematous candidiasis of hard palate

- Candidiasis in the mouth and throat can have varied symptoms, including:
- White patches on the inner cheeks, tongue, roof of the mouth, and throat
- Redness or soreness of buccal mucosa
- Cotton-like feeling in the mouth
- Loss of taste
- Pain while eating or swallowing
- Angular cheilitis

15.4.2 Secondary Candidiasis

Chronic mucocutaneous candidiasis—It includes chronic candidal lesions on the skin, in the mouth, and on other mucous membranes, candid granuloma, candidiasis-endocrinopathy syndrome, and candidiasis thymoma syndrome. Oral and throat candidiasis is secondary to systemic mucocutaneous candidiasis. About 90% of people with chronic mucocutaneous candidiasis have candidiasis in the mouth [17].

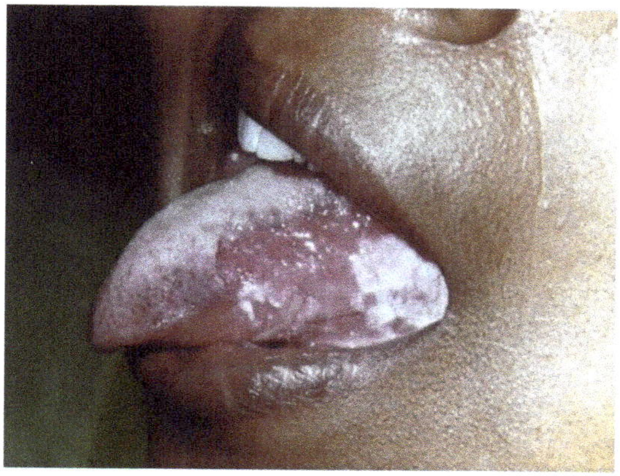

Fig. 15.4 Hyperplastic candidiasis at the lateral border of the tongue [18]

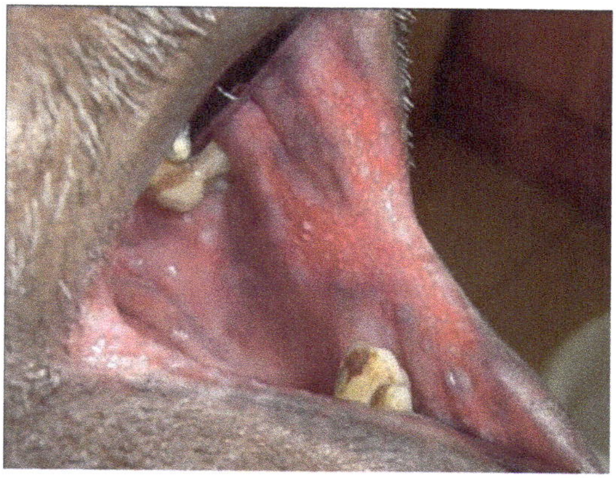

Fig. 15.6 Angular cheilitis on the right and left commissures [20]

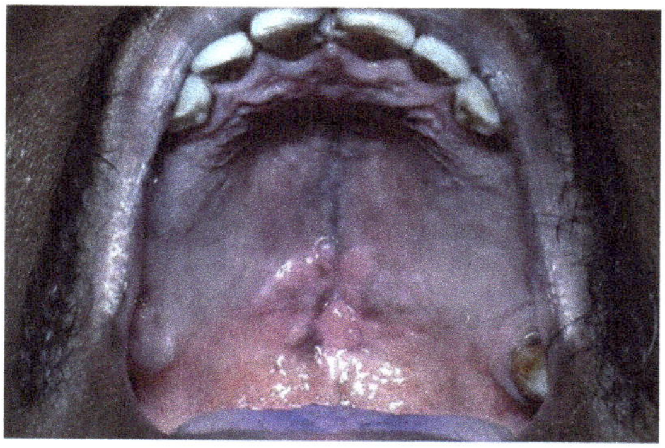

Fig. 15.5 Denture stomatitis of the palate [18]

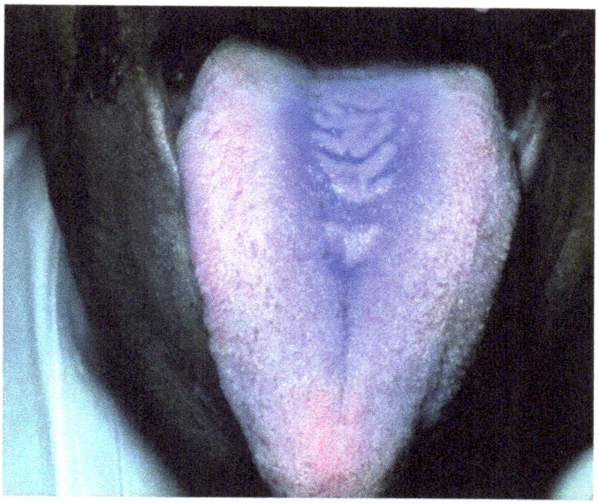

Fig. 15.7 Median Rhomboid glossitis—note the candidal overgrowth [18]

15.5 Candida-Associated Lesions

15.5.1 Denture stomatitis

It is also known as "chronic atrophic candidiasis"; as the name indicates, it is a chronic inflammation of the mucosa typically restricted to the denture-bearing area, seen in association with candidiasis (Fig. 15.5). The lesions are usually asymptomatic, though occasionally patients may complain of burning sensation or soreness. It commonly affects the palate although mandibular mucosa may also be affected.

- Angular cheilitis

This form of candidiasis usually manifests as erythematous or ulcerated fissures, typically affecting unilaterally or bilaterally the commissures of the lip (Fig. 15.6). The factors associated include old age and denture-wearers (due to reduced vertical dimension), vitamin B12 deficiency, and iron deficiency anemia [18, 20].

- Median rhomboid glossitis

Median rhomboid glossitis appears as the central papillary atrophy of the tongue and is typically located around the midline of the dorsum of the tongue (Fig. 15.7). It occurs as a well-demarcated, symmetric, depapillated area arising anterior to the circumvallate papillae [18].

- Linear gingival erythema

It was previously referred to as "HIV-gingivitis" because of its typical occurrence in HIV-associated periodontal diseases. It manifests as a linear erythematous band of 2–3 mm on the marginal gingiva along with petechial or diffuse erythematous lesions on the attached gingiva. The lesions may present with bleeding. In addition to *C. albicans*, *C. dubliniensis* has been reported as an emerging pathogen in this form of candidiasis [18].

(b) Esophageal candidiasis

The patient's history usually includes chemotherapy, the use of broad-spectrum antibiotics or inhaled steroids, the presence of HIV infection or malignancy. Patients may be asymptomatic or may have one or more of the following symptoms:

- Dysphagia
- Odynophagia
- Retrosternal pain
- Epigastric pain
- Nausea and vomiting

Physical examination almost always reveals associated oral candidiasis [17, 19].

(c) Respiratory tract candidiasis

The respiratory tract is frequently colonized with Candida species, especially in hospitalized patients. Approximately 20–25% of ambulatory patients are colonized with Candida species.

Laryngeal candidiasis: It is primarily seen in patients with underlying hematologic or oncologic malignancies. The patient may present with a sore throat and hoarseness. Clinical findings are generally unremarkable, and the diagnosis is frequently made with direct or indirect laryngoscopy.

Candida tracheobronchitis: This is also an uncommon form of invasive candidiasis. Most patients with Candida tracheobronchitis are HIV-positive or are severely immunocompromised. The patient presents with fever, productive cough, and shortness of breath. Physical examination reveals dyspnea and scattered rhonchi. The diagnosis is generally made with bronchoscopy [19].

Candida pneumonia: This rarely develops alone and is associated with disseminated candidiasis in rare cases. The most common form of infection is multiple lung abscesses due to the hematogenous dissemination of Candida species. The high degree of Candida colonization in the respiratory tract greatly complicates the diagnosis of Candida pneumonia. The history reveals risk factors similar to those of disseminated candidiasis, along with reports of shortness of breath, cough, and respiratory distress. Physical examination reveals fever, dyspnea, and variable breath sounds, ranging from clear to rhonchi or scattered rales [19].

(d) Other forms of cutaneous and mucocutaneous candidiasis:

- Genitourinary tract candidiasis includes Vulvovaginal candidiasis, Candida balanitis (penile candidiasis), Candida cystitis, and pyelonephritis.
- Hepatosplenic candidiasis—Usually seen in patients with underlying hematologic malignancy and neutropenia.
- Cutaneous candidiasis syndromes

Generalized cutaneous candidiasis: This is an unusual form of cutaneous candidiasis that manifests as a diffuse eruption over the trunk, thorax, and extremities. The patient has a history of generalized pruritus, with increased severity in the genitocrural folds, anal region, axillae, hands, and feet. Physical examination reveals a widespread rash that begins as individual vesicles that spread into large confluent areas [19, 21].

2. Systemic candidiasis

Systemic candidiasis can be divided into two primary syndromes: Candidemia and disseminated candidiasis (multiorgan infection by Candida species).

(a) Candidemia: Candida species are currently the fourth most commonly isolated organism in blood cultures, and Candida infection is generally considered a nosocomial infection. The patient's history commonly reveals the following:

- Several days of fever that is unresponsive to broad-spectrum antimicrobials; frequently the only marker of infection
- Prolonged intravenous catheterization
- A history of several key risk factors
- Possibly associated with multiorgan infection [19]

Clinical presentation

- Fever
- Macronodular skin lesions (approximately 10%)—Candid granulomas.
- Candidal endophthalmitis (approximately 10–28%)
- Occasionally, septic shock (hypotension, tachycardia, tachypnea) [17, 19, 21]

(b) Disseminated candidiasis

It may lead to life-threatening involvement of multiple organs.

- Candida endophthalmitis–Fundoscopic examination reveals early pinhead-sized off-white lesions in the posterior vitreous with distinct margins and minimal vitreous haze. Classic lesions are large and off-white, similar to a cotton ball, with indistinct borders covered by an underlying haze. Lesions arethree3-dimensional and extend into the vitreous off the chorioretinal surface. They may be single or multiple.
- CNS infections due to Candida species

CNS infections due to Candida species are rare and difficult to diagnose. The two primary forms of infection include exogenous infection and endogenous infection. The exogenous infection results from postoperative infection, trauma, lumbar puncture, or shunt placement. The endogenous infection results from hematogenous dissemination and thus involves the brain parenchyma and is associated with multiple small abscesses (e.g., disseminated candidiasis).

As with other organ infections due to Candida species, patients usually have underlying risk factors for disseminated candidiasis. CNS infections due to Candida species are frequently found in patients hospitalized for long periods in ICUs. The spectrum of this disease includes the following:

- Meningitis
- Granulomatous vasculitis
- Diffuse cerebritis with microabscesses
- Mycotic aneurysms
- Fever unresponsive to broad-spectrum antimicrobials

Candida carditis, arthritis, osteomyelitis, costochondritis, and myositis may also occur [19, 21–23].

15.6 Diagnosis

15.6.1 Microscopy and Culture

Direct microscopy of scrapings from the oral, oesophageal, other mucosal lesions, skin, or sputum is diagnostic. In oropharyngeal candidiasis, oral swabs, oral rinse, or oral smears can be used. Smears are collected by gentle scraping of the lesion with a spatula or tongue blade and the resulting debris is directly applied to a glass slide. Oral swabs are taken if culture is required. Swabs taken from three different oral sites are preferred [21]. Oral rinse involves rinsing the mouth with phosphate-buffered saline for 1 minute and then spitting the solution into a container with a culture medium. Oral rinse technique can distinguish between commensal candidal carriage and candidiasis. A potassium hydroxide smear, Gram stain, or methylene blue is useful for direct demonstration of fungal cells. Hyphae, pseudohyphae, or budding yeast cells are typically demonstrated (Fig. 15.8) [20, 22, 23].

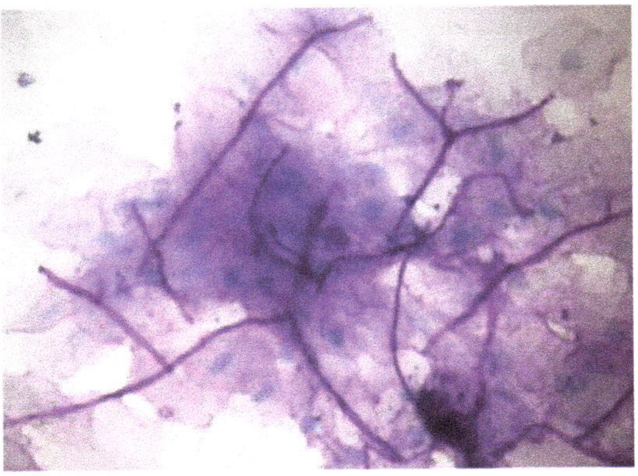

Fig. 15.8 Photomicrograph of the exfoliative smear (40x) showing candidal hyphae [20]

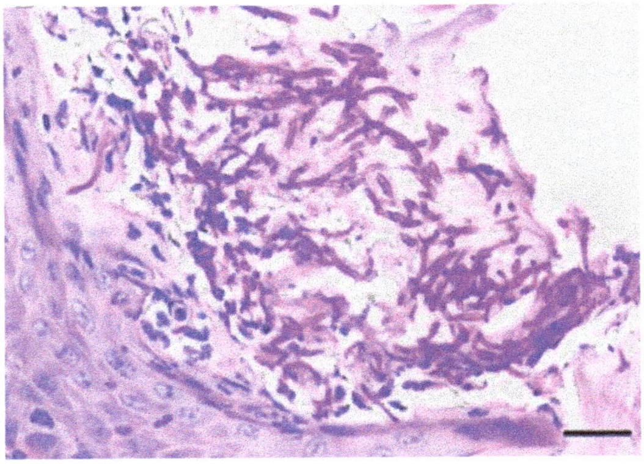

Fig. 15.9 PAS-stained image showing significant accumulation and penetration of *C. albicans* hyphae through the hyperkeratotic surface of the tongue dorsal epithelium. Neutrophilic Munro microabscesses in response to the infection are seen [24]

15.6.2 Histopathology

If candidal leukoplakia is suspected, a biopsy is indicated [22]. Tissue specimen is usually stained with periodic acid-Schiff (Fig. 15.9), which stains carbohydrates in fungal cell walls in magenta. Gram stain is also used as Candida stains are strongly Gram-positive [22, 23].

The histopathologic appearance can be variable depending upon the clinical type of candidiasis. Pseudomembranous candidiasis shows hyperplastic epithelium with a superficial parakeratotic desquamating layer [23]. Hyphae penetrate to the depth of the stratum spinosum and appear as weakly basophilic structures. Polymorphonuclear cells also infiltrate the epithelium, and chronic inflammatory cells infiltrate the lamina propria [23]. Atrophic candidiasis appears as thin, atrophic epithelium, which is non-keratinized. Hyphae are sparse, and inflammatory cell infiltration of the epithelium and the lamina propria is characteristic. Atrophic candidiasis appears like pseudomembranous candidiasis without the superficial desquamating layer [23]. Hyperplastic candidiasis is variable. Usually, there is hyperplastic and acanthotic epithelium with parakeratosis. There is an inflammatory cell infiltrate and hyphae are visible. Unlike other forms of candidiasis, hyperplastic candidiasis may show dysplasia [23, 24].

15.6.3 Candida Species Identification

- *C. albicans*, *C. dubliniensis*, and *Candida stellatoidea* can be identified morphologically via germ-tube formation (hyphae are produced from yeast cells after 2–3 h of incubation) or biochemical assays.
- CHROMagar Candida allows for the presumptive identification of several Candida species by using color reactions in specialized media that demonstrate different colony colors depending on the species of Candida.
- API20C and API32C are biochemical assays that allow for the identification of the different Candida species with more precision. These assays evaluate the assimilation of numerous carbon substrates and generate profiles used in the identification of different fungal species.
- The *C. albicans* peptide nucleic acid (PNA) fluorescence in situ hybridization (FISH) test can be used to identify *C. albicans* in 24–48 h when the probe is added to smears that are made directly from the blood culture bottle and followed by hybridization. A newer version of this test now allows for the simultaneous identification of either *C. albicans* or *C. glabrata* [14, 18, 20].

15.6.4 Endoscopy

- Oesophagoscopy reveals grayish-white pseudomembrane or plaque in mid to distal esophagus; mucosa is erythematous, edematous, ulcerated, or friable ("cottage cheese appearance") It also helps to take brushings or biopsy of the lesion.

15.6.5 Imaging

- Barium swallow esophagogram presents the characteristic manifestations of oesophageal candidiasis. In severe cases, esophageal stenosis may show typical "foamy appearance" and "feather appearance."
- CT and MRI are particularly helpful in disseminated candidiasis showing meningitis, mycotic granulomas, and mycotic aneurysms.

15.6.6 Serology

- The Candida mannan assay yields a sensitivity of 31–90% (less for non-albicans Candida species).
- The Candida heat-labile antigen assay yields a sensitivity of 10–71%.
- The D-arabinitol assay yields a sensitivity of 50% but is not useful for infection with *C. krusei* or *C. glabrata*.
- The enolase assay yields a sensitivity of 55–75%, which improves with serial testing.
- The (1,3)β-D-glucan assay is an amebocyte lysis assay with a sensitivity of 75–100% and a specificity of 88–100%. It is a broad-spectrum assay that detects Aspergillus, Candida, Fusarium, Acremonium, and Saccharomyces species β-D-glucan is a cell wall component in a wide variety of fungi and can be detected based on its ability to activate factor G of the horseshoe crab coagulation cascade. The Fungitell assay may be used in the evaluation of invasive fungal infections caused by the fungi mentioned above. The assay does not detect infections caused by *Cryptococcus neoformans* or Zygomycetes [14, 18, 20].

15.6.7 Molecular Assay

Polymerase chain reaction (PCR) assay and DNA probes appear promising in the rapid diagnosis of Candida infections. The new test, T2Candida, uses polymerase chain reaction (PCR) assay to amplify Candida DNA in blood, with the genetic material hybridizing to superparamagnetic nanoparticles coated with complementary DNA. The nanoparticles aggregate into "microclusters," which greatly alter a T2 magnetic resonance (T2MR) signal. It helps in diagnosing candidemia 25 times faster than blood culture can and quickly identifies the Candida species that is causing the infection [14, 20].

15.6.8 Blood Tests

Systemic candidiasis should be suspected in patients with persistent leukocytosis and either persistent neutropenia or other risk factors and who remain febrile despite broad-spectrum antibiotic therapy. Blood cultures are helpful but yield positive results in only 50–60% of cases of disseminated infection.

15.7 Treatment

The mainstay of treatment is topical antifungal agents and oral Fluconazole. Severe and chronic cases may require IV Amphotericin B followed by oral Fluconazole (Table 15.1) [25].

- Surgical excision of the lesions may be required in cases refractory to anti-fungal medications [24].
- Underlying immunosuppression may be medically manageable once it is identified, and this helps prevent the recurrence of candidal infections.

Table 15.1 Treatment of candidiasis [25]

Severity	Antifungal drug	Dosage/ Duration
First-line agents	Fluconazole (PO or IV)	100–200 mg/7–14 days
	Clotrimazole troches	10 mg five times/7–14 days
	Nystatin suspension (100,000 U/mL)	4–6 ml four times/7–14 days
	Nystatin pastilles (200,000 U each)	1–2 pastilles four times/7–14 days
Second-line agents	Itraconazole solution (PO)	200 mg/28 days
	Posaconazole (PO)	400 mg daily in divided doses
	Voriconazole (PO or IV)	200 mg twice daily
Agents used in refractory cases	Caspofungin (IV)	70 mg loading dose followed by 50 mg daily
	Micafungin (IV)	100–150 mg daily
	Anidulafungin (IV)	100 mg loading dose followed by 50 mg daily
	Amphotericin B oral suspension	500 mg every 6 h
	Amphotericin B deoxycholate (IV)	0.3 mg/kg once

- The candidal load in the mouth can be reduced by improving oral hygiene measures, such as regular toothbrushing and the use of antimicrobial mouthwashes [26]. Since smoking is associated with many forms of oral candidiasis, cessation is beneficial.

15.8 Essential Features

- Usually due to *Candida albicans* or *Candida tropicalis*
- Associated with antibiotic use in nonimmunocompromised; also acid-suppressive therapy, carcinoma, corticosteroids, diabetes mellitus, esophageal motility disorders, gastric surgery, HIV, rheumatic disease, elderly and debilitated patients. Associated with CMV or HSV esophagitis in immunocompromised.
- Candida species produce a wide spectrum of diseases, ranging from superficial mucocutaneous disease to invasive illnesses. Mucocutaneous candidiasis predominantly includes oropharyngeal, oesophageal, respiratory, and genitourinary candidiasis. Systemic form includes candidemia and disseminated candidiasis with multisystem involvement.
- Oropharyngeal candidiasis includes primary, secondary, and associated lesions.
- Primary candidiasis includes Pseudomembranous (Superficial curdy, gray-white membranes that easily wipe off), Erythematous (painful erosions and erythema) or Hyperplastic (nodular) types.
- Candid granuloma is a type of chronic mucocutaneous candidiasis and is often associated with systemic candidiasis (skin lesions, candidiasis-endocrinopathy syndrome, and candidiasis thymoma syndrome)
- Candida-associated Lesions are denture stomatitis, angular chelitis, median rhomboid glossitis, and linear gingival erythema.
- Patients present with cheesy white lesions in the oral cavity/oropharynx with dysphagia, odynophagia, loss of taste, or angular cheilitis.
- Exfoliative smear from oral, esophageal, or genital lesions shows candidal hyphae when stained with gram stain or PAS.
- Histopathologic appearance of inflammatory cell infiltration of the epithelium and the lamina propria is common in all types. Epithelial patterns may show hyperplasia, dysplasia, atrophy, or parakeratosis depending upon the clinical type of candidiasis.
- Mainstay of treatment is topical antifungal agents, oral Fluconazole, improving oral hygiene, and treatment of underlying immunocompromised conditions. Severe and chronic cases may require IV Amphotericin B followed by oral Fluconazole.
- Surgical excision of the nodular/granulomatous lesions may be required in cases refractory to antifungal medications.

References

1. James WD, et al. Andrew's diseases of skin: clinical dermatology. Philadelphia: Saunders Elsevier; 2006. p. 308–11.
2. Patil S, et al. Clinical appearance of oral candida infection and therapeutic strategies. Front Microbiol. 2015; 6:1391. Published online 2015 Dec 17. https://doi.org/10.3389/fmicb.2015.01391.
3. Kordalewska M, Perlin DS. Identification of drug resistant Candida auris. Front Microbiol. 2019; 10:1918. Published online 2019 Aug 20. https://doi.org/10.3389/fmicb.2019.01918
4. CDC. Candida auris. Centers for disease control and prevention. Available at https://www.cdc.gov/fungal/candida-auris/tracking-c-auris.html#world. March 29, 2019; Accessed: April 5, 2019.
5. Scully C. Oral and maxillofacial medicine: the basis of diagnosis and treatment (3rd ed.). Edinburgh: Churchill Livingstone. 2013. p. 254–267.
6. Ghom A, Mhaske S. Textbook of oral pathology. New Delhi: Jaypee Brothers Medical Publishers; 2010. p. 498, 508–514. isbn 9788184484021.
7. Douglas LJ. Adhesion of Candida species to epithelial surface. CRC Crit Rev Microbiol. 1987;15:2–16.
8. Douglas LJ. Adhesion to surfaces. In: Rose AH, Harrison JS, editors. The yeasts, vol. 2. London: Academic Fress Inc; 1987. p. 239–75.
9. Reams MJ, et al. Variability of the adherence of *Candida albicans* strains related to virulence. Sabouraudia. 1984;2:93–8.
10. McCourtie J, et al. Relationship between cell surface com position, adherence, and virulence of *Candida albicans*. Infect Immun. 1984;45:6–12.
11. Ener B, Douglas LJ. Correlation between cell surface hydrophobicity of Candida albicans and adhesion to buccal epithelial cells. FEMS Microbiol Lett. 1992;99:37–42.
12. Hazen RC, et al. Partial biochemical characterization of cell surface hydrophobicity and hydrophilicity of *Candida albicans*. Infect Immun. 1990;58:3469–76.
13. Barrett-Bee R, et al. A comparison of phopholipase activity, cellular adherence and pathogenicity of yeast. J Oen Microbiol. 1985;131:1217–21.
14. Mortazavi, H et al. Oral white lesions: an updated clinical diagnostic decision tree. Dent J (Basel). 2019 Mar; 7(1):15. Published online 2019 Feb 7. doi: https://doi.org/10.3390/dj7010015.
15. Scully C. Oral and maxillofacial medicine: the basis of diagnosis and treatment (2nd ed.). Edinburgh: Churchill Livingstone; 2008. p. 191–199. isbn: 9780443068188.
16. Treister NS, Bruch JM. Clinical oral medicine and pathology. New York: Humana Press; 2010. p. 19, 21, 92, 93. isbn: 978-1-60327-519-4.
17. Soames JV, et al. Oral pathology (3rd ed.). Oxford: Oxford University Press; 1999. p. 147, 193–200. isbn: 978-0192628947.
18. Patil S, et al. Clinical appearance of oral Candida infection and therapeutic strategies. Front Microbiol. 2015; 6: 1391. Published online 2015 Dec 17. https://doi.org/10.3389/fmicb.2015.01391.
19. Pfaller MA, Diekema DJ. Epidemiology of invasive candidiasis: a persistent public health problem. Clin Microbiol Rev. 2007 Jan.;20(1):133–63.
20. Shetti A, et al. Oral candidiasis: aiding in the diagnosis of hiv—a case report. Case Rep Dent. 2011; 2011:929616. Published online 2011 Sep 15. https://doi.org/10.1155/2011/929616.
21. Morgan J. Global trends in candidemia: review of reports from 1995 to 2005. Curr Infect Dis Rep. 2005 Nov.;7(6):429–39.
22. Kerawala C, Newlands C (eds). Oral and maxillofacial surgery. Oxford: Oxford University Press. 2010. p 446, 447. isbn: 9780199204830.
23. Kumaraswamy KL, et al. Oral biopsy: oral pathologist's perspective. J Cancer Res Ther. 2012, Apr–Jun; 8 (2): 192–198. https://doi.org/10.4103/0973-1482.98969. PMID 22842360.
24. Vila T, et al. Oral candidiasis: a disease of opportunity. J Fungi (Basel) 2020 Mar; 6(1):15. Published online 2020 Jan 16. https://doi.org/10.3390/jof6010015.
25. Thompson GR, et al. Oropharyngeal candidiasis in the era of antiretroviral therapy. Oral Surg. Oral Med Oral Pathol Oral Radiol Endod. 2010;109:488–95. https://doi.org/10.1016/j.tripleo.2009.11.026.
26. Shah N, et al. Surgical management of chronic hyperplastic candidiasis refractory to systemic antifungal treatment. J Lab Physician. 2017;9(2):136–9.

Histoplasmosis

16

Abstract

Histoplasmosis is a fungal infection acquired by inhalation of *Histoplasma capsulatum* microconidia. Microconidia are inhaled and deposited in the terminal bronchioles and alveoli of the lung. Clinical manifestations of histoplasmosis depend on the size of the inoculum and the patient's immunological status/underlying conditions. Low level of exposure in the healthy host typically leads to asymptomatic infection, while the acute syndrome usually follows heavy inoculums. Acute pulmonary histoplasmosis causes widespread inflammation of respiratory tract, presenting with acute rhinitis, pharyngitis, tonsillitis, laryngitis, and tracheobronchitis. Chronic pulmonary histoplasmosis manifests as lung parenchymal disease with cavitation and interstitial fibrosis. Acute disseminated histoplasmosis with multisystem involvement is seen in immunocompromised individuals. Chronic histoplasmosis is associated with ulcerative, fungating lesions and granulomas in the upper respiratory tract. It presents as nasal and oral granuloma formation with cartilage and bone destruction, granuloma of the larynx and rarely involves middle ear and mastoid. Definite diagnosis is reached by isolating the fungus in special cultures, while alternate methods include detection of yeast forms in diseased tissues or detecting serum antibodies or specific antigens. Treatment consists of intravenous amphotericin B for 1 week followed by oral itraconazole for 6–12 weeks along with surgical excision of the granulomatous mass.

Synonyms Cave disease, Darling disease, Ohio valley disease, reticuloendotheliosis, spelunkers lung, African histoplasmosis (var duboisii) [1, 2]

16.1 Background

Histoplasmosis was discovered in 1905 by "Samuel T Darling" [1]; till then, many cases of histoplasmosis were mistakenly attributed to tuberculosis. It is caused by the ubiquitous and potentially virulent fungus *Histoplasma capsulatum* [2]. The spores are inhaled through the respiratory tract, and the disease potentially affects the lungs. Histoplasmosis is often asymptomatic in endemic settings, but infection can result in a spectrum of illnesses, ranging from mild influenza-like illness to acute pulmonary infection and disseminated extrapulmonary disease. Immunocompromised persons and the elderly are at greater risk for disseminated disease [2].

S. V. Nemade, K. J. Shinde, *Granulomatous diseases in Otorhinolaryngology, Head and Neck*,
https://doi.org/10.1007/978-981-16-4047-6_16

16.2 Epidemiology

It is endemic in many parts of the world, namely in the American Midwest, Latin America, and Southern Africa. In the USA, histoplasmosis is generally thought to occur mainly in the Ohio and Mississippi River Valleys. In India, the Gangetic West Bengal is the site of most frequent infections, with 9.4% of the population detected positive. *Histoplasma capsulatum* is isolated from the local soil proving the endemicity of histoplasmosis in West Bengal. The global incidence of histoplasmosis in adults aged 65 years and older varies between 2.4 and 6.5 cases per 100,000 population [2]. Rates are highest in the Midwest, with an estimated 6.1–6.5 cases per 100,000 population [2]. It shows no gender predilection [1, 3, 4].

16.3 Etiopathogenesis

Histoplasma capsulatum is found in soil, often associated with decaying bat guano or bird droppings. Its spores are inhaled through the respiratory tract. In the alveoli, macrophages ingest these microconidia. They survive inside the phagosome. As the fungus is thermally dimorphic, these microconidia are transformed into yeast. It grows and multiply inside the phagosome. The macrophages travel in lymphatic circulation and spread the disease to different organs [1].

Within the phagosome, the fungus has an absolute requirement for thiamine. Cell-mediated immunity for histoplasmosis develops within 2 weeks. If the patient has strong cellular immunity, macrophages, epithelial cells and lymphocytes surround the organisms and contain them and eventually calcify to form granuloma. In immunocompromised individuals, the organisms disseminate to different organs such as bone, spleen, liver, adrenal glands and mucocutaneous membranes, resulting in progressive disseminated histoplasmosis. Chronic lung disease can manifest [3–5].

16.4 Clinical Features

ENT involvement is commonly seen in acute disease with widespread inflammation of upper respiratory mucosa manifesting as acute rhinitis, pharyngitis, tonsillitis, laryngitis, and acute otitis media. The most involved sites are the oral cavity, the larynx, and the pharynx (Figs. 16.1 and 16.2) [8]. In the case of chronic granulomatous infection, it presents as nasal and oral granuloma formation with cartilage and bone destruction, granuloma of the larynx (Fig. 16.3) and rarely involves middle ear and mastoid. In this stage, it is frequently mistaken for malignant neoplasm [1], other granulomatous diseases, and benign nasal tumors [6, 7, 9, 10].

Clinical presentation of Histoplasmosis [6, 7, 10, 11]:

Types	Symptoms
Asymptamatic	No symptoms
Acute pulmonary histoplasmosis	Unspecified respiratory symptoms such as cough, dyspnoea, fever, myalgia, weakness, shivering, etc.
Chronic pulmonary histoplasmosis	Common in individuals with underlying pulmonary disease such as pulmonary emphysema, cavitation, interstitial fibrosis Symptoms are chronic productive cough, dyspnoea, malaise
Acute disseminated histoplasmosis	Common in immunocompramised patients. Bone marrow involvement (pancytopenia), hepatoslenomegaly, fever. Disease is rapidly progressive and lethal
Subacute hiastoplasmosis	Destructive lesions, intestinal perforation, meningitis, etc.
Chronic histoplasmosis	Lesions involving upper aerodigestive tract, indolent course with granuloma formation
Other presentations	Mediastinal fibrosis, bronchiolitis

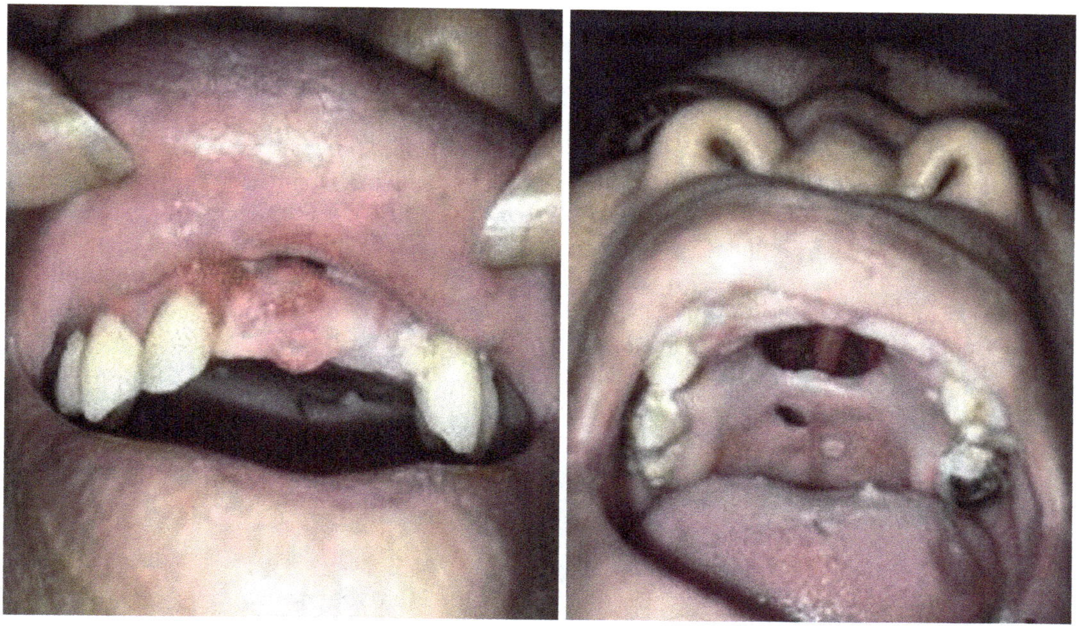

Fig. 16.1 Left: Showing lack of teeth with the gingival ulcer. Right: Bottom view of the face showing nasal tip collapse, hard palate perforation and remaining nasal septum seen through the perforation [6]

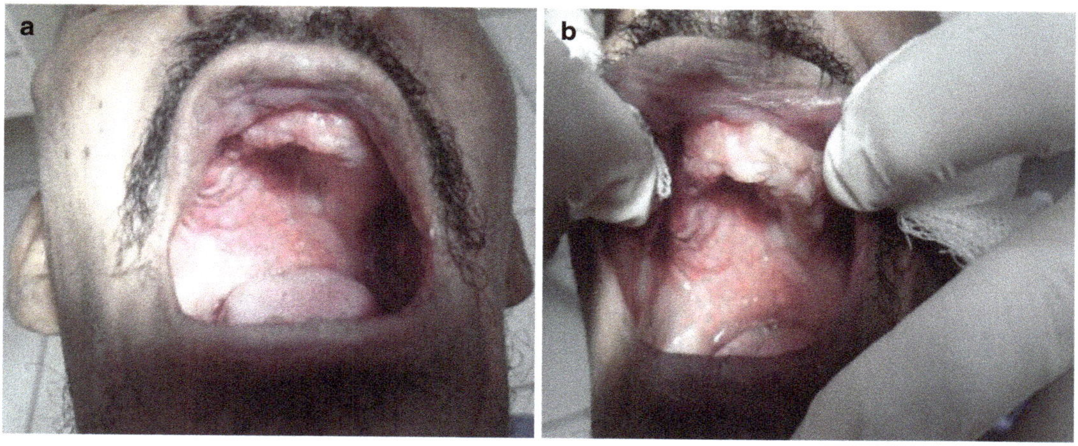

Fig. 16.2 Intraoral lesions in the palate and alveolar ridge regions (**a**, **b**) [7]

16.5 Diagnosis

16.5.1 Microscopy

H. capsulatum is a small spherical or ovoid yeasts measuring 2–6 μm characterized by its ability to make a dimorphic transition to enter host macrophages and to survive intracellularly and proliferate during active infection. Gomori-Grocott stain prominently highlights yeast forms (2–5 μm) with basophilic crescent-shaped nucleus seen within macrophages, often with a pericellular halo (Fig. 16.4) [12].

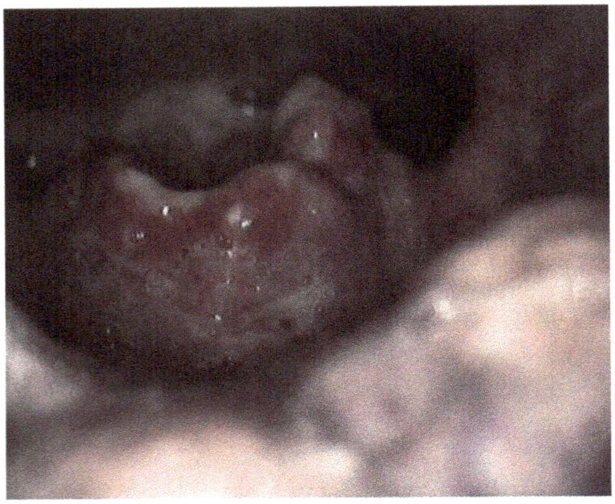

Fig. 16.3 Fiber-optic laryngoscopy showing a vegetative lesion on the lingual surface of the epiglottis [8]

16.5.2 Culture

It is the gold standard diagnostic test. Fungus is isolated from the sputum, blood, sinonasal secretions, or infected organs. It takes from two to four weeks to provide conclusive results. However, it is not useful in severe cases when prompt intervention is required. Sabouraud agar culture is effective in 25–40% of the cases. In chronic aerodigestive lesions—for which the culture is not very effective—Grocott Gomori's SM staining elicits the infectious agent and aids in diagnosis [12, 13]. Characteristic presence of typical yeast cells, some of which are undergoing replication by "budding" is diagnostic [6, 7, 12].

16.5.3 Histopathology

Organism are most easily found within necrotizing granulomas. Histopathologic findings include lymphohistiocytic infiltrate, the presence of variable numbers of primarily intracellular small yeast within histiocytes, lymphoid hyperplasia, infiltrates of eosinophils, neutrophils, and plasma cells. *H. capsulatum* var duboisii yeasts have a thicker wall and are much larger with a diameter up to 15 μm [6, 7, 12] (Fig. 16.5).

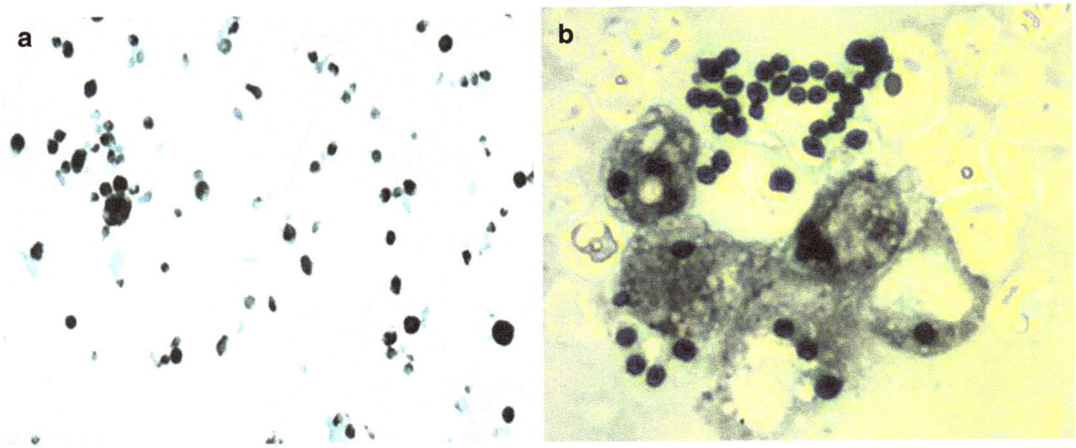

Fig. 16.4 (**a**) Pulmonary histoplasmosis: Bronchoalveolar lavage cytology shows macrophages with numerous intracellular *H. capsulatum* (Gomori-Grocott stain ×400). (**b**) Disseminated histoplasmosis: Extracellular *H. capsulatum* from blood smear (Gomori-Grocott stain ×1500) [12]

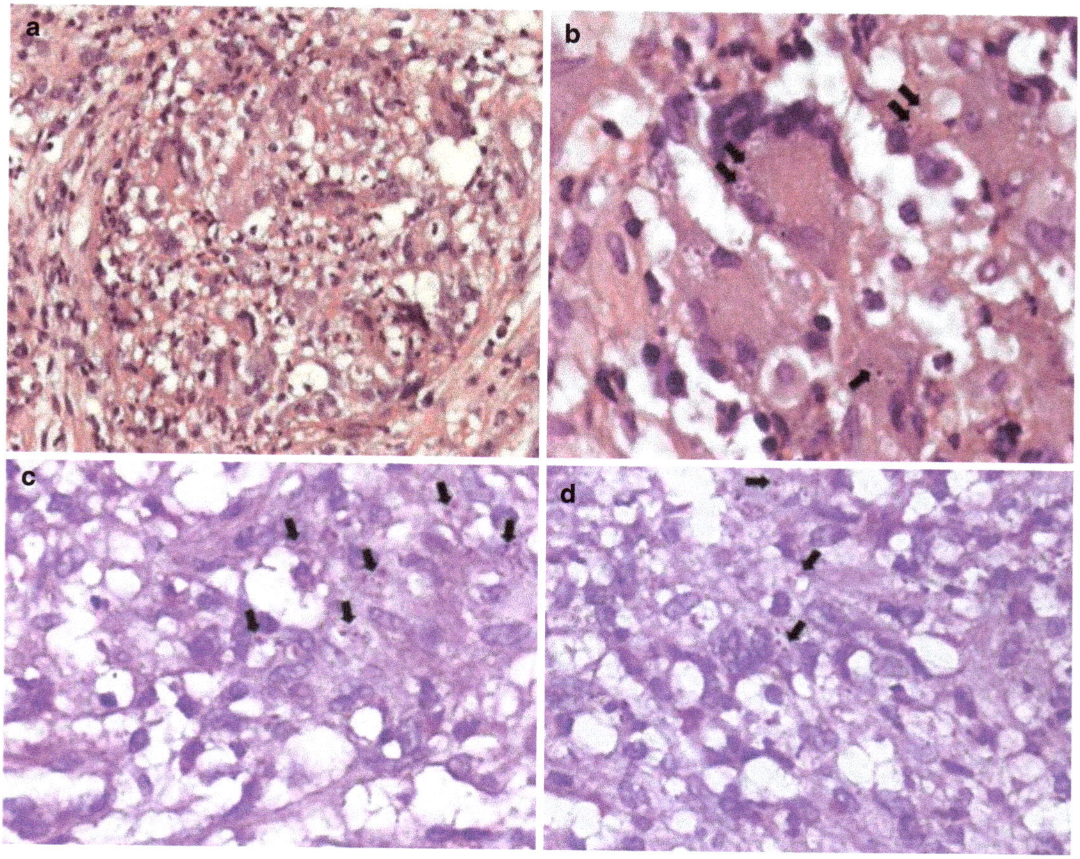

Fig. 16.5 Connective tissue with intense inflammatory infiltrate with a granulomatous pattern, consisting of giant multinucleated inflammatory cells and vacuolated macrophages, with several fungi suggestive of *H. capsulatum*—(hematoxylin-eosin stain; (**a**) ×200, (**b**) ×400). In (**c**) and (**d**), the periodic acid-Schiff (PAS) stain showing vacuolated macrophage with positivity for *H. capsulatum* ((**c, d**) ×400). Note the numerous small rosy dots (arrow) [7]

16.5.4 Serology

- Detection of antigens in blood or urine samples by ELISA or PCR. It is particularly used in disseminated disease.
- Histoplasmosis can also be diagnosed by complement fixation and immunodiffusion tests for the detection of antibodies against Histoplasma in the blood [14].

16.5.5 Imaging

CT scan-Histoplasmosis appears as a conglomerate necrotic mass of low-attenuation, ring-enhancing lymph nodes that simulate an abscess. The early laryngeal lesions usually affect the true vocal folds and epiglottis. Granulomatous masses may be seen in the larynx and pharynx simulating carcinoma. Calcification may be found in the center of a histoplasmoma or in concentric rings and is generally diagnostic. CT scan and MRI scan of PNS help in delineating the extent of granulomas and the bony destruction (Fig. 16.6) [6–8].

HRCT thorax is better than plain radiographs in revealing the pulmonary granulomatous lesions (histoplasmoma) (Fig. 16.7).

16.6 Treatment

In the case of immunocompetent individuals, histoplasmosis is asymptomatic and resolves without any treatment.

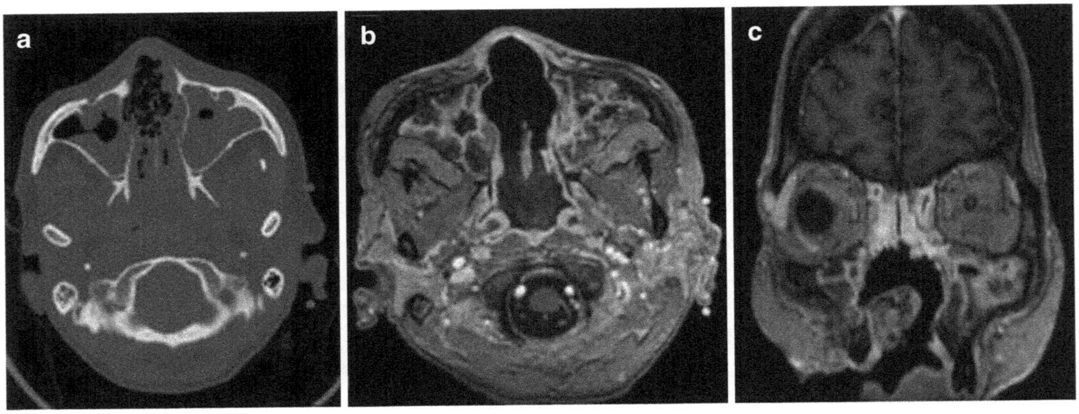

Fig. 16.6 (**a**) Paranasal sinus CT scan showing bony nasal septum destruction and bilateral maxillary sinus opacities; (**b**) and (**c**) Gadolinium-enhanced T1 weighted MRI (**b**: axial section; **c**: frontal section) showing the destruction of bony nasal septum and maxillary sinus walls without enhanced tumor mass [6]

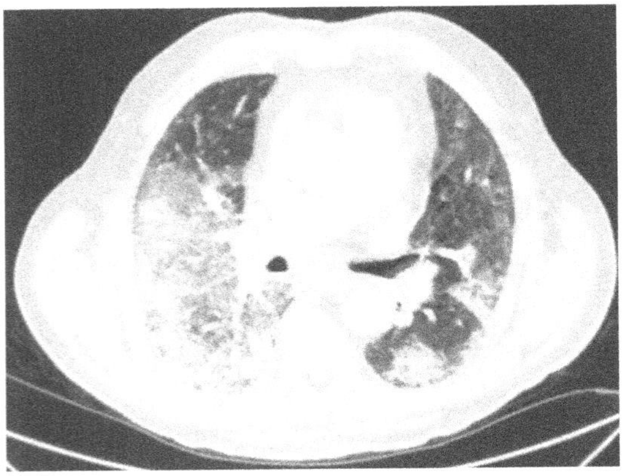

Fig. 16.7 High resolution computed tomography showing bilateral pulmonary opacities [15]

In case of acute severe disease, mild to moderate dissemination and chronic granulomatous changes, IV Liposomal Amphotericin B (3.0–50 mg/kg daily) or deoxycholate mB (07–10 mg/kg daily) for 1–2 weeks, followed by itraconazole (200 mg twice daily for a total of 12 weeks) and Methylprednisolone (0.5–10 mg/kg daily intravenously for 1–2 weeks) is the standard treatment [7, 16, 17].

In case of progressive disseminated histoplasmosis that is moderately severe-to-severe, the preferred treatment is liposomal mB (30 mg/kg daily), mB lipid complex (50 mg/kg daily), or deoxycholate AmB (0.7–10 mg/kg daily) for 1–2 weeks, followed by itraconazole (200 mg twice daily for at least 12 months) [8, 17, 18].

Surgery: Histoplasmosis is not angioinvasive and extensive surgical debridement is not required. Surgical excision of sinonasal granuloma, tympanomastoidectomy for middle ear and mastoid disease, and excision of laryngeal granulomas may be necessary [8, 19, 20].

16.7 Essential Features

- Histoplasmosis is a fungal infection caused by *Histoplasma capsulatum*, a saprophyte that exists in the mycelial form in nature.
- Lungs are the initial site of infection, which occurs after inhalation of spores where Histoplasma converts to a yeast form at body temperature.
- Acute pulmonary histoplasmosis is characterized by widespread inflammation of the respiratory tract presenting with acute rhinitis, pharyngitis, tonsillitis, laryngitis, and tracheobronchitis. Patient often presents with cough and dyspnoea.
- Chronic pulmonary histoplasmosis manifests as lung parenchymal disease with cavitation and interstitial fibrosis.

- Acute disseminated histoplasmosis with multisystem involvement is seen in immunocompromised individuals.
- Chronic histoplasmosis is associated with ulcerative, fungating lesions and granulomas in the upper respiratory tract.
- Microscopy with Gomori's stain elicits typical Yeast forms (2–5 um) with basophilic crescent-shaped nucleus seen within macrophages, often with a pericellular halo. Culture is slow and may take 2–4 weeks for results.
- Organisms are most easily found within necrotizing granulomas. Histopathologic findings include lymphohistiocytic infiltrates, the presence of variable numbers of primarily intracellular small yeast within histiocytes, lymphoid hyperplasia, infiltrates of eosinophils, neutrophils, or plasma cells.
- Detection of *Histoplasma capsulatum* antigen in urine or serum (especially useful in disseminated disease).
- Pharmacotherapy with IV Liposomal Amphoterecin B for 1–2 week followed by oral itraconazole for 6–12 weeks is recommended along with surgical excision of granulomatous mass.

References

1. Darling ST. A protozoan general infection producing pseudotubercles in the lungs and focal necrosis in the liver, spleen and lymphnodes. J Am Med Assoc. 1906;46(17):1283–5.
2. Deepe G. *Histoplasma capsulatum*. Principles and practice of infectious diseases. 5th ed. New York: Churchill Livingston; 2000. p. 2718–33.
3. Sanyal M, Thammayya A. *Histoplasma capsulatum* in the soil of Gangetic plain in India. Indian J Med Res. 1975;63(7):1020–8.
4. Sanyal M, Thammayya A. Skin sensitivity to histoplasmin in Calcutta and its neighbourhood. Indian J Dermatol Venereol Leprol. 1980;46(2):94–8.
5. Rosenberg JD, Scheinfeld NS. Cutaneous histoplasmosis in patients with acquired immunodeficiency syndrome. Cutis. 2003;72(6):439–45.
6. Lehur AC, et al. Case of disseminated histoplasmosis in a HIV-infected patient revealed by nasal involvement with maxillary osteolysis. BMC Infect Dis. 2017;17:328. https://doi.org/10.1186/s12879-017-2419-4.
7. de Freitas Filho SAJ, et al. A case of oral histoplasmosis concomitant with pulmonary tuberculosis. Case Rep Dent. 2019;2019:6895481. https://doi.org/10.1155/2019/6895481.
8. Ahumada F, et al. Subacute histoplasmosis with focal involvement of the epiglottis: importance of differential diagnosis. Case Rep Otolaryngol. 2014;235975:3 p. https://doi.org/10.1155/2014/235975
9. Butt AA, Carreon J. *Histoplasma capsulatum* Sinusites. J Clin Microbiol. 1997;35(10):2649–50.
10. Lucatorto F, Eversole R. Deep mycoses and palatal perfuration with granulomatous Pansinusitis in acquired immunodeficiency syndrome: case reports. Quintessence Int. 1993;24:743–8.
11. Goodwin RA, et al. Disseminated histoplasmosis: clinical and pathological correlations. Medicine. 1980;59:1–33.
12. Alsibai KD, et al. Cytological and histopathological spectrum of histoplasmosis: 15 years of experience in French Guiana. Front Cell Infect Microbiol. 2020;10:591974. https://doi.org/10.3389/fcimb.2020.591974.
13. Som PM, Brandwein M. Inflammatory diseases. In: Som PM, Curtin HD, editors. Head & neck imaging. 4th ed. St. Louis: Mosby Year Book; 2003. p. 193–259.
14. Gerber ME, et al. Histoplasmosis: the otolaryngologist's perspective. Laryngoscope. 1995;105:919–23.
15. Grover K, et al. A rare case of diffuse alveolar hemorrhage secondary to acute pulmonary histoplasmosis. Case Rep Infect Dis. 2015; 821749:4 p. https://doi.org/10.1155/2015/821749
16. Ryan KJ, Ray CG, editors. Sherris medical microbiology. 4th ed. McGraw Hill; 2004. p. 674–6.
17. Wheat LJ, et al. Clinical practice guidelines for the management of patients with histoplasmosis: 2007 update by the infectious diseases society of America. Clin Infect Dis. 2007;45(7):807–25.
18. Moen MD, et al. Liposomal amphotericin B: a review of its use as empirical therapy in febrile neutropenia and in the treatment of invasive fungal infections. Drugs. 2009;69(3):361–92.
19. Wheat LJ, et al. Clinical practice guidelines for the management of patients with histoplasmosis: 2007 update by the Infectious Diseases Society of America. Clin Infect Dis. 2007;45(7):807–25.
20. Kurowski R, Ostapchuk M. Overview of histoplasmosis. Am Famy Physician. 2002;66(12):2247–52.

17 Cryptococcosis

Abstract

Cryptococcosis has been one of the most common opportunistic mycosis caused by *Cryptococcus neoformans*. It is one of the common causes of mortality among HI-infected patients. Exposure usually occurs through inhalation of aerosolised propagules. Cryptococcosis includes three types of infections: Cryptococcal meningitis (most common presentation), Pulmonary cryptococcosis and cutaneous cryptococcosis. Disseminated infection may affect multiple organs. Specifically, in the head and neck, it has been shown to involve the nasopharynx, paranasal sinuses, tonsils, oral cavity and larynx. Mucocutaneous lesions include nodular, granulomatous mass or in the form of superficial or deep ulcers. Laboratory diagnosis of cryptococcosis includes direct microscopic examination, isolation of Cryptococcus from a clinical specimen, and detection of cryptococcal antigen. Early diagnosis and treatment is the key to treatment success. Treatment of cryptococcosis consists of three main aspects: antifungal therapy, intracranial pressure management for cryptococcal meningitis, and restoration of immune function with antiretroviral therapy (ART). Antifungal therapy consists of three phases: induction, consolidation, and maintenance. A combination of two drugs, i.e. amphotericin B plus flucytosine or fluconazole, is preferred in the induction phase. Fluconazole monotherapy is recommended during the consolidation and maintenance phases.

17.1 Background

Cryptococcosis is the most common life-threatening mycosis associated with AIDS worldwide. Exposure usually occurs through inhalation of aerosolised propagules. In the alveoli of normal, healthy individuals, they are quickly phagocytosed by macrophages and are either destroyed or sequestered in granulomas. Poor cell-mediated immunity appears to be the primary problem predisposing to widespread dissemination. The most common clinical presentation is cryptococcal meningitis. Pulmonary and other presentations are less common, and disseminated infection may occur. *C neoformans* has been isolated from virtually every tissue type, including the skin, spleen, liver, kidney, prostate, heart, bone, and eyes. Specifically, in the head and neck, it has been shown to involve the nasopharynx, paranasal sinuses, tonsils, oral cavity and larynx. Clinically, however, the disease has a predilection for the lung, and especially, the CNS [1–3]. Without appropriate treatment, cryptococcosis is fatal. Early diagnosis and treatment is the key to treatment success. Treatment of cryptococcosis

S. V. Nemade, K. J. Shinde, *Granulomatous diseases in Otorhinolaryngology, Head and Neck*,
https://doi.org/10.1007/978-981-16-4047-6_17

consists of three main aspects: antifungal therapy, intracranial pressure management for cryptococcal meningitis, and restoration of immune function with ART. Optimal integration of these three aspects is crucial to achieving successful treatment and reducing mortality [4].

17.2 Epidemiology

Cryptococcosis is a defining opportunistic infection for AIDS and is the second-most common AIDS-defining illness in Africa. Other conditions that pose an increased risk include certain lymphomas (e.g. Hodgkin's lymphoma), sarcoidosis, liver cirrhosis, and patients on long-term corticosteroid therapy.

Distribution is worldwide in soil. The prevalence of cryptococcosis has been increasing over the past 20 years for many reasons, including the increase in the incidence of AIDS and the expanded use of immunosuppressive drugs.

C. gattii has been associated with tropical and subtropical climates, with an outbreak of disease affecting both humans and animals in the Pacific Northwest of the USA, emanating from an initial focus of infection on Vancouver Island, British Columbia, Canada. *C. gattii* has unique features, which distinguish it from *C. neoformans*. *C. gattii* primarily infects immunocompetent hosts, and the organism can cause disease in unusual host species (e.g., horses, ferrets, goats, dolphins) [1, 5, 6].

17.3 Etiopathogenesis

Traditionally, *C. neoformans* is classified into two varieties and five serotypes based on its capsular structure. Patients with AIDS or other immunocompromised states are almost exclusively infected with *C. neoformans* var neoformans (serotypes A, D, AD) while *C. neoformans* var gatti (serotypes B and C) have a propensity to cause disease in immunocompetent hosts and has a limited geographical distribution suggesting that genetic and phenotypic differences are responsible for the different severity of the disease [6, 7]. The major virulence factor is capsular polysaccharide glucuronoxylomannan, which hinders phagocytosis by alveolar histiocytes and inflammatory cell recruitment and migration. Other virulence factors include melanin production (Fontana-Masson stain may be positive; melanin may have antioxidant properties) and enzymes that increase invasiveness [8].

Cryptococcosis is believed to be acquired by inhalation of the infectious propagule from the environment. In the lungs, the organism develops its polysaccharide capsule, responsible for its virulence. Pulmonary infection tends to be asymptomatic, and the lesions are found only on X-ray as was the case with our patient. Reactivation or spread to lymph nodes, blood, CNS, and other tissues may occur with CNS, cutaneous, mucocutaneous, osseous, and visual manifestations [7, 9].

Cryptococcosis includes three types of infections:

- *Cryptococcal meningitis*
- Pulmonary cryptococcosis
- Wound or cutaneous cryptococcosis

Cryptococcal meningitis (infection of the meninges, the tissue covering the brain) is believed to result from dissemination of the fungus from either an observed or unappreciated pulmonary infection [7, 9].

17.4 Clinical Features

17.4.1 CNS Manifestations

It commonly includes meningitis and rarely cryptococcoma (enhancing cortical nodules). The commonest sites for cryptococcoma are the midbrain and basal ganglia [3]. These are typical granulomas. Granulomas in the choroid plexus can result in obstructive hydrocephalus [9–11].

Symptoms include headache, fever, neck stiffness, cranial nerve palsies, lethargy, coma or memory loss over several weeks. Severe headache is seen in more than 75% and fever in 65% of cases of cryptococcal meningitis. Headache may be due to meningeal involvement, raised

ICP or sino-venous thrombosis. Cryptococcal meningitis in immunocompetent individuals is more commonly associated with papilloedema, hydrocephalus, focal deficits, seizures, and cryptococcoma [9, 10].

17.4.2 Pulmonary Cryptococcosis

While the severity of respiratory tract symptoms can vary, lung findings can include nodules, lobar and interstitial infiltrates, hilar lymphadenopathy, effusions, and cavitations [12, 13].

Pulmonary cryptococcosis has clinical manifestations varying from asymptomatic colonization to acute respiratory distress syndrome (ARDS). Common signs and symptoms in HIV-infected patients are coughs, dyspnea, pleuritic chest pain, and constitutional symptoms, such as fever, malaise, and weight loss. Some patients may also have hemoptysis and hypoxemia. In HIV-infected patients, pulmonary cryptococcosis is more severe and has a more acute onset than that in other hosts. There is a higher risk of progression, with ARDS occasionally occurring. Furthermore, pulmonary cryptococcosis in HIV-infected patients is usually a clinical manifestation of disseminated infection [4].

17.4.3 Cutaneous and Mucocutaneous Cryptococcosis

Cryptococcal skin involvement is nonspecific and produces a variety of lesions which may present as papules, nodules, infiltrative plaques, vesicles, pustules, bullae, cellulitis, chancres, purpura, acneiform, herpetiform, Kaposi's sarcoma or basal cell carcinoma like nodules, subcutaneous abscesses, or ulcers [12, 13].

Mucocutaneous lesions include nodular, granulomatous mass or in the form of superficial or deep ulcers. Lesions are usually in the nose, paranasal sinuses or mouth and rarely in the nasopharynx and larynx (Fig. 17.1) [10, 12–14].

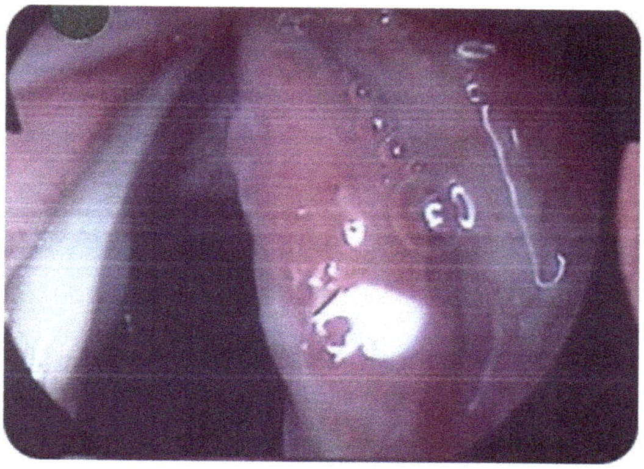

Fig. 17.1 Diffuse erythema and thickening of the right true cord [14]

17.4.4 Other Manifestations

- Cryptococcosis can present as cervical lymphadenitis in HIV-positive patients, although it is far less common than tuberculosis or benign reactive adenopathy. Most often, the manifestation of cutaneous cryptococcosis precedes the onset of more serious systemic or disseminated cryptococcosis by 1–2 weeks [12, 13].
- Ocular manifestations of cryptococcosis are occasionally observed. Photophobia, diplopia, papilledema, ocular palsy, and temporary or permanent visual loss have been reported.

These signs and symptoms are due to inflammation from direct invasion of the yeast or increased intracranial pressure. Visual loss with a rapid onset is usually a result of the former process, while a delayed onset is a result of the latter process [15].

17.5 Diagnosis

Routine diagnosis is made by microbiological culture, histopathological examination or serology. Pulmonary nodules should be worked up with sputum and possibly bronchoscopic examination. Blood culture and cerebrospinal fluid should be analysed to determine dissemination.

Fine-needle aspiration is often employed in the evaluation of neck masses of unknown aetiology. Because of the significant possibility of lymphoma in these cases, an open biopsy is often recommended [10, 12].

17.5.1 Microscopy and Culture

Cryptococcus in clinical specimens appears as encapsulated spherical or oval yeasts without pseudohyphae or hyphae. The size of the yeast ranges from 5 to 10 μm (Fig. 17.2). In tissues, the yeast usually shows a large capsule. Occasional narrow-based budding may be seen. A number of techniques can be employed to visualize the yeast. India ink staining shows a clear halo of a capsule around the yeast within a black background. India ink staining is usually applied to cerebrospinal fluid (CSF) and is not suitable for other specimens, e.g. urine, sputum, or bronchoalveolar lavage. Gomori Silver Methanamine (GMS) stain also highlights the yeast. In HIV-infected patients, the sensitivity of this test is over 80% [17].

Cryptococcus can be cultured from most sites in standard fungal media in the absence of cycloheximide. It can also grow in bacterial media. Colonies appear on solid media as white-to-cream opaque mucoid colonies, usually within 3 days. Delayed growth up to 4 weeks may be observed if patients have already received antifungal therapy. Identification of species can be done by biochemical methods, molecular methods, or matrix-assisted laser desorption/ionization time-of-flight (MALDI-TOF) mass spectrometry [16, 18].

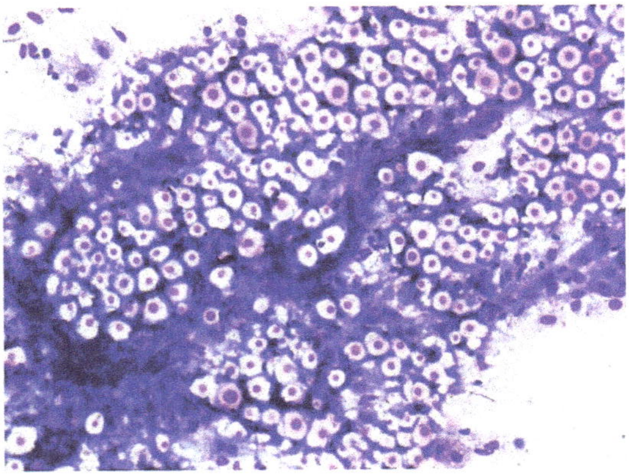

Fig. 17.2 Numerous yeast cells surrounded by halos with endothelial cells and epithelioid cells (MGG, 100×) [16]

17.5.2 Histopathology

Cervical lymph node biopsy, skin lesion biopsy or biopsy of nodular lesions in the upper airway reveals either gelatinous or granulomatous pathology. Gelatinous lesions show numerous cryptococci with minimal inflammatory reaction. Granulomatous lesions show fewer crytococci with a marked inflammatory response comprising of lymphocytes, mononuclear cells, and occasional giant cells [13]. The organism can be seen with haematoxylin and eosin (H and E) (Fig. 17.3a, b), May-Grunwald Giemsa and other special stains such as Gomori's methenamine silver (GMS) (Fig. 17.4a, b), Periodic acid-Schiff (PAS) (Fig. 17.5a, b), and Mucicarmine stains. Special stains help to outstand typical budding fungi [14, 19, 20].

17.5.3 Differentiation Between *C. neoformans* and *C. gattii*

- Matrix-assisted laser desorption/ionization time of flight mass spectrometry (MALDI—TOF MS) can distinguish *C. neoformans* from *C. gattii*.
- *C. gattii* develops deep blue colonies on canavanine glycine bromothymol blue (CGB) media [21].

17.5.4 Serology

Serological tests are most often used, especially in cases of CNS involvement. Latex agglutination and enzyme immunoassay tests for serum antigen are highly sensitive and specific (>90%). HIV-positive patients with cryptococcosis have higher rates of CNS and extrapulmonary infections, more positive blood cultures and higher

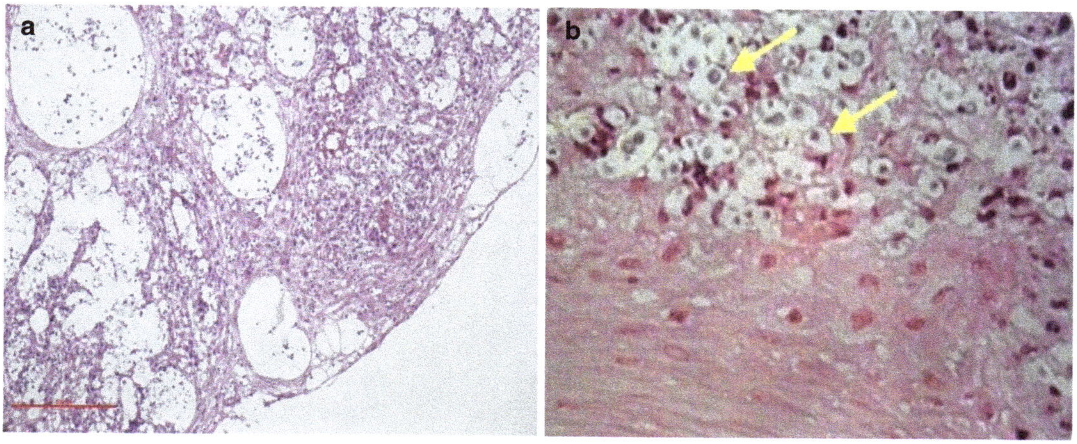

Fig. 17.3 (**a**) Hematoxylin and eosin (H&E) histopathology of the left aryepiglottic folds demonstrating squamous cell proliferation, acute inflammation, and scattered round-shaped microorganisms surrounded by clear halos. Magnification ×100 [19]. (**b**) Numerous encapsulated cryptococcal organisms (arrows) in vocal cord subepithelial stroma, H&E stain, 400× [14]

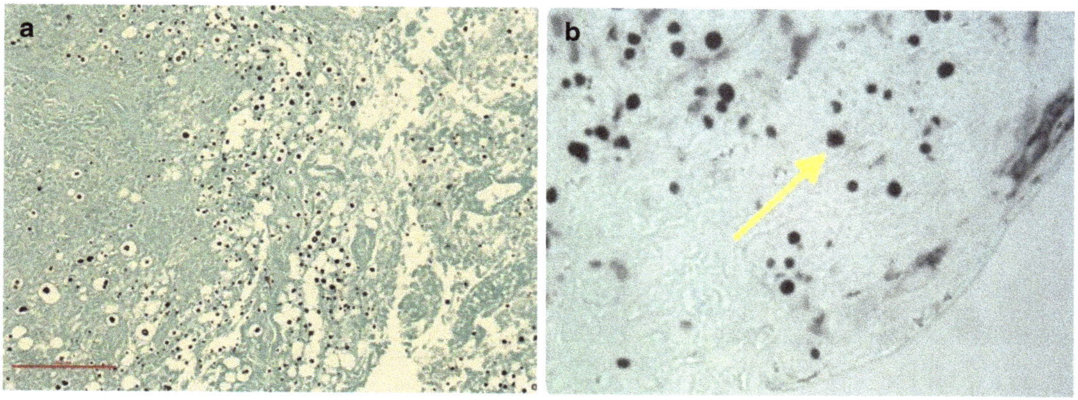

Fig. 17.4 (**a**) Grocott methenamine silver (GMS) histochemical stain identifying the tissue sample as positive for fungal organisms. Magnification ×200 [19]. (**b**) Encapsulated cryptococcal organisms (arrow), methenamine silver stain positive, 400× [14]

polysaccharide antigen titers when compared with non-HIV infected individuals [22, 23].

17.5.5 Imaging

- A chest X-ray and HRCT thorax demonstrates diffuse interstitial infiltrate in pulmonary disease. In pulmonary cryptococcosis, chest imaging findings are various and non-specific, including local or diffuse infiltration, nodules, hilar lymphadenopathy, cavitation, and pleural effusion (Fig. 17.6) [4].
- Cervical lymphadenopathy is better demonstrated on CT neck with contrast which reveals numerous diffuse hypodense rim-enhancing lymph nodes [6, 7].
- In CNS disease, CT or MRI brain is usually normal or may reveal diffuse atrophy, meningeal enhancement, abscess, intraventricular, or intraparenchymal crytpococcoma, gelatinous pseudocyst and/or hydrocephalus [7].

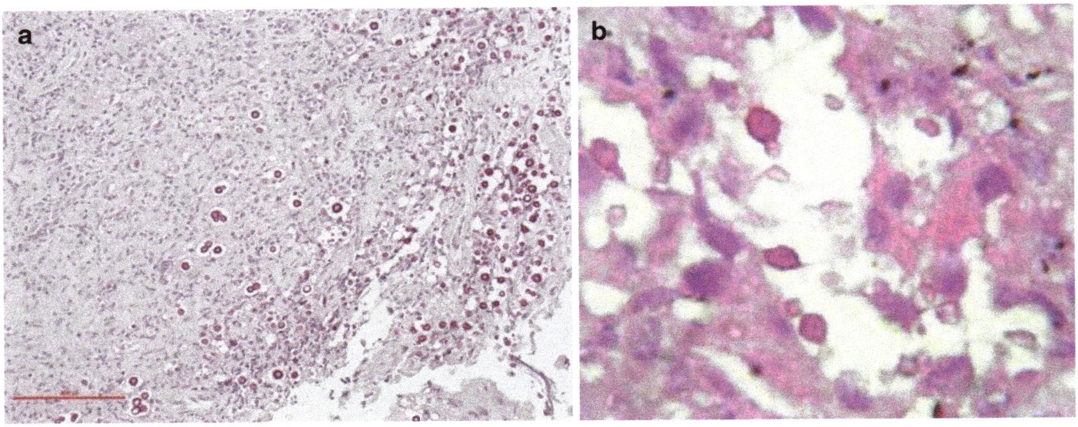

Fig. 17.5 (**a**) PAS stain highlighting the cryptococcus (×200) [19]. (**b**) PAS stain highlighting the cryptococcus (×400). Biopsy taken from laryngeal Cryptococcus lesion [20]

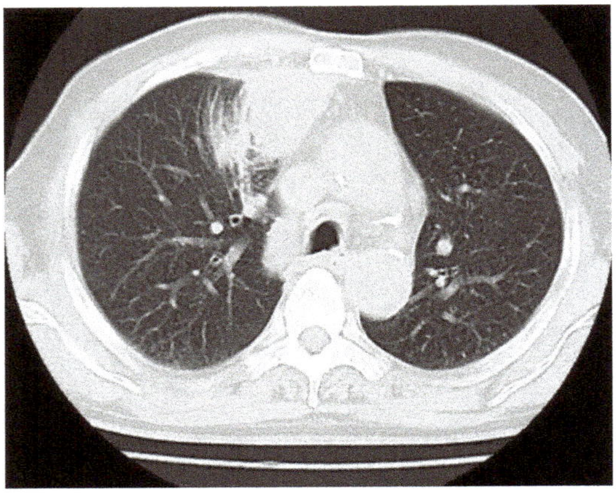

Fig. 17.6 Spiral CT of the thorax showing an irregular mass lesion in the anterior and superior mediastinum [16]

17.5.6 Blood Culture

Initial blood cultures are usually negative. A complete blood count may also be negative for bandaemia (increased levels of band cells which are immature white blood cells released by bone marrow into the blood) or leucocytosis in the initial phase [13].

17.5.7 CSF Analysis

CSF usually reveals a lymphocytic pleocytosis with raised protein and low sugar levels. In cases of cryptococcal meningitis, India ink stain is positive in around 50% HIV-negative cases and in more than 90% of patients with AIDS. Latex agglutination test and enzyme immunoassay for CSF cryptococcal antigen are around 90% sensitive and specific [1]. CSF fungal culture is, however, the gold standard for diagnosis of cryptococcal meningitis and is positive in almost 100% of cases [6, 23].

17.6 Treatment

- Induction therapy: Intravenous liposomal Amphotericin B (3–4 mg/kg/day; as high as 6 mg/kg/day) or Amphotericin B deoxycholate (0.7–1 mg/kg/day) is to be combined with oral Flucytosine(100 mg/kg/day) for 14 days. Patients with HIV infection often have a greater burden of disease and higher mortality (30–70% at 10-weeks), but the recommended therapy even in HIV co-infection is with Amphotericin B and oral Flucytosine. Where Flucytosine is not available, Fluconazole (≥800 mg/day, preferably 1200 mg/day) should be used with Amphotericin B.
- Liposomal Amphotericin B serves as an alternative to amphotericin B deoxycholate, with less nephrotoxicity and infusion reaction.

- Consolidation therapy: After initial induction treatment as above, oral Fluconazole (400 mg/day) is given for at least 8 weeks.
- Maintainance therapy: Consolidation therapy is followed by lower dose Fluconazole (200 mg/day) for 6–12 months [4, 24].

For cerebral cryptococcoma, induction treatment for ≥6 weeks and consolidation and maintenance treatment for 6–18 months should be considered. [24] Symptomatic treatment is necessary for raised intracranial pressure and seizure prevention.

Anti-retroviral therapy in AIDS patients is usually deferred until cryptococcosis starts improving with antifungal treatment [11, 25].

In cryptococcal meningitis, intracranial pressure rises along with CSF fungal burden and is associated with morbidity and mortality. Aggressive control of intracranial pressure should be done. Management options include therapeutic lumbar puncture, lumbar drain insertion, ventriculostomy, or ventriculoperitoneal shunt. Medical treatments such as corticosteroids, mannitol, and acetazolamide are ineffective and should not be used. ART has proven to have a great impact on survival rates among HIV-infected patients with cryptococcosis. The time to start ART in HIV-infected patients with cryptococcosis has to be deferred until 5 weeks after the start of antifungal therapy. In general, any effective ART regimen is acceptable. Potential drug interactions between antiretroviral agents and amphotericin B, flucytosine, and fluconazole are minimal. Of most potential clinical relevance is the concomitant use of fluconazole and nevirapine. Concomitant use of these two drugs should be cautious, and patients should be monitored closely for nevirapine-associated adverse events, including hepatotoxicity. Overlapping toxicities of antifungal and antiretroviral drugs and immune reconstitution inflammatory syndrome are not uncommon. Early recognition and appropriate management of these consequences can reinforce the successfully integrated therapy in HIV-infected patients with cryptococcosis.

17.7 Essential Features

- Cryptococcosis is the most common life-threatening mycosis associated with AIDS worldwide. Most commonly an opportunistic infection, but disease may occur in immunocompetent patients.
- Caused by encapsulated yeast *C. neoformans* or *C. gatti*. *C. neoformans* infection in immunocompromised individuals; however, *C. gattii* infects immunocompetent individuals.
- Diseases range from cutaneous to severe pulmonary and central nervous system disease.
- Cutaneous manifestation are pustules, papules, superficial granulomas or cellulitis.
- Pulmonary disease can be subacute and indolent causing-
  - Cough and dyspnea with or without constitutional symptoms.
  - Pulmonary nodules; old cryptococcomas.
  - Latent infections can reactivate in immunosuppressed
- CNS disease presents with increased intracranial pressure, seizures, and focal neurologic deficits. Spectrum of diffuse meningeal disease and focal lesions, including soap bubble lesions, are characteristic. Meningitis is a major concern in immunocompromised patients.
- Mucocutaneous lesions include nodular, granulomatous mass or in the form of superficial or deep ulcers. Lesions are usually in the nose, paranasal sinuses or mouth and rarely in the nasopharynx and larynx.
- Microscopy reveals variably sized yeasts with thin walls, narrow-based budding and encapsulated by thick mucinous capsule composed of glucuronoxylomannan (GXM).
- Histopathology: Yeasts stain positive with methenamine silver, mucicarmine, Fontana-Masson, and India ink stains. Can distinguish *C. gattii* by deep blue colonies on canavanine glycine bromothymol blue (CGB) media.
- Treatment comprises of induction therapy with liposomal amphotericin B and flucytosine for 14 days, consolidation with high dose

fluconazole for 8 weeks and maintenance with lower dose fluconazole for 6–12 months.

References

1. Mandell G, et al. Principles and practice of infectious diseases. New York: Churchill Livingstone; 2005. p. 2997–3012.
2. Barzan L, et al. Head and neck manifestations during HIV infection. J Laryngol Otol. 1993;107:133–6.
3. Lee KC, Cheung SW. Evaluation of the neck mass in human immunodeficiency virus-infected patients. Otolaryngol Clin N Am. 1992;25:1287–305.
4. Srichatrapimuk S, Sungkanuparph S. Integrated therapy for HIV and cryptococcosis. AIDS Res Ther. 2016;13:42. https://doi.org/10.1186/s12981-016-0126-7.
5. Satishchandra P, et al. Cryptococcal meningitis: clinical, diagnostic and therapeutic overview. Neurol India. 2007;55(3):226–32.
6. Chakrabarti A. Epidemiology of central nervous system mycoses. Neurol India. 2007;55(3):191–7.
7. Jain KK, et al. Imaging features of central nervous system fungal infections. Neurol India. 2007;55(3):241–50.
8. Buchanan KL, Murphy JW. What makes *Cryptococcus neoformans* a pathogen? Emerg Infect Dis. 1998;4(1):71–83. https://doi.org/10.3201/eid0401.980109.
9. Shankar SK, et al. Pathobiology of fungal infections of the central nervous system with special reference to the Indian scenario. Neurol India. 2007;55(3):198–215.
10. Nadkarni TD, et al. A solitary cryptococcal granuloma in an immunocompetent host. Neurol India. 2005;53:365–7.
11. Khwaja GA. Fungal meningitis. Neurosci Today. 1999;3(4):185–96.
12. Quartarolon N, et al. Primary cutaneous cryptococcosis. Acta Dermatovenol Alpina, Pannonica ET Adriatica. 2002;II(4).
13. Garbyal RS, et al. Cryptococcal lymphadenitis: report of a case with fine needle aspiration cytology. Acta Cytol. 2005;49:58–60.
14. Wong DJY, et al. Laryngeal cryptococcosis associated with inhaled corticosteroid use: case reports and literature review. Front Surg. 2017;4:63. https://doi.org/10.3389/fsurg.2017.00063.
15. Ghatalia PA, et al. Reversible blindness in cryptococcal meningitis with normal intracranial pressure: case report and review of the literature. Clin Infect Dis. 2014;59:310–3. https://doi.org/10.1093/cid/ciu216.
16. Suchitha S, et al. Disseminated cryptococcosis in an immunocompetent patient: a case report. Case Rep Pathol. 2012;652351:3 p. https://doi.org/10.1155/2012/652351
17. Guarner J, Brandt ME. Histopathologic diagnosis of fungal infections in the 21st century. Clin Microbiol Rev. 2011;24:247–80. https://doi.org/10.1128/CMR.00053-10.
18. McTaggart LR, et al. Rapid identification of *Cryptococcus neoformans* and *Cryptococcus gattii* by matrix-assisted laser desorption ionization-time of flight mass spectrometry. J Clin Microbiol. 2011;49:3050–3. https://doi.org/10.1128/JCM.00651-11.
19. Mallany HP, et al. Squamous cell proliferation as a reactive mechanism to laryngeal cryptococcus infection: a case report. Cureus. 2021;13(1):e12587. https://doi.org/10.7759/cureus.12587.
20. Sandhu J, et al. Laryngeal cryptococcus: a rare cause of hoarseness in renal allograft recipient. J Nephropharmacol. 2017;6(1):27–9.
21. Burkett A, et al. Cryptococcus neoformans & gatti. PathologyOutlines.com. https://www.pathologyoutlines.com/topic/microbiologycneoformans.html
22. Shoham S, Levitz SM. The immune response to fungal infections. Br J Haematol. 2005;129:569–82.
23. Yao Z, et al. Management of cryptococcosis in non-HIV-related patients. Med Mycol. 2005;43(3):245–51.
24. Perfect JR, et al. Clinical practice guidelines for the management of cryptococcal disease: 2010 update by the Infectious Diseases Society of America. Clin Infect Dis. 2010;50:291–322. https://doi.org/10.1086/649858.
25. Saag MS, et al. Practice guidelines for the management of cryptococcal disease. Clin Infect Dis. 2000;30:710–8.

18 Coccidioidomycosis

Abstract

Coccidioidomycosis consists of a spectrum of diseases, ranging from a mild, self-limited, febrile illness to severe, life-threatening infection. It is considered one of the most virulent primary fungal infections. It is caused by the soil-dwelling fungi, *Coccidioides immitis* and *C. posadasii*, which are present in diverse endemic areas. Climate changes and environmental factors affect the Coccidioides lifecycle and influence infection rates. The incidence of coccidioidomycosis has risen substantially over the past two decades. People with immunodeficiency diseases, diabetics, transplant recipients, and prisoners are particularly vulnerable to disseminated infection. Primary pulmonary coccidioidomycosis may present with mild flu-like symptoms to acute respiratory distress syndrome. Infection may proceed to progressive pulmonary coccidioidomycosis with cavitary or miliary pulmonary lesions. Disseminated coccidioidomycosis shows nodules, papules, abscesses, granulomatous lesions in the head neck region. Direct inoculation of fungus into the skin leads to primary cutaneous coccidioidomycosis. Microscopy, culture, and serological tests aid in diagnosis. Treatment is with oral azole antifungal drugs and amphotericin B.

Synonyms

Valley fever, California fever, desert rheumatism, Coccidiomycosis, Posadas–Wernicke Disease, Coccidioidal Granuloma; San Joaquin Valley fever [1, 2].

18.1 Background

Coccidioidomycosis is a fungal infection, almost always acquired from the environment, that can affect many species of mammals and some reptiles. It is caused by fungus *Coccidioides immitis* or *Coccidioides posadasii*. The causative agent of coccidioidomycosis was first identified by a medical intern, Alejandro Posadas, in Buenos Aires in 1892. Initially, it was mistaken as parasite. Consequently, in 1896, it was given the name Coccidioides (derived from its morphologic appearance of "resembling Coccidia") immitis ("not mild," because it was believed that the organism caused lethal disease). Just a few years later, William Ophuls and Herbert C Moffitt accurately classified *C. immitis* as a fungus [3]. Most infections in people are relatively mild or asymptomatic, but severe or fatal illness also occurs, especially in the elderly or immunocompromised. Coccidioidomycosis is often limited to the respiratory tract. In a small percentage of cases, the fungi disseminate to other tissues from the lungs [4, 5].

S. V. Nemade, K. J. Shinde, *Granulomatous diseases in Otorhinolaryngology, Head and Neck*,
https://doi.org/10.1007/978-981-16-4047-6_18

18.2 Epidemiology

Coccidioides spp. occur in the Western Hemisphere, at latitudes between 40°N and 40°S, from California to Argentina. The distribution of these organisms is patchy. They are endemic in the southwestern USA, including Arizona (where the incidence in humans is particularly high), parts of New Mexico, Texas (west of El Paso), and the central and southern portions of California, especially the San Joaquin Valley. Overall, it is estimated that 70% of all Coccidioidomycosis cases in the USA occur in Arizona, and 25% in California [6].

It has been more common among men than women. Although coccidioidomycosis affects all age groups, the highest incidence rates are consistently documented among adults, typically among those aged 40–60 years. The incidence of coccidioidomycosis in the USA in 2011 (42.6 per 100,000) was almost ten times higher than the incidence reported in 1998 (5.3 per 100,000). In the area, where it is most prevalent, the infection rate is 2–4% [4, 7, 8].

18.3 Etiopathogenesis

Coccidioidomycosis is caused by the dimorphic, soil-borne, ascomycete fungi *Coccidioides immitis* and *C. posadasii* (formerly known as the "California" and "non California" populations of *C. immitis*). *C. immitis* and *C. posadasii* differ in some characteristics, such as their tolerance to heat and salt, but no differences in their pathogenicity have been recognized. These are soil saprophytes that grow in semiarid regions with sandy, alkaline soils. Arthroconidia are produced by the mold form growing in the environment and are dispersed by the wind. After air-borne infection in the lungs, arthroconidia become spherules. As each spherule enlarges, endospores develop inside it. The spherule eventually ruptures and releases the endospores which are disseminated to other parts of the body in the blood or lymph [4, 7].

Initially, coccidioidomycosis begins with Valley fever, which is its initial acute form. Valley fever may progress to the chronic form and then to disseminated coccidioidomycosis. Therefore, Coccidioidomycosis may be divided into the following types [9].

- Acute coccidioidomycosis, sometimes described in the literature as primary pulmonary coccidioidomycosis
- Chronic coccidioidomycosis
- Disseminated coccidioidomycosis, which includes primary cutaneous coccidioidomycosis

Persons that are especially vulnerable to developing severe or disseminated coccidioidomycosis are those with diseases that impair T-cell function. Such conditions include hematologic malignancies, inflammatory arthritis, and diabetes [6].

18.4 Clinical Features

The incubation period for primary pulmonary or cutaneous coccidioidomycosis is usually 1–3 weeks. Disseminated disease or chronic pulmonary coccidioidomycosis can occur months or years after the initial infection [4, 5].

Cutaneous manifestations can be seen in three different types of coccidioidal infection:

- As a part of the acute pulmonary infection and present as an "acute pulmonary exanthema."
- It can reflect the presence of disseminated infection (secondary cutaneous infection).
- It can represent a primary infection due to direct inoculation (primary cutaneous infection).

Despite their variability and heterogeneity, cutaneous manifestations differ between these three forms of the disease. Acute pulmonary disease is associated with reactive skin manifestations that do not contain visible microorganisms. Organism-specific manifestations present with lesions that contain the organism, which can be identified in cultures or histopathology; they result from hematogenous spread of primary pulmonary infection (secondary cutaneous disease) or, very rarely, as a result of direct trauma to the skin (primary cutaneous disease) [6].

18.4.1 Primary Pulmonary Coccidioidomycosis

It can be asymptomatic or so mild that they are unrecognized. In symptomatic cases, the illness is often flu-like, with fever, fatigue, malaise, headache, sore throat, and cough and/or pleuritic chest pain. Overt signs of pneumonia may also be seen. Severe respiratory disease, with high fever, dyspnea, and hypoxemia, is uncommon in healthy people but more frequent in individuals who are immunocompromised. It may progress to acute respiratory distress syndrome or respiratory failure [4, 10].

Ten percent–fifty percent of patients with pulmonary disease develop skin lesions. Erythematous, macular rash may occur in the early stages, and hypersensitivity reactions can cause erythema nodosum or erythema multiforme, reactive interstitial granulomatous dermatitis and Sweet's syndrome. Sweet's Syndrome, also called "acute febrile neutrophilic dermatosis" is characterized by an acute eruption, consisting of painful erythematous, well-demarcated papules and plaques, in association with fever and neutrophilic leukocytosis [6]. Erythema nodosum is characterized by tender, reddened nodules on the lower extremities. Desert rheumatism refers to the immunologic phenomena triad, including fever, arthralgia and erythema nodosum [6, 9, 11].

18.4.2 Progressive Pulmonary Coccidioidomycosis

In this, the clinical signs do not resolve but develop into chronic and progressive disease. The patients present symptoms that last for more than 3 months (persistent cough, hemoptysis, and weight loss) [12]. Nodular or cavitary lesions, cavitary lung disease with fibrosis, or miliary pulmonary dissemination may be seen. Even when the lungs are extensively involved, the disease usually remains limited to the respiratory tract [4, 11]. Mass lesions can be seen in chronic infection, usually well demarcated, often with central cavitation [12]. Fungus ball (mycetoma) is usually found in 28% of cases with cavity lesions [11, 12].

18.4.3 Disseminated Coccidioidomycosis

Disseminated coccidioidomycosis occurs in a small percentage of cases, and may develop weeks, months or years after the primary infection. It is usually acute and can be rapidly fatal without treatment, but it may also progress more slowly with periods of remission and recurrence. The skin, regional lymph nodes, bones, and joints are most often affected in humans, but virtually any tissue or organ including the visceral organs and testes may be involved. The clinical signs vary with the affected tissues. A wide variety of lesions, including nodules, papules, pustules, furuncles, verrucous (wart-like) plaques, abscesses, granulomatous lesions or ulcerations, may be seen when the fungus disseminates to the skin. The head, neck, and chest are most often involved. Lymph nodes that are infected may become necrotic and ulcerate or drain. Dissemination to the musculoskeletal system can result in osteomyelitis, septic arthritis, and/or synovitis. Arthritis usually affects only one joint, often a weight-bearing joint such as the knees, but it can be migratory. Subcutaneous abscesses and sinus tracts can develop near the affected bones and joints. Septic shock can also be seen [10, 11]. In people, dissemination to the central nervous system usually results in coccidioidal meningitis. The symptoms may include fever, headache, and signs of meningeal irritation. Cognitive impairment or personality changes are possible, and inflammation can result in complications of vasculitis, stroke, or hydrocephalus [10, 11].

18.4.4 Primary Cutaneous Coccidioidomycosis

Primary cutaneous coccidioidomycosis, the result of direct inoculation into the skin, is rare. The initial lesion may be a chancriform ulcerated nodule or plaque (Fig. 18.1). The infection spreads along the lymphatic vessels and may be accompanied by regional lymphadenopathy. The lesions often heal spontaneously within a few weeks if the person is immunocompetent [9, 11].

18.5 Diagnosis

18.5.1 Microscopy and Culture

Microscopic visualization of the fungus in respiratory secretions, pleural fluid, tissues, or exudates. Organisms are rarely found in cerebrospinal fluid (CSF) in cases of meningitis. In the body, coccidioides spp. form spherules, double-walled structures that vary widely in abundance and size. Most spherules are 20–80 μm in diameter, but some can be as large as 200 μm. They contain endospores, small, 2–5 μm globular structures that develop into new spherules when they are released (Figs. 18.2 and 18.3). Spherules containing endospores are diagnostic, while spherules without endospores are presumptive evidence for coccidioidomycosis. The calcofluor white (CFW) fluorescent stain, potassium hydroxide (KOH) wet mounts, Grocott-Methenamine silver (GMS) stain, Periodic Acid-Schiff (PAS) stain (Fig. 18.3) or Hematoxylin-Eosin (H&E) stain can be used to visualize the organism (Fig. 18.4) [14–16].

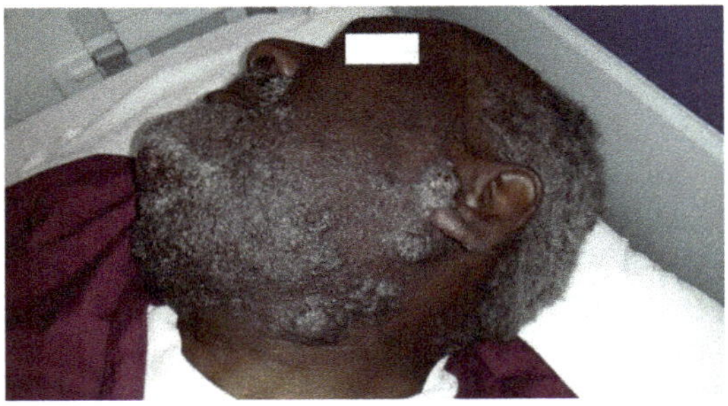

Fig. 18.1 Facial lesions from coccidioides infection [13]

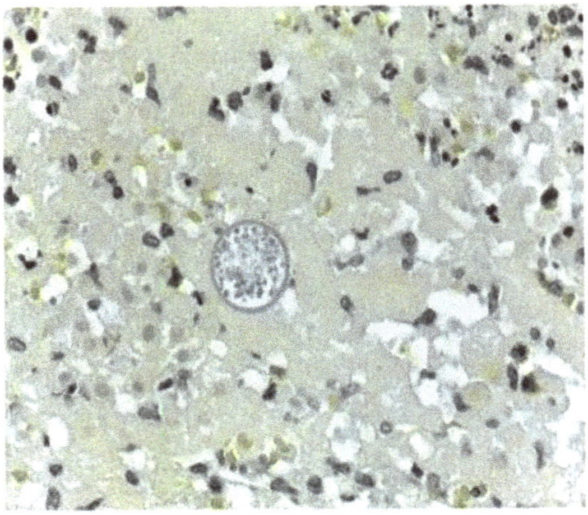

Fig. 18.2 30 μm large endospore-containing spherule, floating in necrotic debris (original magnification ×630) [14]

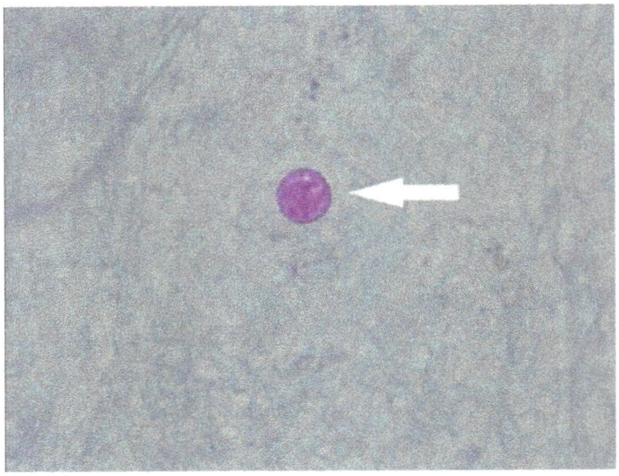

Fig. 18.3 PAS stain of coccidioides spherules [13]

Coccidioidomycosis can also be diagnosed by culturing affected body fluids, exudates, or tissue specimens. *C. immitis* and *C. posadasii* can grow on most fungal media such as Sabouraud agar, brain-heart infusion agar, potato dextrose or potato flakes agar, with or without cycloheximide, as well as on many media used to isolate bacteria. Growth can be fast, from 2–7 days, or take up to 2–3 weeks. They grow at room temperature as a white, cottony mold [17]. Lactophenol cotton blue stains show septate hyphae with alternating barrel-shaped arthroconidia. It is Biosafety level 3 pathogen, hence laboratory personnel should be

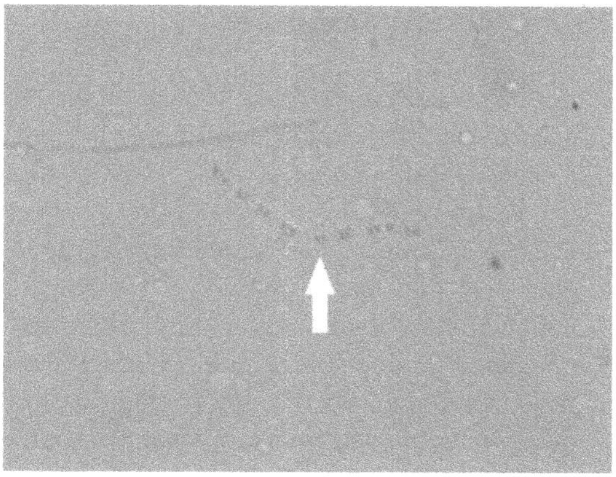

Fig. 18.4 *Coccidioides arthroconidia* [13]

aware of the diagnosis for necessary precautions to be taken.

Complete blood count: Eosinophilia is usually found in 27% of cases [18, 19].

18.5.2 Serology

Serologic tests identifying anticoccidioidal antibodies (IgM and IgG) are the most frequently employed assays for the diagnosis and prognosis of coccidioidomycosis. Specific IgM can usually be detected within 1–3 weeks after infection [18].

These tests are highly specific and relatively sensible. They include tube precipitin (TP) and complement fixation (CF) assays, as well as immunodiffusion tube precipitin (IDTP) and immunodiffusion complement fixation (IDCF), which are variants of these assays that employ immunodiffusion in agar [20].

18.5.3 The Coccidioidin or Spherulin Skin Test

Skin testing is a diagnostic method that can evaluate the overall incidence of coccidioidomycosis in endemic areas. However, its use is limited, since a positive skin test does not distinguish between current or previous infection [21].

18.5.4 Molecular Assay

Molecular techniques such as in situ hybridization (ISH) and polymerase chain reaction (PCR) may assist in the diagnosis of coccidioidomycosis. They are not widely available, and their sensitivity has not been determined (it may range from 80 to 98%, depending on the specimen site) [22].

18.5.5 Imaging

Chest X-ray and CT chest delineate specific changes in various types of infections [23]-

- Acute infection resembles acute bacterial pneumonia, including consolidation (75%), nodular opacities (20%), hilar adenopathy (20%), pleural effusion (15–20%), solitary pulmonary nodule may be seen.
- Chronic pulmonary coccidioidomycosis: chronic cavitary lesion can be seen radiographically in 2% of cases, up to 11% by CT scan. Grape skin sign is classic finding showing very thin-walled cavitary lesion that develops in lung parenchyma previously affected by consolidation followed by central necrosis.
- Disseminated infection: miliary nodules from hematogenous spread.

18.6 Treatment

Three important factors that must be taken into consideration when treating coccidioidomycosis are the severity of pulmonary infection, the presence or absence of dissemination, and the patient's individual risk factors. Treatment modalities range from observation to antifungal drugs, depending on the severity of the disease and risk factors for dissemination [24, 25].

Primarypulmonarycoccidioidomycosis[19,25]-

- Immunocompetent patients without risk factors for dissemination are treated with fluconazole or itraconazole at doses of 400 mg per day, for 3–6 months.

- Patients with immunosuppression/risk factors for dissemination are treated with fluconazole or itraconazole at doses of 400 mg per day for 4–12 months.

Chronic pulmonary coccidioidomycosis [25]-

- Fluconazole or itraconazole at doses of 400 mg per day for 12–18 months or more are indicated, according to clinical response.
- Severe or refractory infections may be treated with amphotericin B, deoxycholate (0.5–1 mg/kg/day) and liposomal (2–5 mg/kg/day) forms. Posaconazole and voriconazole have been successful in treating some cases.

Disseminated, meningeal forms of coccidioidomycosis [25]-

- Lifelong treatment with antifungal therapy such as fluconazole 400 mg per day (with initial doses of up to 1000 mg per day) or itraconazole 400–600 mg per day. Intrathecal amphotericin has also been indicated.

Disseminated, non-meningeal forms of coccidioidomycosis [25]:

- Fluconazole or itraconazole at doses of 400 mg per day for 3–6 months, with the alternative of using amphotericin B in severe or rapidly progressing cases.

Primary cutaneous coccidioidomycosis [6, 25]-

- Itraconazole at doses of 400 mg per day for 6 months gives excellent response.

Surgical excision or debridement may occasionally be employed in disseminated cases or enlarging pulmonary cavitary lesions [19, 24].

18.7 Essential Features

- Coccidioidomycosis is a fungal infection caused by dimorphic, soil-borne fungus *Coccidioides immitis* or *Coccidioides posadasii*.
- Primary pulmonary coccidioidomycosis presents with flu-like symptoms, sore throat, cough and/or pleuritic chest pain in immunocompetent individuals. Acute respiratory distress syndrome or respiratory failure may occur in individuals who are immunocompromised—sometimes associated with erythema nodosum.
- Progressive pulmonary coccidioidomycosis: Nodular or cavitary lesions with lung parenchymal fibrosis or miliary pulmonary dissemination may be seen.
- Disseminated coccidioidomycosis shows nodules, papules, abscesses, granulomatous lesions in the head neck region. Common extrathoracic sites: skin, joints, bones, and meninges.
- Direct inoculation of fungus into the skin leads to primary cutaneous coccidioidomycosis with ulcerated nodules and regional lymphadenopathy.
- Microscopy of secretions showing spherules containing endospores is diagnostic.
- Necrotizing granulomatous inflammation with characteristic spherules is evident on histopathology.
- Serologic testing for anticoccidioidal IgG, IgM is also helpful.
- In situ hybridization (ISH) and polymerase chain reaction (PCR) assist in the diagnosis of coccidioidomycosis.
- The coccidioidin or spherulin skin test: It does not differentiate between past and current infection.
- HRCT thorax helps to reveal the lung parenchymal lesions. CT PNS delineates sinonasal granulomatous lesions.

- Treatment is with oral azole antifungal drugs (Fluconazole or iatroconazole).
- Amphotericin B is reserved for severe or refractory infections.
- Surgical resection of the long-standing pulmonary cavitary lesion may be required.

References

1. Malo J, et al. Update on the diagnosis of pulmonary coccidioidomycosis. Ann Am Thor Soc. 11(2):243–53. https://doi.org/10.1513/AnnalsATS.201308-286FR.
2. Rapini RP, Bolognia JL, Jorizzo JL. Dermatology: 2-Volume Set. St. Louis: Mosby; 2007. ISBN: 978-1-4160-2999-1.
3. Brown J, et al. Coccidioidomycosis: epidemiology. Clin Epidemiol. 2013;5:185–97. https://doi.org/10.2147/CLEP.S34434
4. Nguyen C, et al. Recent advances in our understanding of the environmental, epidemiological, immunological, and clinical dimensions of coccidioidomycosis. Clin Microbiol Rev. 2013;26(3):505–25.
5. Thompson GR 3rd. Pulmonary coccidioidomycosis. Semin Respir Crit Care Med. 2011;32:754–63.
6. Garcia SC, et al. Coccidioidomycosis and the skin: a comprehensive review. An Bras Dermatol. 2015;90(5):610–9. https://doi.org/10.1590/abd1806-4841.20153805.
7. Kolivras K, Comrie A. Modeling valley fever (coccidioidomycosis) incidence on the basis of climate conditions. Int J Biometeorol. 2003;47(2):87–101.
8. Barker BM, Jewell KA, Kroken S, Orbach MJ. The population biology of coccidioides: epidemiologic implications for disease outbreaks. Ann N Y Acad Sci. 2007;1111:147–63.
9. Galgiani JN, et al. Coccidioidomycosis. Clin Infect Dis. 2005;41:1217–23.
10. Ampel NM. Coccidioidomycosis in persons infected with HIV-1. Ann N Y Acad Sci. 2007;1111:336–42.
11. Acha PN, Szyfres B (Pan American Health Organization [PAHO]). Zoonoses and communicable diseases common to man and animals. Volume 1. Bacterioses and mycoses. 3rd ed. Washington, DC: PAHO; 2003. Scientific and Technical Publication No. 580. Coccidioidomycosis; p. 320–5.
12. Chiller TM, et al. Coccidioidomycosis. Infect Dis Clin N Am. 2003;17(1):41–57.
13. Gerstein W, Ilieva V. *Coccidioides immitis* soft tissue infection mimicking pseudofolliculitis barbae. Clin Case Rep. 2018;6(4):758–9. https://doi.org/10.1002/ccr3.1421
14. Baek O, et al. Peritoneal and genital coccidioidomycosis in an otherwise healthy Danish female: a case report. BMC Infect Dis. 2017;17:105. https://doi.org/10.1186/s12879-017-2212-4
15. Shubitz LF, Dial SM. Coccidioidomycosis: a diagnostic challenge. Clin Tech Small Anim Pract. 2005;20(4):220–6.
16. Sutton DA. Diagnosis of coccidioidomycosis by culture: safety considerations, traditional methods, and susceptibility testing. Ann N Y Acad Sci. 2007;1111:315–25.
17. Welsh O, et al. Coccidioidomycosis. Clin Dermatol. 2012;30:573–91.
18. Saubolle MA, McKellar PP, Sussland D. Epidemiologic, clinical, and diagnostic aspects of coccidioidomycosis. J Clin Microbiol. 2007;45(1):26–30.
19. Saubolle MA. Laboratory aspects in the diagnosis of coccidioidomycosis. Ann N Y Acad Sci. 2007;1111:301–14.
20. Laniado-Laborín R, et al. Coccidioidomycosis: an update. Curr Fungal Infect Rep. 2012;6:113–20.
21. DiCaudo DJ. Coccidioidomycosis: a review and update. J Am Acad Dermatol. 2006;55:929–42.
22. Ampel NM. The diagnosis of coccidioidomycosis. F1000 Med Rep. 2010;2:pii: 2.
23. Jude CM, et al. Pulmonary coccidioidomycosis : pictorial review of chest radio-graphic and CT findings. Radiographics. 2014;34:912–25.
24. Blair JE. State-of-the-art treatment of coccidioidomycosis: skin and soft-tissue infections. Ann N Y Acad Sci. 2007;1111:411–21.
25. Wollina U, et al. Successful treatment of relapsing disseminated coccidioidomycosis with cutaneous involvement with posaconazole. J Dtsch Dermatol Ges. 2009;7:46–9.

19 Blastomycosis (North American Blastomycosis)

Abstract

Blastomycosis is caused by *Blastomyces dermatitidis* that belong to a group of thermally dimorphic fungi that can infect healthy and immunocompromised individuals. Following inhalation of mycelial fragments and spores into the lungs, Blastomyces convert into pathogenic yeast, which facilitates evasion of host immune defenses to cause pneumonia and disseminated disease. The clinical manifestations of blastomycosis are broad, ranging from asymptomatic infection to acute respiratory distress syndrome and death. Extrapulmonary dissemination to the skin, bone, and central nervous system, nose, and throat can occur. While culture and non-culture diagnostic tests are available, a high index of clinical suspicion is essential for prompt diagnosis. Clinical diagnosis is supported by imaging modalities and laboratory identification of the fungi. Treatment is with polyene or azole antifungal agents, with selection influenced by disease severity, site of infection and immunosuppression.

Synonyms
North American Blastomycosis.

19.1 Background

Blastomycosis is a pulmonary disease caused by inhaling spores of the dimorphic fungus *Blastomyces dermatitidis*; though the fungi may spread hematogenously, causing extrapulmonary disease. Human blastomycosis was first reported by Gilchrist in 1894 in a case of cutaneous disease first mistakenly attributed to the protozoan disease. Four years later, in 1898, Gilchrist and Stokes isolated the causative agent, a fungus they called. The first case of canine blastomycosis was reported by Meyer in 1912 [1]. The clinical spectrum of pulmonary blastomycosis is diverse, ranging from subclinical infection, acute pneumonia resembling bacterial community-acquired pneumonia, chronic pneumonia mimicking tuberculosis or malignancy, and acute respiratory distress syndrome. The most common extrapulmonary manifestation is in the skin but may involve Ear Nose Throat. Clinical diagnosis is supported by imaging modalities and laboratory identification of the fungi. Treatment is with itraconazole, Fluconazole, or Amphotericin B [1, 2].

19.2 Epidemiology

Overall, blastomycosis is uncommon. Most cases occur in the United States and Canada. In North America, Blastomyces is endemic to the

S. V. Nemade, K. J. Shinde, *Granulomatous diseases in Otorhinolaryngology, Head and Neck*,
https://doi.org/10.1007/978-981-16-4047-6_19

midwestern, south-central, and southeastern regions of the United States and four Canadian provinces from Saskatchewan to Quebec [3]. In states where blastomycosis is reportable, yearly incidence rates are approximately 1–2 cases per 100,000 population [1, 2, 4]. It shows no age or gender predilection. Blastomyces dermatitidis (also called North American blastomycosis) is endemic to Canada and the upper Midwest of the United States, particularly in moist wooded areas near this region's many lakes, rivers, and streams [4].

19.3 Etiopathogenesis

B. dermatitidis is a thermally dimorphic fungus that grows in a mycelial form at room temperature and in the culture at 25 °C. The conidia are easily aerosolized (2–10 m in diameter) and inhaled into the lungs.Human exposures occur during outdoor activities when fungal microhabitats existing in soil with high organic content are disturbed. Inhaled airborne fungal spores result in primary lung infection. It initiates a granulomatous reaction mediated by neutrophils, monocytes, and macrophages. This host response is usually capable of destroying the conidia and inhibiting the conversion of mycelia to yeast. However, conidia that overwhelm host defenses rapidly convert to the yeast form and become more resistant to destruction [3, 5]. This generally occurs 2–4 weeks after incubation. It may be limited to pulmonary infection or may show haematogenous widespread dissemination of the disease [5, 6]. The most common extrathoracic site is the skin, followed by bone, the male genitourinary system, oral cavity and the central nervous system (CNS) [5].

19.4 Clinical Features

19.4.1 Acute Pulmonary Blastomycosis

It manifests with fever, chills, and cough, similar to bacterial pneumonia. It is often treated as pneumonia and sputum or tissue culture is obtained only after the patient fails to respond to therapy.

19.4.2 Chronic Pulmonary Blastomycosis

It is the most common presentation. Patients present with intermittent low-grade fever, mild persistent productive cough, chest pain, and hemoptysis. General symptoms of malaise, fatigue, and weight loss are also often present. These symptoms have been mistakenly diagnosed as tuberculosis or atypical pneumonia [7].

19.4.3 Fulminant Blastomycosis

It is rare, manifesting as fever, chills, dyspnoea. Rapid systemic dissemination and progression to acute respiratory distress syndrome result within 1 week, often leading to death. Patients often require ventilator assistance within a few days of admission. The fulminant manifestation occurs in both immunocompetent and immunocompromised patients [5, 6, 8, 9].

Other system manifestations: [5, 9–11]

- Nose and paranasal sinuses: Sinonasal granulomas extending to the nasopharynx and diffuse destruction of the skull base may occur.
- The middle ear and mastoid involvement causing temporal bone destruction are possible.
- Oral cavity, oropharynx, and larynx: The common manifestation is leucoplakia not responding to steroids and local treatment. Laryngeal leucoplakia is mostly mistaken as malignancy [12].
- Bone and joint: Bone involvement has been reported in up to 25% of extrathoracic cases. Joint swelling or osteomyelitis is the common features that cause joint or bone pain. Temporal bone involvement may be associated with otitis media and mastoiditis. Skull base involvement may be associated with nasopharyngeal granulomas.

- Skin: It is believed to occur in 20%–40% of cases of disseminated disease. Cutaneous lesions may appear verrucous (warty) or ulcerative. It may include a rash, sores, or nodules (small elevated areas on the skin) (Figs. 19.1 and 19.2) [12]. Primary cutaneous Blastomycosis is rare and occurs following direct inoculation of the organism into the skin. Secondary cutaneous lesions occur in the course of disseminated disease. Skin lesions are commonly located on the face, neck, and extremities.

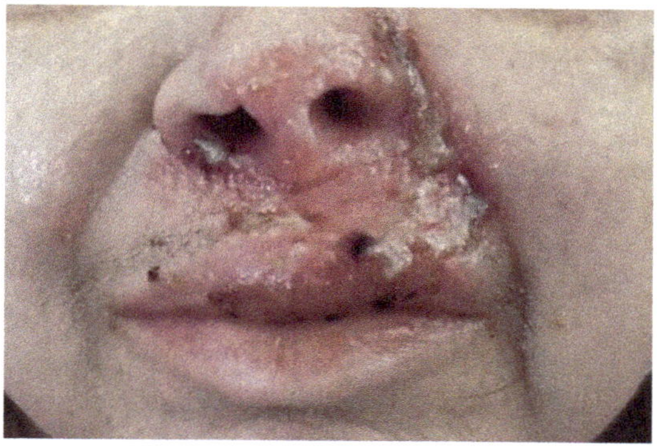

Fig. 19.1 Fungating nasal and upper lip lesion showing cutaneous disseminated blastomycosis on nose [12]

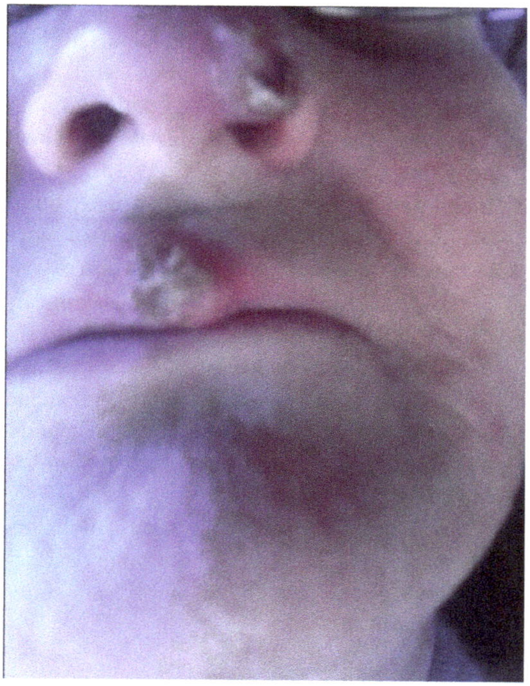

Fig. 19.2 Blastomycosis lesion on left ala of nose and middle of the upper lip [12]

- Central nervous system: Involvement of the CNS occurs in 5%–10% of cases of blastomycotic dissemination. The most common manifestation is epidural abscess followed by meningitis. It is usually seen in immunocompromised patients.
- Genital lesions: Usually seen in males. Prostatitis and epididymo-orchitis are the most common forms of genitourinary involvement.

19.5 Diagnosis

19.5.1 Microscopy and Culture

Microscopy and culture of infected material such as nasal secretions, swab taken from ulcers, infected material from skin lesions, synovial fluid, CSF is useful in the identification of fungus.

At microscopy, the mycelia possess branching hyphae with right-angled conidiophores ending in single round conidia. Many other fungal mycelial forms share this appearance with *B. dermatitidis*, thus, and this appearance is not specific. *B. dermatitidis* converts to a yeast form within tissues and in the culture at 37 °C. At gross examination, yeast colonies appear cream or tan with buttery wrinkled surfaces. At the microscopic examination, the yeast cells possess thick double refractile cell walls. Reproducing cells are characterized by single broad-based budding. These features are typical of blastomycosis [5, 9]. Culture is definitive when positive [7].

19.5.2 Histopathology

Biopsy of sinonasal granulomatous mass, oral, or laryngeal lesions may reveal mixed inflammatory reaction with clusters of polymorphonuclear leucocytes, and granulomas, usually non-caseating, with epithelioid histiocytes and foreign body giant cells (Fig. 19.3). As granulomas form, number of organisms tends to decrease. Infection of the skin and mucosal surface is characterised by prominent pseudoepitheliomatous hyperplasia that histologically may resemble squamous cell carcinoma. Histological similarities of laryngeal lesions with tuberculous laryngitis and squamous cell carcinoma make the diagnosis difficult [7, 9]. The organisms are best demonstrated by PAS and Silver Methenamine stains (Figs. 19.4 and 19.5).

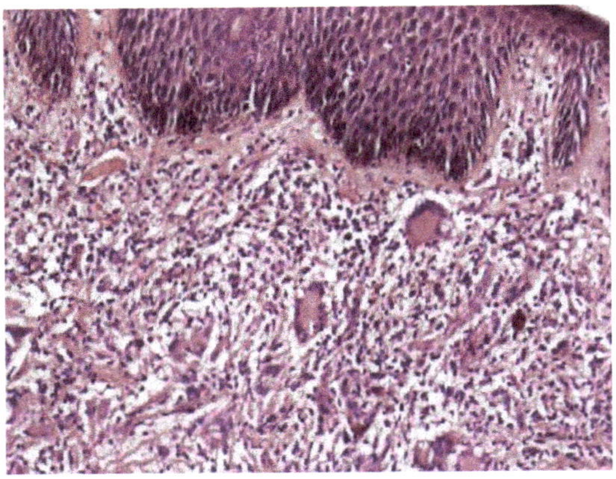

Fig. 19.3 Blastomycosis granuloma (H&E stain) [12]

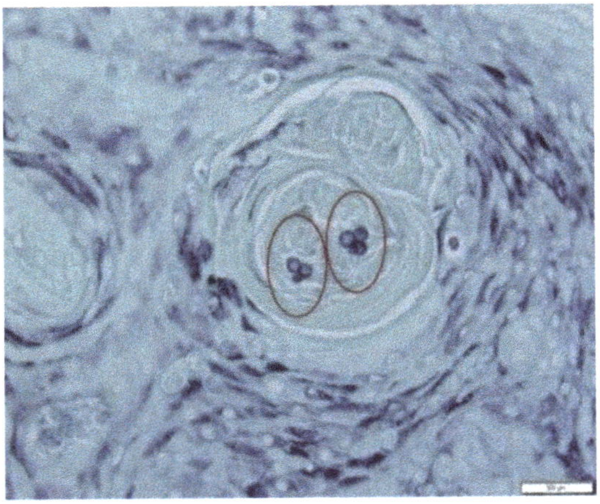

Fig. 19.4 Grocott's methenamine silver (GMS) stain showing budding cells of blastomycosis (red circles) [12]

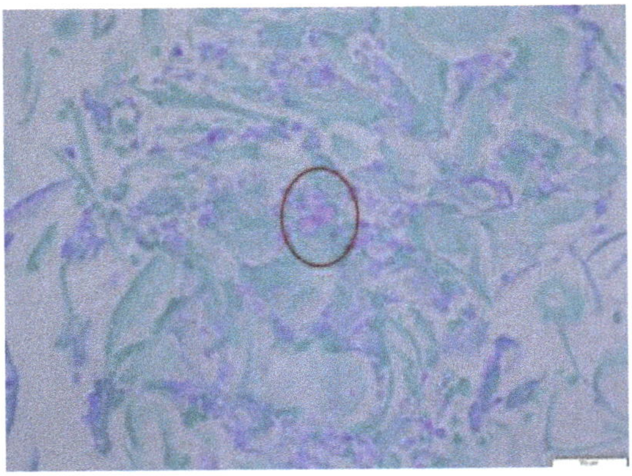

Fig. 19.5 Periodic acid-Schiff (PAS) stain showing blastomycosis with characteristic broad-based budding (red circle) [12]

19.5.3 Imaging

- X-ray Chest and CT thorax-Airspace consolidation is the most common radiologic manifestation of blastomycosis. Other features may be paramediastinal or parahilar mass. Unlike Histoplasmosis, Blastomycotic infections rarely have parenchymal or lymph node calcifications. Lymph node enlargement is also rare. Identification of intermediate-sized nodules (0.5–3 cm) in combination with other manifestations such as consolidation should raise suspicion for fungal disease and may help make the diagnosis [7, 11, 13, 14]. In Interstitial disease, the pattern is usually bilateral and diffuse; it often accompanies a more focal area of consolidation, a mass, or a cavity. The pattern usually has a "tree-in-bud" appearance at CT. Miliary disease has a relatively low reported prevalence (11%–28% in small series) and is usually associated with acute and severe clinical manifestations. Cavitary lesions are uncommon but may occur simulating cavitary tuberculosis [13].
- CT paranasal sinuses and brain-Involvement of paranasal sinuses, skull base bone destruction, along with intracranial spread, are better delineated [14].

19.5.4 Serology

Complement fixation test for antibody detection, using yeast phase antigens have sensitivity of 57%, while immunodiffusion using purified *B. dermatidis* A antigen has a sensitivity of 65–80% [14]. Urine antigen test: It is useful, but cross-reactivity with Histoplasma is high [13, 14].

19.5.5 Molecular Assay

PCR assay use identical primer pair sequences targeting the putative promoter region of the BAD1 (earlier known as WI-1) gene, which codes for an important adhesin molecule and virulence factor. It results in the identification of four haplotypes of *B. dermatitidis*. The recent development of a TaqMan real-time PCR assay using a specific region of the BAD1 promoter encompasses all known haplotypes of *B. dermatitidis* [7, 13, 15].

19.6 Treatment

Treatment of blastomycosis depends on the severity of the infection.

- Mild to Moderate Disease:
  Itraconazole: 200 mg orally three times a day for 3 days, followed by 200 mg orally once a day or two times a day for 6–12 months is used. Fluconazole appears less effective, but 400–800 mg orally once a day may be tried in itraconazole-intolerant patients with the mild disease [13, 14, 16].
- Severe, Disseminated, and Fulminant Infection:
  IV liposomal Amphotericin B 3–5 mg/kg once a day or amphotericin B deoxycholate 0.7–1.0 mg/kg once a day for 1–2 weeks or until improvement is noted. Therapy is changed to oral itraconazole once patients improve; dosage is 200 mg three times a day for 3 days, then 200 mg two times a day for ≥ 12 months [16].

Voriconazole, Isavuconazole, and Posaconazole are active against *B. dermatitidis*, but clinical data are limited, and the role of these drugs has not yet been defined [16].

19.7 Essential Features

- Blastomycosis is caused by inhaling spores of the dimorphic fungus Blastomyces dermatitidis.
- Acute pulmonary blastomycosis presents with consolidative pneumonia.
- Chronic pulmonary blastomycosis is the most common presentation. Grossly often resembles tuberculosis. May present as nodules resembling carcinoma, common in upper lobes. ENT manifestations are common in the form of nasal/ nasopharyngeal granuloma. Middle ear of mastoid disease with temporal bone destruction may occur. Oral cavity or laryngeal leucoplakia may be mistaken for malignancy.
- Fulminant blastomycosis presents with ARDS. May also infect skin and bone.
- At microscopy, the mycelia possess branching hyphae with right-angled conidiophores ending in single round conidia.
- Histopathology reveals mixed acute and granulomatous inflammation caused by large budding yeasts (15–10 μm) with broad-based buds and refractile walls, easily seen with H&E stain. PAS and GMS stains prominently stand out from the fungus.
- Mild to moderate disease is treated with oral itraconazole.
- Severe, disseminated, and fulminant infection is treated with IV Amphotericin B followed by oral itraconazole.

References

1. Seyedmousavi S, et al. Blastomycosis in mammals. Emerg Epizootic Fungal Infect Anim. 2017:159–176. https://doi.org/10.1007/978-3-319-72093-7_8
2. Bradsher RW. Blastomycosis. Infect Dis Clin N Am. 2003;17:21–40.

3. McBride JA, et al. Clinical manifestations and treatment of blastomycosis. Clin Chest Med. 2017; 38(3):435–49. https://doi.org/10.1016/j.ccm.2017.04.006
4. Crampton TL, et al. Epidemiology and clinical spectrum of blastomycosis diagnosed at Manitoba hospitals. Clin Infect Dis. 2002;34:1310–6.
5. Kuzo RS, Goodman LR. Blastomycosis. Semin Roentgenol. 1996;31(1):45–51.
6. Sriram PS, et al. A 19-year- old man with non-resolving pneumonia. Chest. 2004;125:330–3.
7. Zinreich SJ, et al. Fungal sinusitis: diagnosis with CT and MR imaging. Radiology. 1988;169:439–44.
8. Failla PJ, Cerise FP. Blastomycosis: pulmonary and pleural manifestations. South Med J. 1995;88(4):405–10.
9. Gerwin JM, Myer CM. Intranasal blastomycosis. Am J Otolaryngol. 1981;2:267–73.
10. Berkowitz I, Diamond TH. Disseminated blastomyces demartidis infection on a non-endemic area. S Afr Med 717–718.
11. Som PM, et al. Chronically obstructed sinonasal secretions: observations on T1 and T2 shortening. Radiology. 1989;172:515–20.
12. Kuzel AR, et al. Cutaneous, intranasal blastomycosis infection in two patients from Southern West Virginia: diagnostic dilemma. Cureus. 2018;10(1):e2095. https://doi.org/10.7759/cureus.2095
13. Brown LR, et al. Roentgenologic features of pulmonary blastomycosis. Mayo Clin Proc. 1991;66:29–38.
14. Patel RG, et al. Clinical presentation, radiographic findings, and diagnostic methods of pulmonary blastomycosis: a review of 100 consecutive cases. South Med J. 1999;92(3):289–95.
15. Sidamonidze K, et al. Real-time pcr assay for identification of blastomyces dermatitidis in culture and in tissue. J Clin Microbiol. 2012;50(5):1783–6. https://doi.org/10.1128/JCM.00310-12.
16. Kaplan W, Clifford MK. Blastomycosis. I. A review of 198 collected cases in veterans administration hospitals. Am Rev Respir Dis. 1964;89:659–72.

Paracoccidioidomycosis (South American Blastomycosis) 20

Abstract

Paracoccidioidomycosis (PCM) is a systemic granulomatous disease that can affect any organ in the body; however it predominantly affects the organs rich in mononuclear phagocyte system cells—lungs, the mucous membrane of the upper aerodigestive tract, skin, lymphatic system, and adrenal glands. It is caused by thermally dimorphic fungi of the *Paracoccidioides brasiliensis*. It occurs in mucocutaneous form, lymphatic, and visceral forms. In mucocutaneous form, ulcers may involve the nose, oral cavity (Angular-Pupo stomatitis). Ulcers typically have a granular base and mulberry-like appearance. It is associated with granulomas in the upper respiratory tract. In lymphatic form, painless lymphadenopathy involving cervical, supraclavicular, axillary, or hilar nodes is common. Pulmonary involvement is most common in visceral form. Culture shows characteristic "steering wheel" appearance of multiple budding yeasts and "mickey mouse" form (fungi with exogenous sporulation). Histopathology reveals well-formed granulomas composed of cohesive clusters of histiocytes and organized centrally with peripheral admixed lymphocytes with occasional eosinophils and/or neutrophils. The morphology of the fungus can be seen on routine hematoxylin-eosin sections. Detection of IgG antibodies with ELISA and PCR are highly sensitive tests. Oral itraconazole (200 mg per day for 6 months) is the drug of choice.

Synonyms

South American Blastomycosis [1, 2].

20.1 Background

Paracoccidioidomycosis (PCM) is progressive mycosis predominantly affecting organs rich in mononuclear phagocyte system cells—lungs, the mucous membrane of the upper aerodigestive tract, skin, lymphatic system, and adrenal glands. It is caused by *Paracoccidioides brasiliensis*. The two earliest cases of PCM were reported in 1908 by Adolpho Lutz, who described the clinical manifestations and anatomopathological findings of the disease and isolated its aetiological agent in pure cultures [3]. Symptoms are skin ulcers, nasal and paranasal sinus granulomas, oral ulcers, adenitis, and abdominal organ involvement. Diagnosis is by clinical and microscopic evaluation and confirmed by culture. Treatment is with azoles (e.g. itraconazole), Amphotericin B, or Sulfonamides [1, 2, 4].

S. V. Nemade, K. J. Shinde, *Granulomatous diseases in Otorhinolaryngology, Head and Neck*,
https://doi.org/10.1007/978-981-16-4047-6_20

20.2 Epidemiology

More than 15,000 cases of paracoccidioidomycosis have been recorded since 1930. Paracoccidioidomycosis occurs only in discrete foci in South and Central America, most often in men aged 20 to 50, especially coffee growers of Colombia, Venezuela, and Brazil. An estimated 10 million people in South America are infected.

Although a relatively unusual opportunistic infection, paracoccidioidomycosis sometimes occurs in immunocompromised patients but infrequently occurs in those with AIDS [1, 2].

20.3 Etiopathogenesis

Although specific natural sites for *Paracoccidioides brasiliensis* remain undefined, it is presumed to exist in soil as a mold, with infection due to inhalation of conidia (spores produced by the mycelial form of the fungus). Conidia convert to invasive yeasts in the lungs and are assumed to spread to other sites via blood and lymphatics. It leads to disseminated granulomatous inflammation [2, 4].

Paracoccidioidomycosis manifests as-

- An acute/subacute form that usually affects patients of <30 years of age and manifests as disseminated disease (involving the lymph nodes, liver, spleen, and bone marrow).
- An adult form that results from reactivation and that can cause chronic pulmonary disease with pulmonary fibrosis, emphysema, and bullae, nasal and paranasal sinus granulomas, laryngeal granulomas, nasopharyngeal granulomas [4, 5].

20.4 Clinical Features

Most people who inhale conidia of *P. brasiliensis* develop an asymptomatic pulmonary infection. Occasionally it may manifest as acute pneumonia, which may spontaneously resolve. Clinically apparent infections can become chronic and progressive but are not usually fatal. There are three patterns:

- Mucocutaneous Form: Infections most often involve the face, especially at the nasal and oral mucocutaneous borders. It presents as nasal/oral ulcers (Angular-Pupo stomatitis). The ulcer typically has a fine granular base, mulberry-like appearance and surrounding hyperemia (Figs. 20.1, 20.2, and 20.3). Yeasts are usually abundantly present within pinpoint lesions throughout granular bases of slowly expanding ulcers. In 25% of patients, it is associated with cutaneous papules, ulcers, nodules, plaques, and verrucous lesions [5, 7]. The ulcers predominate in the oral cavity. In the oropharynx, lesions affect more frequently the soft palate and anterior and posterior pillars, followed by the lateral and posterior walls, uvula, tongue, and tonsil area. Hypopharyngeal lesions are distributed uniformly among the lateral, anterior and posterior walls and the pyriform sinus, and hyperemia with moriform lesions are the predominant lesion types. All the areas of the larynx may be affected, more frequently the ventricular fold, arytenoid area, vocal cords and the free portion of the epiglottis, followed by the laryngeal surface of the epiglottis, aryepiglottic fold, subglottic area and the laryngeal-ventricle space. Swelling, granular lesions, hyperemia, and moriform lesion, are the most common lesion types, having similar prevalences [3]. In severe cases, it may form granulomas in the nasopharynx or oropharynx.

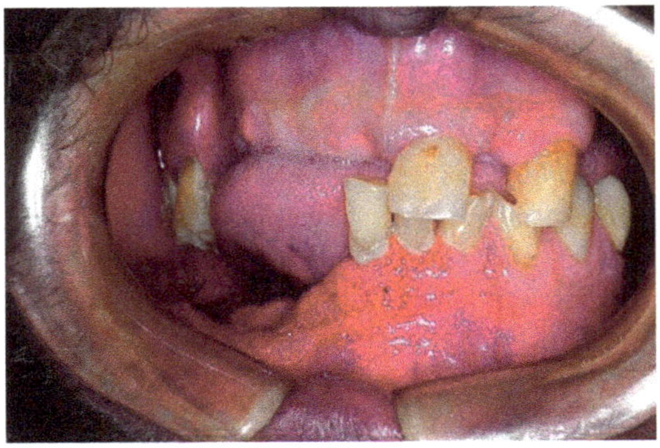

Fig. 20.1 A granulomatous ulcer with hemorrhagic dots and moriform aspect was observed in the posterior mandibular alveolar ridge and in the right jugal mucosa [3]

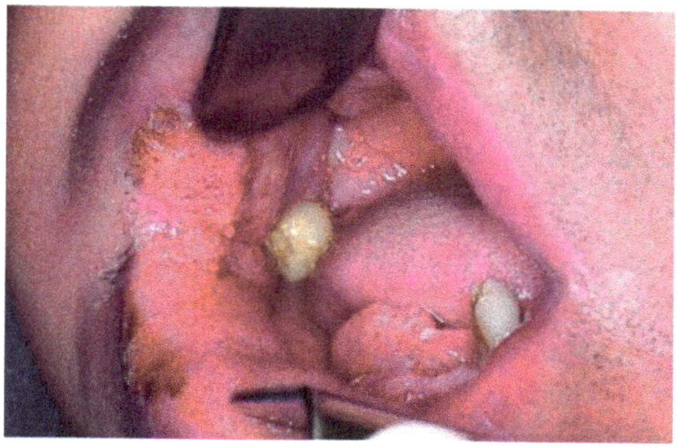

Fig. 20.2 Ulcerated lesion in the jugal mucosa, lips, and buccal commissure [3]

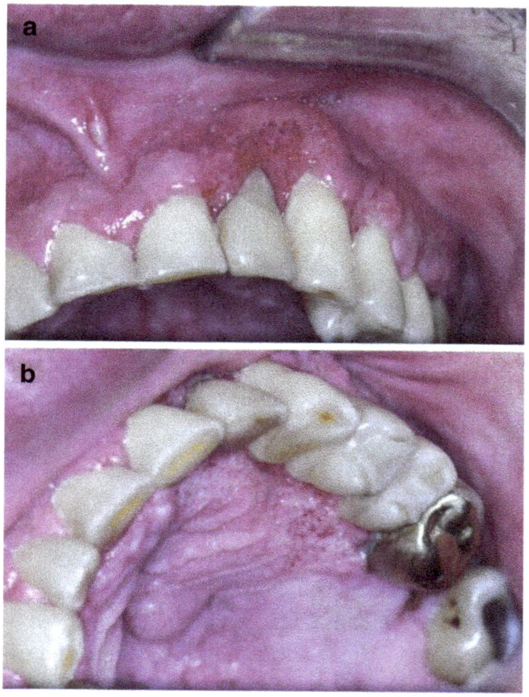

Fig.20.3 (**a**) Erythematous and irregular ulcer, with granular surface, located in the buccal gingiva. (**b**) Moriform ulcer in palatine gingiva [6]

Hoarseness, pain, and difficulty swallowing, burning in the throat, the feeling of a lump or a wound in the mouth and dyspnoea are the most common clinical manifestations. The mucous ulcers may be very painful, especially when eating hot or very salty foods. Regional lymphadenopathy may be associated with ulcers [3, 8].

- Lymphatic Form: Paracoccidioides may spread to the lymph nodes via the hematogenous or lymphatic routes. The fungus is drained from organ lesions to the regional lymph nodes and then spreads to other lymph nodes via the lymphatic system. Cervical, supraclavicular, or axillary nodes enlarge but are usually painless (Fig. 20.4). Lymph nodes may become necrotic and form cutaneous ulcers (Fig. 20.5). Lung infection is associated with hilar lymphadenopathy [6].
- Visceral Form: Lung involvement is particularly relevant due to the occurrence of residual fibrosis as well as because the lungs are the portal of entry for *P. brasiliensis* in almost all of the patients [6]. Typically, focal lesions cause enlargement mainly of the liver, spleen, and abdominal lymph nodes, sometimes causing abdominal pain.

The overall presentation of Paracoccidioidomycosis is often mixed, involving combinations of all three patterns [6, 7, 9].

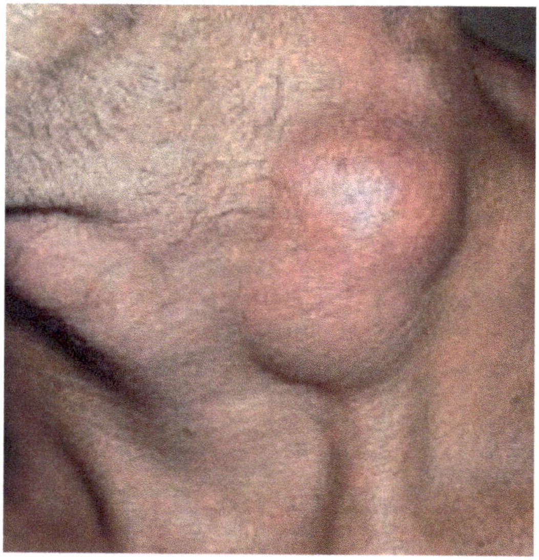

Fig. 20.4 Cervical lymph node involvement by paracoccidioidomycosis

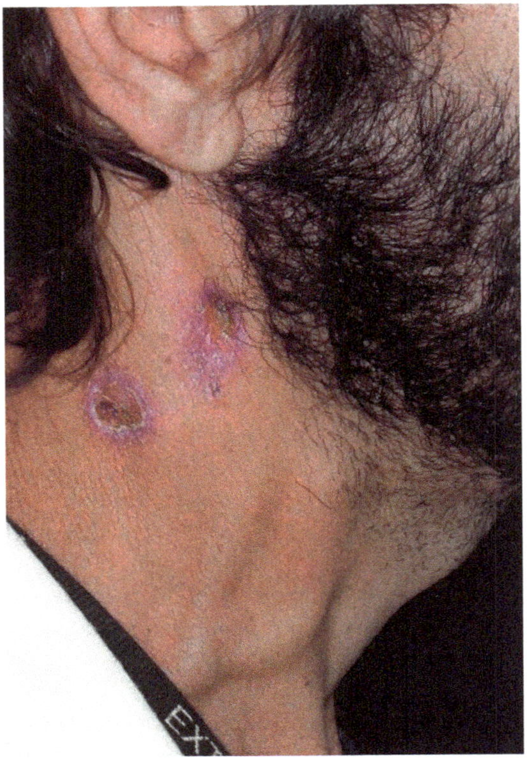

Fig. 20.5 Ulcerated lesion in the right cervical/submandibular region [3]

20.5 Diagnosis

20.5.1 Microscopy and Culture

Culture is diagnostic, although observation of large (often >15 μm) yeasts that form characteristic multiple buds (steering wheel) in specimens provides strong presumptive evidence. Culture of sputum, upper respiratory secretions, and skin lesions are helpful in the diagnosis.

Because culturing *P. brasiliensis* can pose a severe biohazard to laboratory personnel, the laboratory should be notified of the suspected diagnosis. *P. brasiliensis* should be cultured in one of the following culture media: Mycosel (BBL) or Mycobiotic Agar (Difco), SABHI (Difco), Sabouraud agar or yeast extract agar.

Another useful technique is the cell block preparation of sputum in paraffin, followed by staining of sections with hematoxylin-eosin (HE) and methenamine silver (Gomori-Grocott). Methenamine silver stains the fungus wall, thus revealing the presence of fungi with characteristic exogenous sporulation that gives rise to the so-called "mickey mouse" form, strongly suggestive of *P. brasiliensis*. In addition, the "steering wheel" form can be observed, which is pathognomonic for this fungus species (Fig. 20.6). Methenamine silver staining does not allow for assessing the inflammatory response in tissues [6].

20.5.2 Histopathology

Tissue collected through biopsy and stained using the H&E and methenamine silver methods are used to establish the histopathological diagnosis of disease. Hematoxylin and eosin staining revealed multiple well-formed granulomas composed of cohesive clusters of histiocytes and organized centrally with peripheral admixed lymphocytes; however, some eosinophils and/or neutrophils may be detected. The histiocytes characterized by broad, foaming cytoplasm called epithelioid, and giant cells are occasionally observed in inflammatory infiltrate. Both cells may engulf a relatively small number of *P. brasiliensis* forms in granulomas; however, they may also course freely within the connective tissue. Moreover, necrosis is not frequently observed but may occur in some cases [10]. The histopathological examination has a sensitivity of 97% for the diagnosis of paracoccidioidomycosis (Fig. 20.7) [6, 11].

20.5.3 Serology

Antibody testing-Use of polysaccharide antigen in the complement fixation test (CFT), detection of IgG antibodies with ELISA are commonly used tests. Other tests are indirect immunofluorescence (IIF), dot-blotting, and Western blotting [10].

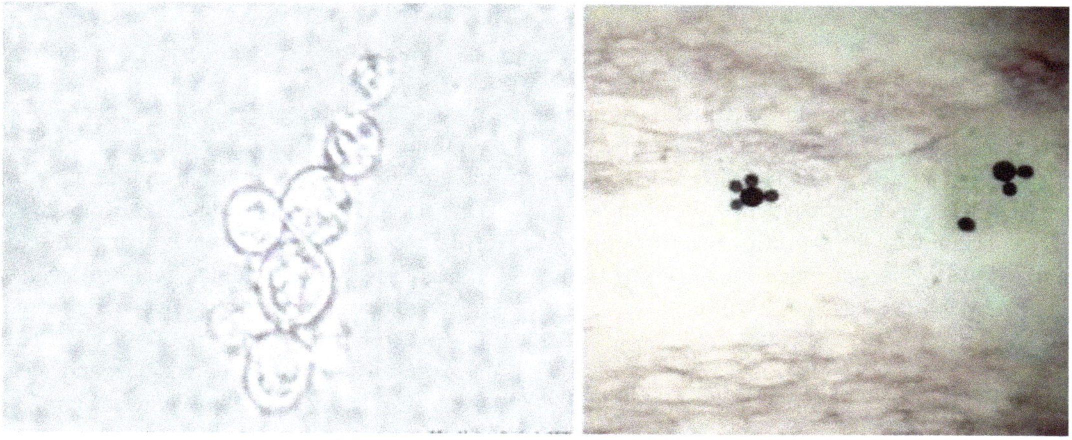

Fig. 20.6 (Left) 10% KOH preparation of sputum showing multiple budding yeast forms, with birefringent walls; (Right)-cell-block preparation of sputum (GMS, ×400) showing the "mickey mouse" and "steering wheel" [3]

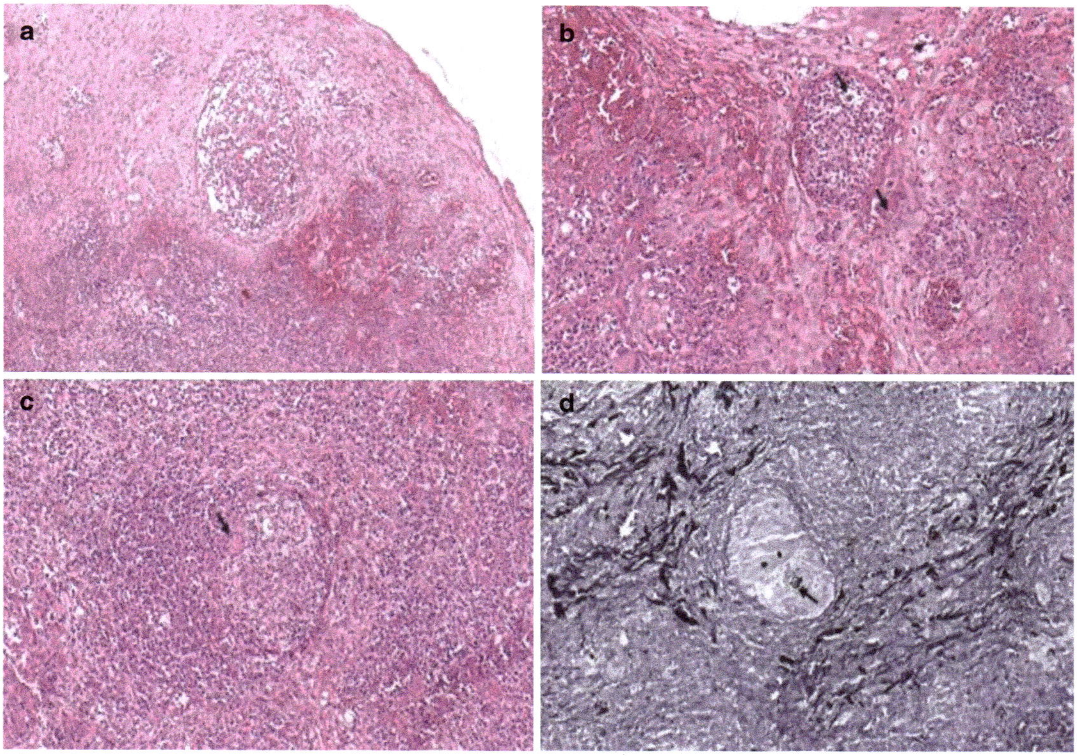

Fig. 20.7 (**a**) Epithelial hyperplasia with the presence of microabscess (hematoxylin-eosin, original magnification, ×100). (**b**) Intraepithelial microabscess with the presence of extracellular yeasts and inside of the multinucleated giant cell (arrows) (hematoxylin-eosin, original magnification, ×200). (**c**) Severe chronic inflammatory reaction with formation of granuloma. Multinucleated giant cells are observed (arrow) (hematoxylin-eosin, original magnification, ×200). (**d**) Yeasts showing globous aspect, with multiple buddings of "mickey mouse" appearance (Gomori-Grocott, original magnification, ×200) [6]

20.5.4 Molecular Assay

PCR and nested PCR allows for confirming the etiology of disease through the identification of DNA fragments specific to *P. brasiliensis*, with no need to culture the fungus [11, 12].

Nested PCR helps to detect *P. brasiliensis* DNA fragments through the use of primers derived from the gene that encodes gp43 and detection of a 196-base pair (bp) sequence [3].

20.5.5 Imaging

Radiography—In active disease, chest radiography reveals interstitial infiltrates (in 64% of cases), or mixed lesions with linear and nodular infiltrate [9, 13, 14].

Computed Tomography—CT neck reveals lymphadenopathy with heterogenous echotexture (Fig. 20.8). High resolution Computerised axial tomography of the chest represents a major contribution to the understanding of PCM lung lesions. In untreated patients, nodules predominate, especially small nodules. Other findings include septum thickening, thick lines, alveolar opacities, blocks of fibrosis, bronchial wall thickening, bronchiectasis, and cavities without fluid content [3, 10].

20.6 Treatment

- Antifungal Drugs:
  Azoles are highly effective. Oral itraconazole (200 mg per day) is generally considered the drug of choice. Therapy is given for 6 months. Oral itraconazole has a cure rate of 95% [15, 16]. Itraconazole is considered superior to ketoconazole because of shorter treatment course, lower toxicity profile, and lower relapse rate (3–5%). Fluconazole is not typically used because of its lower response rates and more frequent relapse. Voriconazole, a newer azole agent, has in vitro activity against the yeast cells of *P. brasiliensis* and has been shown in open-label trials to be an effective agent. Another newer azole, posaconazole, has been used with reported success in this disease [12].

  IV Amphotericin B (liposomal AmB-2–5 mg/kg/day or AmB deoxycholate-0.5–1 mg/kg/day) can also eliminate the infection and is often used in very severe cases as the initial therapy followed by oral azole therapy [12].
- Sulfonamides (Sulfamethoxazole-Trimethoprim):
- Trimethoprim-sulfamethoxazole (TMP-SMX) is typically dosed as one double-strength tablet (160 mg trimethoprim, 800 mg sulfa-

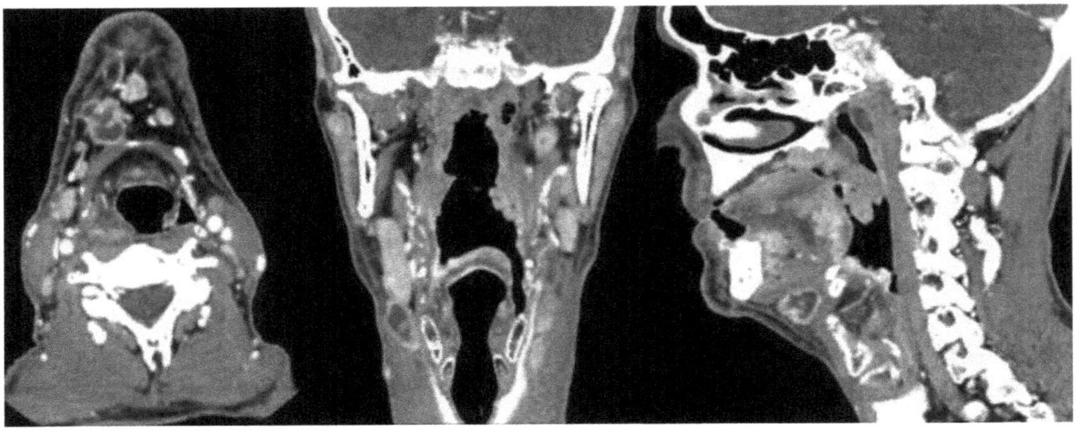

Fig. 20.8 Computed tomography cuts showing lymph node enlargement as a hypodense and heterogeneous image in the right submandibular region [3]

methoxazole) twice daily (8–10 mg/kg/day [based on trimethoprim] for children) [10, 15–17]. Compared to itraconazole in a recent study, TMP-SMX treatment was associated with a 51% cure rate (vs. 95% for itraconazole) with a treatment duration of 4–5 years (vs. 6–12 months for itraconazole) [10].

- β-glucan was found to behave as a powerful inducer of the production of tumor necrosis factor alpha (TNF-α) and interferon-gamma (IFN-γ) in B LB/c mice these findings may account for the adjuvant effects of β-glucan in the treatment of PCM. For this reason, β-glucan should be indicated for treatment of severe forms of the disease, provided the patient's TNF-α levels can be monitored, as it is harmful to patients in excess [18].
- In the past, PCM treatment was divided into two phases: initial treatment, in which amphotericin B was used until a clinical cure was achieved and/or cumulative dose limits were reached, and complementary treatment, in which sulphonamides derivatives were initiated and used until a serological cure was achieved. Currently, both azoles and SMX are used throughout the course of treatment [10]. In general, clinical cure occurs in a relatively short time and gives patients the false impression that they are fully healed. For this reason, they should be made aware of the risk of recrudescence and of the consequent need for prolonged treatment and periodical assessment.

20.7 Essential Features

- Paracoccidioidomycosis (South American Blastomycosis) is progressive mycosis of the lungs, skin, mucous membranes, lymph nodes, and adrenal glands caused by *Paracoccidioides brasiliensis*.
- Mucocutaneous Form: Ulcers may involve the nose, oral cavity (Angular-Pupo stomatitis). Ulcers typically have a granular base and mulberry-like appearance; associated with cutaneous papules, ulcers, nodules, plaques, and verrucous lesions. Ulcers may also involve the oropharynx, hypopharynx, and larynx. In severe cases, granulomas may form in the upper respiratory tract.
- Lymphatic Form—Painless lymphadenopathy involving cervical, supraclavicular, axillary, or hilar nodes is common.
- Visceral Form—Pulmonary involvement is commonly followed by focal lesions in liver, spleen, and abdominal lymph nodes.
- Culture of sputum, upper respiratory secretions, and skin lesions on Mycosel (BBL) or Mycobiotic Agar (Difco), SABHI (Difco), Sabouraud agar or yeast extract agar typically show multiple budding yeasts (steering wheel appearance).
- Cell block (paraffin block) stained with methenamine silver shows "mickey mouse" form (fungi with exogenous sporulation).
- Histopathology reveals well-formed granulomas composed of cohesive clusters of histiocytes and organized centrally with peripheral admixed lymphocytes; with occasional eosinophils and/or neutrophils. The morphology of the fungus can be seen on routine hematoxylin-eosin sections. GMS stain can be helpful to highlight the organism.
- Serology: Complement fixation test (CFT), detection of IgG antibodies with ELISA are commonly used tests.
- PCR is highly sensitive to classify the organism.
- HRCT thorax is particularly helpful in pulmonary lesions.
- Oral itraconazole (200 mg per day for 6 months) is the drug of choice.

References

1. Marques-da-Silva SH, et al. Occurrence of Paracoccidioides lutzii in the Amazon region: description of two cases. Am J Trop Med Hyg. 2012;87(4):710–4.
2. Lupi O, et al. Tropical dermatology: fungal tropical diseases. J Am Acad Dermatol. 2005;53(6):931–51. quiz 952-4
3. Antonio Dionizio De Albuquerque Neto, et al. Treatment of paracoccidioidomycosis in the maxillofacial region: a report of 5 cases. Case Rep

Otolaryngol. 2018;2018:1524150. https://doi.org/10.1155/2018/1524150
4. Brazão-Silva MT, et al. Paracoccidioidomycosis: a series of 66 patients with oral lesions from an endemic area. Mycoses. 2011;54(4):e189–95.
5. Bellissimo-Rodrigues F, et al. Endemic paracoccidioidomycosis: relationship between clinical presentation and patients' demographic features. Med Mycol. 2013;51(3):313–8.
6. Reydson-Alcides-de Lima Souza, et al. Oral paracoccidioidomycosis in a non-endemic region from Brazil: a short case series. J Clin Exp Dent. 2019;11(10):e865–e870. https://doi.org/10.4317/jced.56199
7. Azenha MR, et al. A retrospective study of oral manifestations in patients with paracoccidioidomycosis. Braz Dent J. 2012;23(6):753–7.
8. Weber S, et al. Complete perforation of hard palate in a paracoccidioidomycosis (PBM) patient. Rev Soc Bras Med Trop. 2000;33(Suppl 1):460–1.
9. Pereira RM, et al. Fatal disseminated paracoccidioidomycosis in a two-year-old child. Rev Inst Med Trop Sao Paulo. 2004;46(1):37–9.
10. Rinaldo Poncio Mendes, et al. Current perspectives from Brazil. Open Microbiol J. 2017;11:224–82. https://doi.org/10.2174/1874285801711010224
11. Moreto TC, et al. Accuracy of routine diagnostic tests used in paracoccidioidomycosis patients at a university hospital. Trans R Soc Trop Med Hyg. 2011;105(8):473–8. https://doi.org/10.1016/j.trstmh.2011.03.001.
12. Queiroz-Telles F, et al. An open-label comparative pilot study of oral voriconazole and itraconazole for long-term treatment of paracoccidioidomycosis. Clin Infect Dis. 2007;45(11):1462–9.
13. de Almeida SM, et al. Central nervous system paracoccidioidomycosis: clinical features and laboratorial findings. J Infect. 2004;48(2):193–8.
14. Freitas RM, et al. Pulmonary paracoccidioidomycosis: radiology and clinical-epidemiological evaluation. Rev Soc Bras Med Trop. 2010;43(6):651–6.
15. Borges SR, et al. Itraconazole vs. trimethoprim-sulfamethoxazole: a comparative cohort study of 200 patients with paracoccidioidomycosis. Med Mycol. 2014;52(3):303–10.
16. Travassos LR, et al. Treatment options for paracoccidioidomycosis and new strategies investigated. Expert Rev Anti-Infect Ther. 2008;6(2):251–62.
17. Ollague JM, et al. Paracoccidioidomycosis (South American blastomycosis) successfully treated with terbinafine: first case report. Br J Dermatol. 2000;143(1):188–91.
18. Marcondes-Machado J. Avaliação dos níveis séricos de IL-12p40, α-TNF e γ-IFN em camundongos B LB/c tratados pela β-1,3 poliglicose, com ou sem infecção aguda pelo Toxoplasma gondii. Botucatu, SP: Faculdade de Medicina da Universidade Estadual Paulista; 2001. livre-docência.

21 Leishmaniasis

Abstract

Leishmaniasis is a vector-borne tropical disease caused by different species of protozoan parasites of the genus Leishmania. It is transmitted through the bites of female insect vectors, the phlebotomine sand flies. The clinical manifestations of leishmaniasis in humans depend on complex interactions between the virulence characteristics of the infecting Leishmania species and the immune responses of its host. The disease can manifest in three major clinical forms. The cutaneous form is associated with erythematous and odematous ulcers. The auricular ulcer is typically known as chiclero's ulcer with perichondritis. The mucocutaneousform includes granulomatous changes and destruction in the upper airway. Visceral leishmaniasis or kala-azar is highly fatal if untreated. There are other forms also which include diffuse cutaneous leishmaniasis (DCL) and post kala-azar dermal leishmaniasis (PKDL), and these are often linked to host immune status. Smear stained with Leishman stain or Giemsa stain reveals amastigotes. Histopathology identifies parasites along with granulomatous infiltrate. Fluorescent antibody tests or PCR using species-specific primers are also useful. For treatment of leishmaniasis the most commonly used drugs have been pentavalent antimonials, oral miltefosine, amphotericin B, liposomal amphotericin B and paromomycin. Currently, the only means to treat and control leishmaniasis is by rational medications and vector control.

Synonyms
Leishmaniosis.

21.1 Background

Physicians in the Indian subcontinent would describe it as kala-azar (pronounced kala-azar, the Urdu, Hindi, and Hindustani phrase for "black fever," kala meaning black and azar meaning fever or disease). Some fifteenth- and sixteenth-century texts from the Inca period and from Spanish colonials mention "valley sickness," "Andean sickness," or "white leprosy," which are likely to be the cutaneous form.

Leishmaniasis is caused by protozoan parasites belonging to the genus Leishmania. The infection is transmitted by the bite of phlebotomine sandflies, and a wide range of domestic and wild vertebrates and humans serve as reservoirs of infection. The infecting Leishmania species determines the clinical presentation of disease, of which there are three dominant clinical forms: cutaneous leishmaniasis, mucocutaneous leishmaniasis (MCL), and visceral leishmaniasis [1, 2]. The mucocutaneous disease is a chronic

S. V. Nemade, K. J. Shinde, *Granulomatous diseases in Otorhinolaryngology, Head and Neck*,
https://doi.org/10.1007/978-981-16-4047-6_21

inflammatory process involving the nasal, pharyngeal, and laryngeal mucosa, which can lead to extensive tissue destruction. The disease affects some of the poorest people on earth and is associated with malnutrition, population displacement, poor housing, an immunocompromised condition and lack of financial resources [1–3].

21.2 Epidemiology

Leishmaniasis is endemic throughout the Middle East, North Africa, parts of Europe, and Central and South America [1, 2]. The worldwide prevalence is 4–12 million. The annual global incidence is 0.2–0.4 million cases of visceral leishmaniasis (VL) and 0.7–1.2 million cases of cutaneous leishmaniasis (CL) [3]. In some 98 countries [4]. About 2 million new cases and between 20 and 50 thousand deaths occur each year. Over 90% of mucocutaneous leishmaniasis cases occur in Bolivia, Brazil, Ethiopia, and Peru. It shows no age or gender predilection [4].

21.3 Etiopathogenesis

Leishmaniasis is transmitted by the bite of infected female phlebotomine sandflies, which can transmit the protozoa Leishmania. The sandflies inject the infective stage, metacyclic promastigotes, during blood meals. Metacyclic promastigotes that reach the puncture wound are phagocytized by macrophages and transform into amastigotes. Amastigotes multiply in infected cells and affect different tissues, depending in part on the host and in part on which Leishmania species is involved.

Mucocutaneous disease is a chronic inflammatory process involving the nasal, pharyngeal, and laryngeal mucosa, which can lead to extensive tissue destruction. MCL develops as a complication of cutaneous leishmaniasis, parasites disseminating from the primary cutaneous lesion via lymphatic vessels and blood to reach the upper respiratory tract mucosa. Such metastatic spread more commonly occurs with species belonging to the *L. viannia* subgenus (formerly known as the *L. braziliensis* complex), which are present in tropical forested areas of central and South America [1, 2].

21.4 Clinical Features

The symptoms of leishmaniasis are skin sores which erupt weeks to months after the person is bitten by infected sand flies.

Leishmaniasis may be divided into the following types: [5, 6]

A. Cutaneous Leishmaniasis
   It is the most common form, which causes an open sore at the bite sites, which heals in a few months to a year and a half, leaving an unpleasant-looking scar. Diffuse cutaneous leishmaniasis produces widespread skin lesions which resemble leprosy and may not heal on its own (Fig. 21.1) [2, 4]. The erythematous, oedematous ulcer with bleeding bed covered with fibrin is characteristic feature and may mimic carcinoma (Fig. 21.2). The ulcer on the auricle is called as chiclero's ulcer (Fig. 21.2). It may be complicated with bacterial perichondritis with cartilage destruction and deformity (Fig. 21.3). When the ear is affected (chiclero's or gum tree harvester's ulcer), it results in mutilations in the form of notches or clefts.
B. The Mucocutaneous Leishmaniasis (MCL)-
   It causes both skin and mucosal ulcers with damage primarily of the nose and mouth [3, 8, 9]. It is almost always secondary to skin lesions, generally appear months or years after the resolution of lesions on the skin. There seems to be a predilection for the nose, leading to the appearance of septal granuloma resulting in perforation of the nasal septum (Fig. 21.4). Therefore, the most common complaints in these cases are nasal obstruction, epistaxis, rhinorrhea, and nasal crusts. There may be the partial or total destruction of the nasal pyramid with the fall of the tip of the nose for the destruction of the septum and the cartilaginous framework, producing the so-called "bulldog face." Granulomatous ulcer-

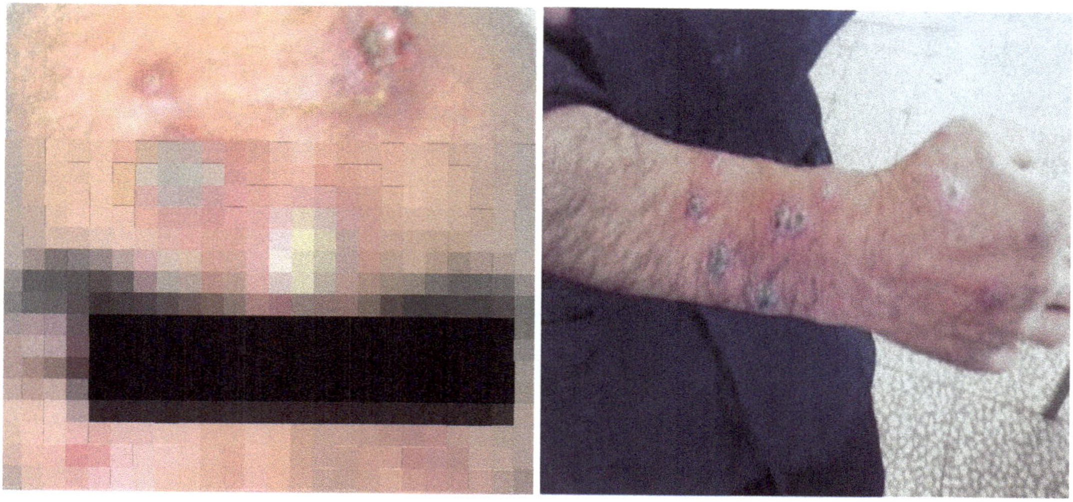

Fig. 21.1 Patient with lesions on the face, right eyelid, and some lesions on the hands [7]

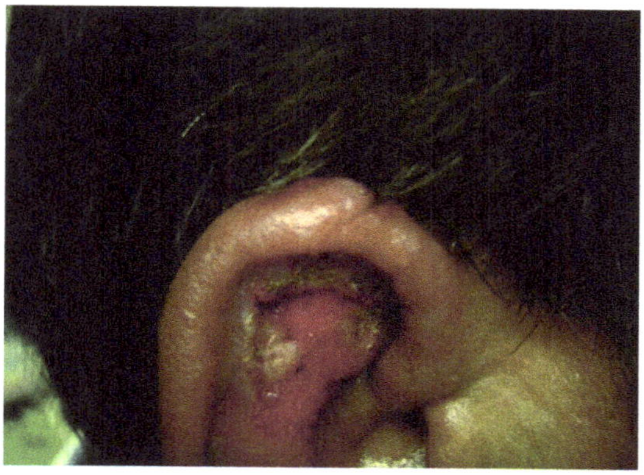

Fig. 21.2 Chiclero's ulcer with bleeding bed and periphery covered by fibrin [5, 6]

ations in the oral mucosa, pharynx, and larynx presents with sore throat, hoarseness of voice, coughing, dyspnoea due to glottis edema, and drooling [10, 11]. The oral cavity and pharyngeal lesions mainly involve the posterior portion of the hard palate and the soft palate (Fig. 21.5). These granulomatous lesions are irregular, called "cobble street," and in some cases, the uvula may be destroyed [10, 11].

C. Visceral Leishmaniasis or Kala-Azar ("Black Fever")-

It is potentially fatal if untreated. Manifestations can occur few months to years after infection [2, 12]. Parasites spread throughout the reticu-

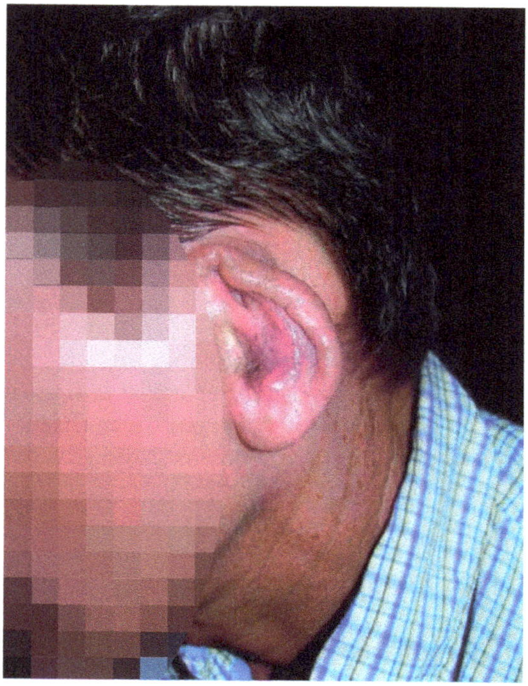

Fig. 21.3 Atrophic stage of chiclero's ulcer with scarring of the ear and deformity [6]

loendothelial system, causing fever, malaise, hepatosplenomegaly, anorexia, pancytopenia, hypergammaglobulinemia. It usually spares skin except for irregular areas of dark pigmentation (kala-azar means black sickness).

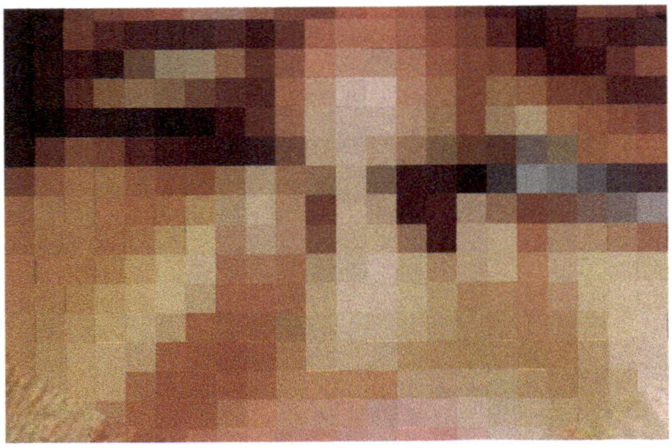

Fig. 21.4 Nasal septum perforation secondary to granuloma on the septum.. Instrument passing through the perforation [10]

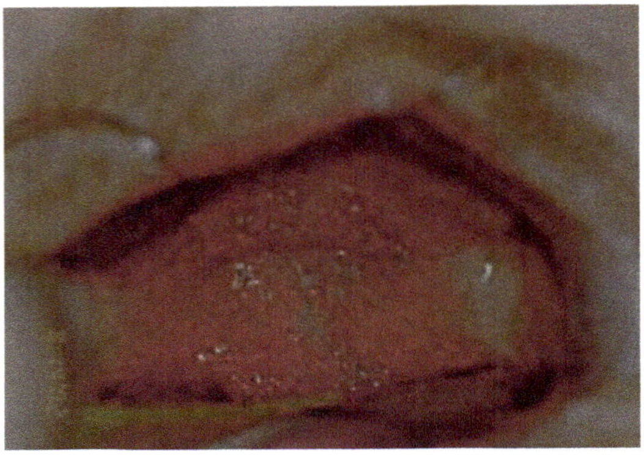

Fig. 21.5 Granulomatous Lesion on palate extending to the pharynx [10]

Leishmaniasis is considered one of the classic causes of a markedly enlarged spleen (splenomegaly); it may even become larger than the liver in severe cases [2, 12].

21.5 Diagnosis

21.5.1 Microscopy

Leishmaniasis is diagnosed by direct visualization of the amastigotes (Leishman–Donovan bodies). Buffy-coat preparations of peripheral blood or aspirates from bone marrow, spleen, lymph nodes, or skin lesions should be spread on a slide to make a thin smear and stained with Leishman stain or Giemsa stain (pH 7.2) for 20 min. Amastigotes are seen within blood and spleen monocytes or, less commonly, in circulating neutrophils and in aspirated tissue macrophages (Figs. 21.6 and 21.7). They are small, round bodies 2–4 μm in diameter with indistinct cytoplasm, a nucleus, and a small, rod-shaped kinetoplast (Fig. 21.8). Occasionally, amastigotes may be seen lying free between cells [7, 12, 13].

21.5.2 Histopathology

Biopsy from skin lesions, upper respiratory lesions, mucocutaneous lesions or viscera such as

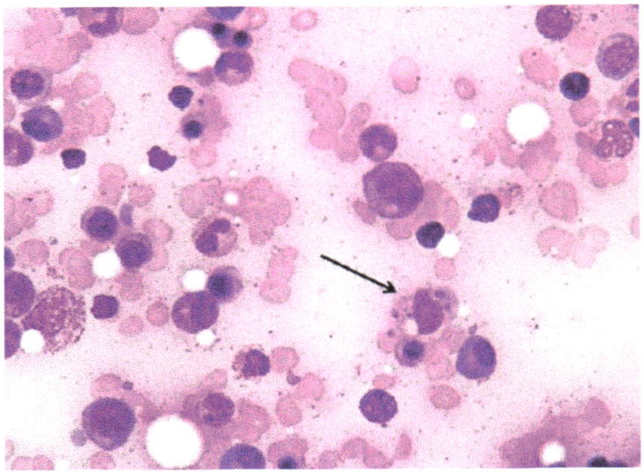

Fig. 21.6 Bone marrow aspirate smear: Amastigote form of Leishmania (arrow) (×400 Giemsa)

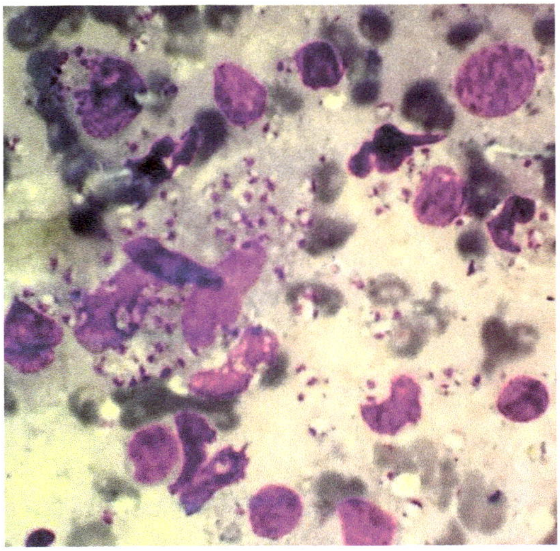

Fig. 21.7 Direct smear from skin lesions positive for leishman bodies (Giemsa stain) [7]

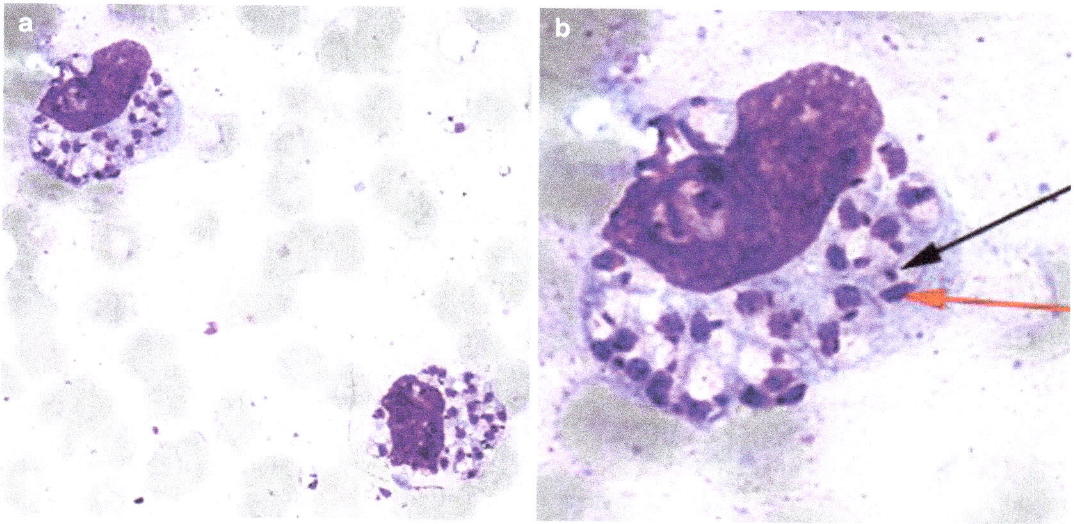

Fig. 21.8 (**a**) and (**b**) Light-microscopy examination of a stained bone marrow specimen from a patient with visceral leishmaniasis—showing a macrophage (a special type of white blood cell) containing multiple Leishmania amastigotes (the tissue stage of the parasite). Note that each amastigote has a nucleus (red arrow) and a rod-shaped kinetoplast (black arrow). Visualization of the kinetoplast is important for diagnostic purposes

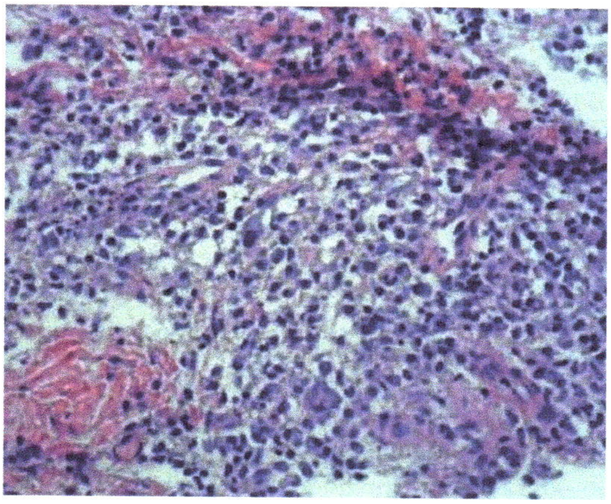

Fig. 21.9 Inflammatory process with lymph-plasmacytic predominance and possible leishmaniasis [10]

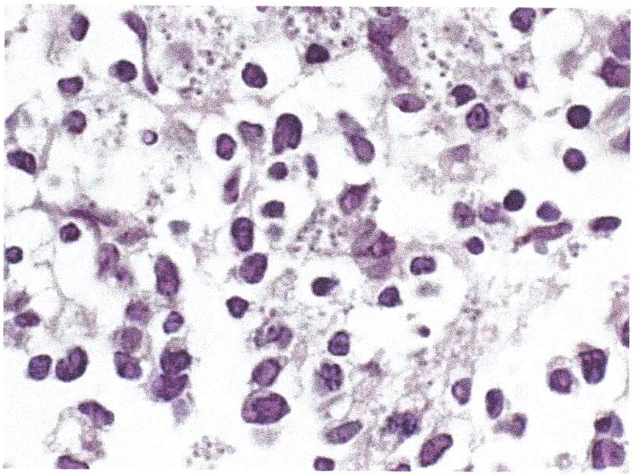

Fig. 21.10 Needle biopsy of a lymph node showing histiocytes containing abundant Leishmania amastigotes (H-E ×1000)

spleen or liver may reveal typically dense granulomatous infiltrate and contains histiocytes and plasma cells (Fig. 21.9) predominantly. In the early stages, numerous amastigotes typically distend histiocytes and impart quite a characteristic diagnostic morphology (Fig. 21.10).

21.5.3 Serology

Specific leishmanial antigens prepared from cultures have been used in a number of tests. Serologic detection of antibodies to recombinant K39 antigen using a direct agglutination test

(DAT), immunofluorescence assay (IFA), or enzyme-linked immunosorbent assay (ELISA) has been shown to be highly sensitive and specific in diagnosing visceral leishmaniasis and post-kala-azar dermal leishmaniasis. A nitrocellulose dipstick test has also been used with K39 testing. DAT detects the specific immunoglobulin M (IgM) antibody at an early stage and has been found to be useful in the detection of both clinical and subclinical leishmaniasis infections [14, 15].

Electrophoresis—In visceral leishmaniasis, an elevated serum immunoglobulin level with polyclonal spike may be present on serum plasma electrophoresis (SPEP). The visceral disease was traditionally diagnosed based on the addition of formaldehyde to a serum sample (aldehyde test), which would increase the viscosity secondary to excessive immunoglobulins.

Cellulose acetate electrophoresis is a well-standardized method for determining the species of parasites grown from clinical samples. Although this test is standardized, it requires experience and special facilities; therefore, it is available only in highly specialized diagnostic facilities [16].

21.5.4 Molecular Assay

Several different polymerase chain reaction (PCR) tests are available for the detection of Leishmania DNA. With this assay, a specific and sensitive diagnostic procedure is finally possible. The most sensitive PCR tests use minicircle kinetoplast DNA found in the parasite.

Polymerase chain reaction is also used to differentiate *L. viannia* subgenus infections, which are associated with the greatest risk of MCL [5]. The different species of the parasite can be differentiated by isoenzyme analysis, DNA sequence analysis, or monoclonal antibodies [12, 13].

21.5.5 Montenegro Skin Test

The Montenegro skin test is a tool for determining the degree of exposure and immunity to the parasite. It is also known as Leishmanin Skin Test. Injection of killed promastigotes (Montenegro test) or preparations made from killed promastigotes induce a DTH reaction in individuals with prior exposure to Leishmania. 5-mm area of induration over 48–72 h suggests past infection.

In active visceral leishmaniasis, the test is almost always negative, and a positive result usually appears 2–24 months after clinical recovery. Thus this test has no role in the diagnosis of the acute disease [17].

21.5.6 Imaging

CT and MRI have role particularly in the visceral form of the disease that typically reveals hepatosplenomegaly and multiple hypoechoic nodular splenic lesions that appear hypodense on CT. T2-weighted MRI sequences show a markedly inhomogeneous intensity of the parenchyma, seemingly caused by multiple ill-defined and heterogeneous hypointense nodules [18].

21.6 Treatment

The treatment of leishmaniasis depends on several factors, including the type of disease, concomitant pathologies, parasite species and geographic location. Leishmaniasis is a treatable and curable disease, which requires an immunocompetent system because medicines will not get rid of the parasite from the body, thus the risk of relapse if immunosuppression occurs [19, 20].

The effective treatment with satisfactory clinical and microbiological results for all clinical forms of leishmaniasis is achieved with current intravenous pentavalent antimonials ($Sb5+$) in the form of sodium stibogluconate (SSG; Pentostam, UK) or meglumine antimoniate (Glucantime, France). Trivalent antimonials are prescribed parenterally (repodral and anthiomaline) in a dose of 2–3 mL (0.02–0.03 g) on alternate days for 12–20 days, pentavalents such as meglumine (glucantime) in a dose of 10–60 mg/kg for 12 days to 3 weeks (or until clinical and parasitological evidence of cure), and SSG (Pentostam) in a dose of 20 mg/kg per day for 30 days, not necessarily consecutive; this periodicity can be determined by the onset of side effects. The drug should be diluted in 200 mL of 5% dextrose and delivered in 1 h. Intravenous administration is used only in hospitalized patients, as intramuscular injection is very painful, but it is the only feasible alternative for treatment on a large scale. For treatment of the mucocutaneous forms, the duration of a parenteral therapeutic regimen with antimonials is 28 days, achieving a cure rate of about 75% [11].

In patients resistant to pentavalent antimonials, Paromomycin, an antiparasitic agent, is an effective treatment for leishmaniasis. It is given in the dose of 15–20 mg/kg/day for 21 days.

For visceral leishmaniasis in India, South America, and the Mediterranean, liposomal Amphotericin B (7.5 mg/kg) is the recommended treatment and is often used as a single dose [19]. Rates of cure with a single dose of Amphotericin have been reported as 95% [19]. In India, almost all infections are resistant to pentavalent antimonials. Oral Fluconazole or Itraconazole appears effective against certain species such as *L. major* and *L. tropica* [20]. Miltefosine is orally and topically active alkyl-phosphocholine compound with potential ant-neoplastic activity. Dose of 50 mg 2 times a day (<45 kg weight patient) or three times a day (>45 kg weight patient) for 28 days is effective against both visceral and cutaneous leishmaniasis [11, 21].

Radiofrequency thermotherapy had a cure rate of 87% particularly in cutaneous lesions [20, 22].

21.7 Essential Features

- Vector-borne protozoal disease. Human infection through bite of Phlebotomus sand fly (smaller than mosquitoes); rarely through blood contamination.
- Occurs in three forms: cutaneous, mucocutaneous (may be disseminated), and visceral.
- Cutaneous form—It is usually restricted to face, scalp, arms, or other exposed areas. It can be localized or disseminated (in the immunocompromised state favoring invasion by parasite).
- Mucocutaneous form—Occurs when the primary infection becomes disseminated to the upper respiratory tract, produces lesions of oral, pharyngeal, or nasal mucosa with ulceration, granulomas, and destruction.
- Visceral form—Also known as "kala-azar" is a potentially fatal disease; parasites spread throughout the reticuloendothelial system, causing fever, malaise, hepatosplenomegaly, anorexia, pancytopenia, hypergammaglobulinemia.
- Usually spares skin except for irregular areas of dark pigmentation (kala-azar means black sickness).
- Amastigotes are detectable within macrophages/monocytes. Smear stained with Leishman stain or Giemsa stain reveals amastigotes. Kinetoplast—like a second, small nucleus is a helpful morphologic feature.
- Intradermal delayed hypersensitivity test (Montenegro skin test) suggests past infection, hence no role in the diagnosis of acute infection.
- Histopathology with H&E stain identifies parasites along with granulomatous infiltrate and contains histiocytes and plasma cells predominantly.
- Fluorescent antibody tests using the patient's serum or by PCR using species-specific primers are useful.
- Pentavalent antimonials give effective and satisfactory clinical and microbiological results for all clinical forms of leishmaniasis.
- In patients resistant to pentavalent antimonials, Paromomycin is used with equal efficacy.
- For visceral leishmaniasis, single dose of Amphotericin B (7.5 mg/kg) is the recommended treatment. Miltefosine is an effective alternative to Amphoterecin B.

References

1. Herwaldt BL. Leishmaniasis. Lancet. 1999;354:1191–9.
2. Dedet JP, Pratlong F. Leishmaniasis. In: Cook GC, Zumla A, editors. Manson's tropical diseases. 21st ed. London: Saunders; 2003. p. 1339–64.

3. Okwor I, Uzonna J. Social and economic burden of human Leishmaniasis. Am J Trop Med Hyg. 2016;94(3):489–93. https://doi.org/10.4269/ajtmh.15-0408.
4. Barrett MP, Croft SL. Management of trypanosomiasis and leishmaniasis. Br Med Bull. 2012;104:175–96.
5. David C, et al. Fifteen years of cutaneous and mucocutaneous leishmaniasis in Bolivia: a retrospective study. Trans R Soc Trop Med Hyg. 1993;87:7–9.
6. Torres-Guerrero E, et al. Leishmaniasis: a review. Version 1. F1000Res. 2017;6:750. https://doi.org/10.12688/f1000research.11120.1
7. Doroodgar M, et al. Unusual presentation of cutaneous leishmaniasis: ocular leishmaniasis. Case Rep Infect Dis. 2017;3198547:4 p. https://doi.org/10.1155/2017/3198547
8. Rosbotham JL, et al. Bryceson AD. Imported mucocutaneous leishmaniasis. Clin Exp Dermatol. 1996;21:288–90.
9. Bensoussan E, et al. Comparison of PCR assays for diagnosis of cutaneous leishmaniasis. J Clin Microbiol. 2006;44(4):1435–9.
10. Casalle N, et al. Mucocutaneous leishmaniasis with rare manifestation in the nasal mucosa and cartilage bone septa. Case Rep Infect Dis. 2020;2020:8876020. https://doi.org/10.1155/2020/8876020
11. Ramos-E-Silva M, De Moura Castro Jacques C. Leishmaniasis and other dermatozoonoses in Brazil. Clin Dermatol. 2002;20(2):122–34. https://doi.org/10.1016/s0738-081x(01)00251-6.
12. Lohuis PJ, et al. Leishmania braziliensis presenting as a granulomatous lesion of the nasal septum mucosa. J Laryngol Otol. 1997;111:973–5.
13. De Bruijin MHL, Barker DC. Diagnosis of New World leishmaniasis: specific detection of species of the *Leishmania braziliens* is complex by amplification of kinetoplast DNA. Acta Trop. 1992;52:45–58.
14. Monno R, et al. Recombinant K39 immunochromatographic test for diagnosis of human leishmaniasis. Future Microbiol. 2009;4(2):159–70.
15. Kubar J, Fragaki K. Recombinant DNA-derived leishmania proteins: from the laboratory to the field. Lancet Infect Dis. 2005;5(2):107–14.
16. Srivastava S, et al. Possibilities and challenges for developing a successful vaccine for leishmaniasis. Parasit Vectors. 2016;9:277. https://doi.org/10.1186/s13071-016-1553-y.
17. de Fátima Antonio L, et al. Montenegro skin test and age of skin lesion as predictors of treatment failure in cutaneous leishmaniasis. Rev Inst Med Trop Sao Paulo. 2014;56(5):375–80. https://doi.org/10.1590/S0036-46652014000500002.
18. Clem A. A current perspective on leishmaniasis. J Global Infect Dis. 2010;2:124–6.
19. Pirmez C, et al. Use of PCR in diagnosis of human American tegumentary leishmaniasis in Rio de Janeiro, Brazil. J Clin Microbiol. 1999;37:1819–23.
20. Dorlo TP, et al. Miltefosine: a review of its pharmacology and therapeutic efficacy in the treatment of leishmaniasis. J Antimicrob Chemother. 2012;67(11):2576–97. https://doi.org/10.1093/jac/dks275.
21. Singer C, et al. Imported mucocutaneous leishmaniasis in New York city. Report of a patient treated with amphotericin B. Am J Med. 1975;59:444–7.
22. SVCB G, CHN C. Treatment of cutaneous leishmaniasis with thermotherapy in Brazil: an efficacy and safety study. An Bras Dermatol. 2018;93(3):347–55. https://doi.org/10.1590/abd1806-4841.20186415.

Part III

Idiopathic Granulomatous Diseases

Sarcoidosis

22

Abstract

Sarcoidosis is a multisystem granulomatous disease of unknown etiology. The hallmark is the presence of non-caseating granulomas affecting multiple organs. 10–15% of patients with sarcoidosis demonstrate head and neck manifestations as sinonasal, oropharynx, hypopharynx, skin, eye, salivary glands, neck, larynx, bone, and even intracranial granulomatous infiltration. Systemic complaints of fever, weight loss and fatigue are common. About 90% of patients have pulmonary granulomas with frequent involvement of lymph nodes, skin, liver, eye, central nervous system and heart. Owing to the high variability in clinical manifestations, it can be challenging to diagnose sarcoidosis. Diagnosis of sarcoidosis is based on three elements clinical and radiographic manifestations; exclusion of diseases with similar presentation and identification of non-caseating granulomas on histopathology. Chest X-ray and computed tomography are the most commonly used imaging techniques. Fluorine-18 fluorodeoxyglucose positron emission tomography can also be used to evaluate extrapulmonary manifestations of sarcoidosis or to guide the biopsy site. Blood tests provide supportive information through detection of high serum levels of angiotensin-converting enzyme or soluble interleukin 2 receptor (sIL-2R), which is a marker for increased activation of T cells. Corticosteroids are the mainstay of therapy. In refractory cases, immunosuppressants and TNF inhibitor therapy are implemented.

Synonyms

Benign lymphogranuloma, Besnier Boeck disease, Besnier-Boeck-Schaumann syndrome [1, 2].

22.1 Background

Sarcoidosis is a multisystemic disorder of unknown cause that is characterized by the formation of immune granulomas in involved organs [2]. A prevailing hypothesis is that various unidentified antigens, either infectious or environmental, could trigger an exaggerated immune reaction in genetically susceptible hosts. The clinical expression of sarcoidosis is protean, in particular as regards the number and sites of involved organs. The lung and the lymphatic system are predominantly affected, but virtually every organ may be affected. Otolaryngologic manifestations are identified in 10–15% of patients, the most common being cervical adenopathy. There is a possibility to involve nearly every subsite: sinonasal, oropharynx, hypopharynx, skin, eye, salivary glands, neck, larynx, bone, and even intracranial infiltration [1–3].

S. V. Nemade, K. J. Shinde, *Granulomatous diseases in Otorhinolaryngology, Head and Neck*, https://doi.org/10.1007/978-981-16-4047-6_22

22.2 Epidemiology

The ethnic distribution of sarcoidosis is vast, and a variation has been noticed worldwide. It shows a range of incidence of 5–65 cases per 100,000 population. There is a female predominance, and the age at presentation ranges from 20 to 40 years with a peak at 20–29 years. Sarcoidosis affects the respiratory tract in 80–90% of cases, and the most common presentation is as an incidental finding. Global incidence varies between 10 and 50/1,00,000 population [2–4].

22.3 Etiopathogenesis

The cause of the disease is not known; however, both genetic and environmental factors seem to play a role [1]. As yet, no bacterial, fungal, or viral antigen has been consistently isolated from the sarcoidosis lesions. Sarcoidosis is neither a malignant nor an autoimmune disease.

Sarcoidosis is caused by a granulomatous reaction, an example of a cell-mediated immune response caused by an initial reaction to an unidentified antigen. T cells play a central role in the development of sarcoidosis, as they likely propagate an excessive cellular immune reaction. For example there is an accumulation of CD4 cells accompanied by the release of interleukin (IL)-2 at sites of disease activity. This may manifest clinically by an inverted CD4/CD8 ratio. Pulmonary sarcoidosis is frequently characterized by a $CD4^{+}/CD8^{+}$ ratio of at least 3.5 in bronchoalveolar lavage fluid (BALF). Macrophages initially identify the antigen, and in cohort, with cytokine activity and T cell stimulation, an immune response is mounted, leading to macrophage-giant cell creation. These giant cells mass together, walling off the offending antigen from the rest of the body, a classic feature seen in granulomas [2, 5]. Moreover, both tumor necrosis factor (TNF) and TNF receptors are increased in this disease.

In addition to T cells, B cells also play a role. There is evidence of B cell hyperreactivity with immunoglobulin production.

Soluble HLA class I antigens levels in serum and BALF are higher in patients with sarcoidosis. Active sarcoidosis has also been associated with plasma hypergammaglobulinemia [2].

22.4 Clinical Features

Presentation depends on the extent and severity of the disease and the organ involved. Approximately 5% of cases are asymptomatic and incidentally detected by chest radiography. Systemic complaints of fever, anorexia, weight loss and arthralgias occur in 45% of cases. Pulmonary complaints—dyspnea on exertion, cough, chest pain, and hemoptysis (rare)—occur in 50% of cases [5–7].

The disease follows two patterns:

1. Acute Sarcoidosis: It has a sudden onset, typically undergoes spontaneous remission within 2 years, and is more common in whites. Lofgren's syndrome, which is characterized by bilateral hilar lymphadenopathy, ankle arthritis, erythema nodosum, and constitutional symptoms, may be the presenting picture [8] and carries a very good prognosis. ENT manifestations in this type are limited to cervical lymphadenopathy.
2. Chronic Sarcoidosis: It shows a gradual onset and organ-specific symptoms. Symptoms are mainly attributed to the progression of the granulomatous disease to an irreversible fibrosis, and carry tendency towards symptomatic relapses. Ear Nose Throat manifestations are common in this.

   Ten percent–fifteen percent of patients with sarcoidosis demonstrate head and neck manifestations as sinonasal, oropharynx, hypopharynx, skin, eye, salivary glands, neck, larynx, bone, and even intracranial infiltration [2].

Sinonasal Sarcoid—It shows varied presentation from mucosal ulcers, small granulomas (Fig. 22.1) to extensive sinonasal mass with bony erosions. Common symptoms are rhinorrhea, nasal obstruction, epistaxis, anosmia/hyposmia, and epiphora due to sinonasal granulomatous mass.

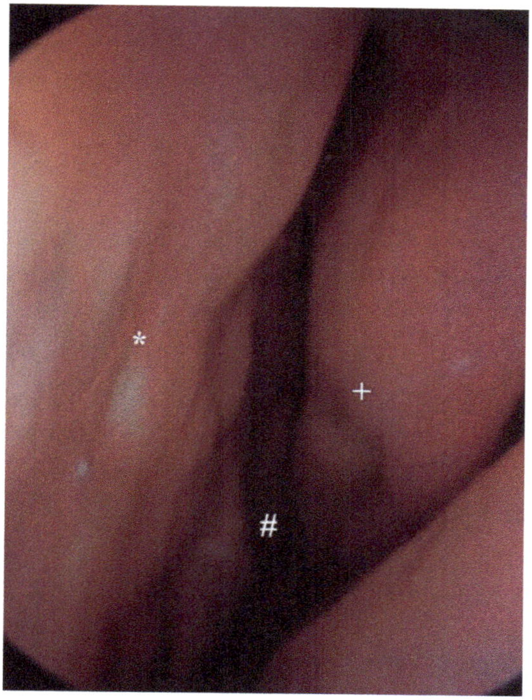

Fig. 22.1 Involvement of the nasal mucosa in sarcoidosis, left nasal cavity (choanal #, nasal septum*, medial nasal concha+) Small granulomas are seen involving nasal septum and medial nasal concha [9]

Laryngeal sarcoid—Isolated laryngeal sarcoidosis is found in only 0.5% of patients. Lesions vary from mucosal ulcers to granulomatous obstructive lesions involving the epiglottis, false vocal cords, true vocal cords and subglottic region [10].

Otological sarcoid—Sensorineural hearing impairment can be secondary to granulomatous meningitis involving the posterior fossa-causing VIII cranial nerve and brainstem dysfunction [11].

Rarely, pinna, external auditory canal, middle ear, and temporal bone may be involved. Otitis media may occur secondary to sinonasal disease and lead to conductive hearing loss [12].

Salivary Gland sarcoid—There is sparse literature regarding salivary gland involvement in sarcoidosis. Reports estimate that 6% of patients can have parotid gland manifestations ranging from xerostomia to facial nerve palsy. The most common presentation, however, is a painless enlargement of the gland. This can at times be associated with Heerfordt's syndrome, also known as uveoparotid fever and sarcoidosis syndrome, characterized by mild fever, painless parotid gland enlargement, cranial nerve involvement, and uveitis. There have been additional reports of chronic bilateral parotid swelling that present with a hard elastic subcutaneous tumor demonstrating sarcoidosis [13].

22.4.1 Other System Involvement

Ocular Manifestations—About 30–60% of sarcoidosis patients develop intraocular inflammatory signs, and bilateral granulomatous uveitis is the most common presentation [14].

Cutaneous Manifestation—Erythema nodosum is the typical nonspecific lesion, which is commonly associated with Lofgren's syndrome. Maculopapular lesions and subcutaneous nodules are associated with systemic disease remission, while plaques and lupus pernio are distinct hallmarks of chronic disease [15].

Neurologic Manifestations (Rare)—Cranial nerve palsies and hypothalamic/pituitary dysfunction may occur. Lymphocytic meningitis is the most common neurologic manifestation [4, 7]. Granulomatous involvement of the brain parenchyma is one of the most serious complications of sarcoidosis. However, attributing neurologic dysfunction to sarcoidosis is challenging, particularly in the absence of identifiable granulomatous disease in other organs. Symptoms of headache, nausea, and ataxia raise suspicion for cerebellar or brainstem involvement. Visual impairment, diplopia, and seizures may also occur. The brainstem is frequently affected, often with granulomatous infiltration of the hypothalamus and pituitary, leading to dysfunction of the hypothalamic-pituitary axis. Leptomeningeal involvement may yield an appearance of aseptic meningitis, and involvement of the spinal cord may result in myelopathy. Spinal cord involvement tends to occur in older patients with sarcoidosis and can be difficult to distinguish from cervical spondylosis. Neuropsychiatric symptoms are uncommon [16].

Endocrine Manifestations—Diabetes insipidus is the most frequently reported endocrine disorder, followed by hyperprolactinemia. Hormonal deficiencies associated with hypothalamic-pituitary sarcoidosis frequently include hypogonadism and diabetes insipidus [15].

Cardiac Manifestations—Cardiac arrest and sudden death may occur. The incidence rate of ventricular tachyarrhythmias requiring implantable cardioverter-defibrillator therapy is estimated to be 15% per year in those patients with cardiac involvement [3, 15].

22.5 Diagnosis

The diagnosis of sarcoidosis begins with clinical suspicion based on history, which is supported with imaging and is finally confirmed with tissue biopsy.

22.5.1 Laboratory Studies

- Serum markers such as serum amyloid A (SAA), soluble interleukin-2 receptor (sIL-2R), lysozyme, angiotensin-converting enzyme (ACE), and the glycoprotein KL-6 have been reported to be markers of sarcoidosis [17].
- Hypercalcemia or hypercalciuria may occur (non-caseating granulomas [NCGs] secrete 1,25 vitamin D). Hypercalcemia is seen in about 10–13% of patients, whereas hypercalciuria is three times more common. An elevated alkaline phosphatase level could suggest hepatic involvement. ACE levels may be elevated.
- Elevated 1, 25-dihydroxyvitamin D levels are associated with protracted treatment in sarcoidosis.

22.5.2 Imaging

- Chest radiography staging system- [18].
  - Stage 0 is normal chest radiography findings.
  - Stage I is bilateral hilar lymphadenopathy (BHL).
  - Stage II is BHL and parenchymal infiltrates.
  - Stage III is parenchymal infiltrates alone.
  - Stage IV is fibrosis.

Air trapping is a common feature in sarcoidosis that can be supported with imaging studies and correlates with evidence of small airways disease on pulmonary function tests [18, 19].

- CT Scan—CT paranasal sinuses (PNS) help to delineate the extent of granulomas and the bony destruction (Fig. 22.2). High-resolution CT (HRCT) scanning of the chest may identify active alveolitis or fibrosis (Fig. 22.3c). It may reveal enlargement of paratracheal and hilar nodes. In parotid involvement, a CT scan typically shows bilateral inhomogeneous parotid gland enlargements with multiple and punctuate small hypodense lesions (Fig. 22.3a, b) [20, 21].
- On Gallium-67 (Ga-67) scintigraphy, the typical uptake patterns of both lambda and panda signs are observed in the case of parotid sarcoidosis. Increased uptake is observed in bilateral paratracheal and hilar nodes along with bilateral parotid glands (Fig. 22.4) [21].

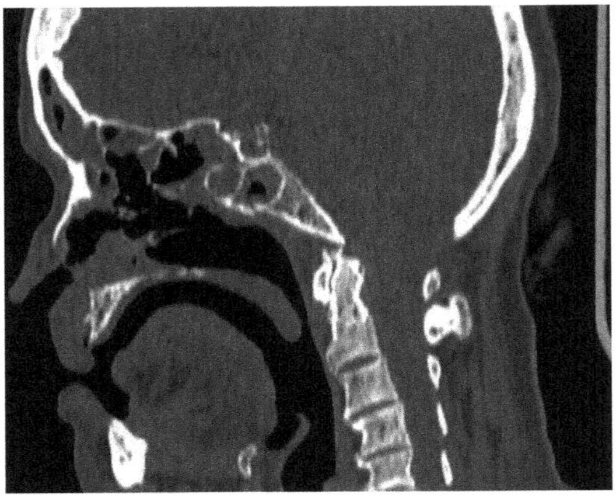

Fig. 22.2 CT PNS (sagital view) of biopsy-proven sinonasal sarcoidosis showing granulomatous mass in the nasal cavity with destruction of palate and nasal septum

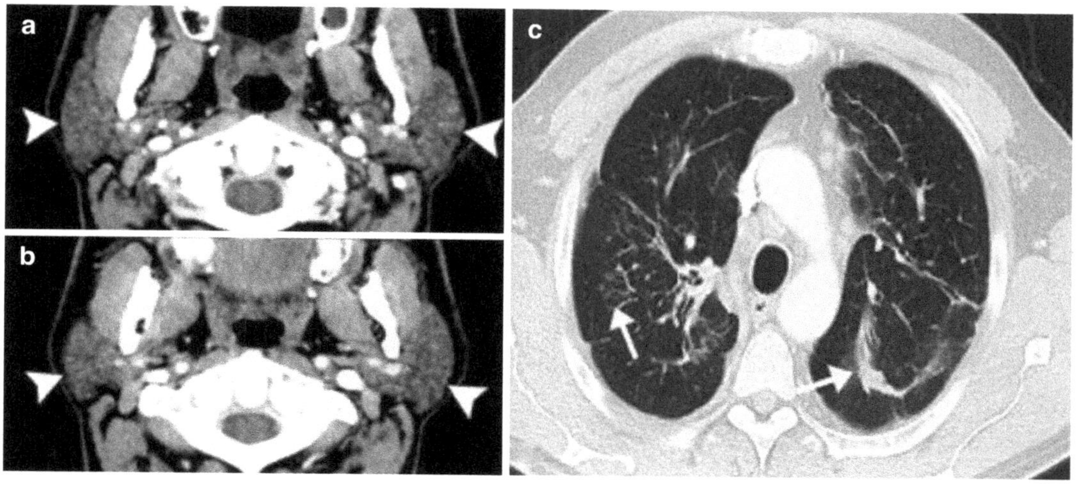

Fig. 22.3 Parotid gland sarcoidosis. On enhanced-CT images, parotid glands show inhomogeneous pattern (white arrowheads) (**a** and **b**) with multiple and punctuate small hypodense lesions. (**c**) shows typical pattern of thoracic disease on CT acquisitions [20]

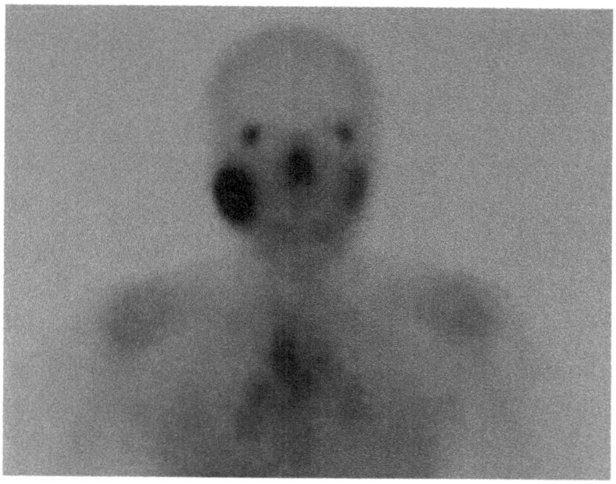

Fig. 22.4 A Gallium-67 scintigraphy demonstrating the typical uptake patterns of panda and lambda signs [21]

- MRI—It is particularly helpful in neurosarcoidosis. A variety of lesions can be seen on brain MRI, including enhancing parenchymal lesions, leptomeningeal thickening or enhancement, and dural involvement. Periventricular white matter lesions may be easily mistaken for lesions from multiple sclerosis [16].
- Whole-body F (18)-fluorodeoxyglucose positron emission tomography (FDG-PET) scanning appears to be of additional value to assess inflammatory activity in patients with persistent symptoms in the absence of signs of serological inflammatory activity and to detect extrathoracic lesions [22]. Whole-body FDG-PET scanning is of value in identifying occult and reversible granulomas in patients with sarcoidosis [23, 24].

22.5.3 Histopathology

The hallmark of sarcoidosis is the development of epithelioid granulomas—biopsy from cervical lymphadenopathy, skin lesions, lung biopsy. Transbronchial biopsy of lung and hilar lymph nodes via fiberoptic bronchoscopy has a high diagnostic yield [25]. The central histologic finding is the presence of non-caseating granulomas (NCGs) (Fig. 22.5) with special stains negative for fungus and mycobacteria. Granulomas in different organs tend to conform to a similar histologic pattern, consisting of a dense collection of epithelioid macrophages and CD4+ T cells, with fewer CD8+ T cells restricted to the periphery [26, 27].

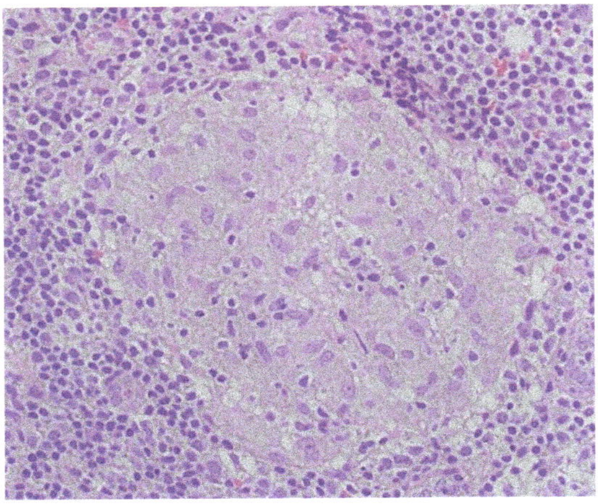

Fig. 22.5 Granuloma without necrosis in a lymph node of a person with sarcoidosis [26]

22.5.4 Other Tests

- Evaluation for neurosarcoidosis typically includes a lumbar puncture. Cerebral spinal fluid analysis may reveal an increased cell count with a lymphocytic pleocytosis, increased protein levels, and oligoclonal bands [16].
- Pulmonary function tests.
- Cardiopulmonary exercise test.
- Kveim–Siltzbach reaction is an earlier tool used in the diagnosis of sarcoidosis. Suspected patients are injected intradermally with a mixture of sarcoid positive lymph or spleen tissue, and, within 2–4 weeks, a clear local nodular granulomatous reaction should appear. When initially implemented, it was found that 80% of patients demonstrated a positive reaction to the test.

22.6 Treatment

Most patients (>75%) require only symptomatic therapy with NSAIDs. Approximately 10% of patients need treatment for the extrapulmonary disease, while 15% of patients require treatment for persistent pulmonary disease.

22.6.1 First-Line Therapy

Corticosteroids are the mainstay of therapy. Generally, prednisolone given daily and then tapered over a 6-month course is adequate for pulmonary disease. Earlier recommendations suggested an initial dose of 1 mg/kg/day of prednisone; however, more recent expert opinions endorse a lower dose (40 mg/day) [5–7]. Topical corticosteroids are effective for ocular disease and sinonasal sarcoidosis or used as an adjuvant to systemic steroid therapy [5–7].

22.6.2 Second-Line Therapy

Noncorticosteroid agents are being increasingly tried. Common indications for the initiation of such agents include steroid-resistant disease, intolerable adverse effects, or patient desire not to take corticosteroids.

- Nonsteroidal anti-inflammatory drugs (NSAIDs) are preferred for the treatment of arthralgias and other rheumatic complaints. Patients with stage I sarcoidosis often require only occasional treatment with NSAIDs with no steroid therapy [28].
- Methotrexate (MTX) has been a successful alternative to prednisone and is a steroid-sparing agent [29].
- Chloroquine and hydroxychloroquine are antimalarial drugs with immunomodulating properties, which have been used for cutaneous lesions, hypercalcemia, neurological sarcoidosis, and bone lesions. Chloroquine has also been shown to be efficacious for the treatment and maintenance of chronic pulmonary sarcoidosis [5, 6, 28].
- Cyclophosphamide has been rarely used with modest success as a steroid-sparing treatment in patients with refractory sarcoidosis [30].
- Azathioprine is another second-line therapy, which is best used as a steroid-sparing agent

rather than as a single-drug treatment for sarcoidosis [30, 31].

- Chlorambucil is an alkylating agent that may be beneficial in patients with progressive disease unresponsive to corticosteroids [32].
- Cyclosporine is a fungal cyclic polypeptide with lymphocyte-suppressive properties and may be of limited benefit in skin sarcoidosis or in progressive sarcoidosis resistant to conventional therapy [33].

22.6.3 Third-Line Therapy

It is preserved for refractory cases.

- Infliximab [34] and thalidomide [20] have also been used for refractory sarcoidosis, particularly for cutaneous disease. Infliximab appears to be an effective treatment for patients with systemic manifestations such as lupus pernio, uveitis, hepatic sarcoidosis, and neurosarcoidosis.
- Tumor necrosis factor (TNF)-inhibitor therapy: Efficacy of anti-TNF agents, such as pentoxifylline and infliximab, in treating this disease is usually limited to patients with systemic manifestations such as lupus pernio, uveitis, hepatic sarcoidosis, and neurosarcoidosis [31, 35].

This approach is successful in ~50% of treated patients in whom the granulomas resolve with no or little remaining organ damage. However, 20–25% of all diagnosed patients develop chronic disease with pulmonary fibrosis. Current therapies target inflammatory pathways and have little effect on fibrosis. This is a major limitation because fibrosis results in increased morbidity and mortality and the need for lung transplantation [31].

22.6.4 Surgical Management

- Lung transplantation is a viable option for patients with stage IV sarcoidosis. Transplantation in such patients should be strongly considered when the forced vital capacity falls below 50% predicted and/or the forced expiratory volume in 1 s falls below 40% predicted [28, 31].
- Endoscopic excision of sinonasal granulomatous mass, functional endoscopic sinus surgery for sinusitis.
- Laryngeal sarcoidosis with airway obstruction may warrant temporary tracheostomy till the completion of pharmacotherapy. Supraglottoplasty using CO_2-laser excision of granulomatous lesions is a technique that removes involved mucosa and allows suturing to promote primary healing of mucosal surfaces [26]. Excision of the involved salivary gland may be required in severe disease [13].

Long-Term follow-up is mandatory to monitor pulmonary function and chest radiography every 6–12 months. Progression or resolution of the disease should be assessed [4, 5].

22.7 Essential Features

- Sarcoidosis is a multisystem granulomatous disease of unknown etiology.
- The hallmark of this disease is the presence of non-caseating granulomas affecting multiple organs.
- Systemic complaints of fever, weight loss and fatigue are common.
- Lofgren's syndrome of acute sarcoidosis is characterized by bilateral hilar lymphadenopathy, cervical lymphadenopathy, ankle arthritis, and erythema nodosum.

- Ten percent–fifteen percent of patients with chronic sarcoidosis demonstrate head and neck manifestations as sinonasal, oropharynx, hypopharynx, skin, eye, salivary glands, neck, larynx, bone, and even intracranial granulomatous infiltration.
- About 30–60% of sarcoidosis patients develop intraocular inflammatory signs and bilateral granulomatous uveitis.
- Endocrine manifestations—Diabetes insipidus is the most frequently reported endocrine disorder, followed by hyperprolactinemia.
- Serum markers such as serum amyloid A (SAA), soluble interleukin-2 receptor (sIL-2R), lysozyme, angiotensin-converting enzyme (ACE), and the glycoprotein KL-6 have been reported to be markers of sarcoidosis.
- Histopathological evidence of non-caseating granulomas is the hallmark of diagnosis.
- Chest X-ray and computed tomography are the most commonly used imaging techniques.
- Nuclear techniques, such as the fluorine-18 fluorodeoxyglucose positron emission tomography, can also be used to evaluate extrapulmonary manifestations of sarcoidosis or to guide the biopsy site.
- Corticosteroids are the mainstay of therapy. In refractory cases, immunosuppressants and TNF inhibitor therapy are implemented

References

1. Sverrild A, et al. Heredity in sarcoidosis: a registry-based twin study. Thorax. 2008;63(10):894–6.
2. Mrowka-Kata K, et al. Sarcoidosis and its otolaryngological implications. Eur Arch Otorhinolaryngol. 2010;267(10):1507–14. https://doi.org/10.1007/s00405-010-1331-y.
3. Schwartzbauer HR, Tami TA. Ear, nose, and throat manifestations of sarcoidosis. Otolaryngol Clin N Am. 2003;36(4):673–84.
4. Dastoori M, et al. Sarcoidosis: a clinically orientated review. J Oral Pathol Med. 2013;42(4):281–9.
5. Baltzan M, et al. Randomized trial of prolonged chloroquine therapy in advanced pulmonary sarcoidosis. Am J Respir Crit Care Med. 1999;160(1):192–7.
6. Zic JA, et al. Treatment of cutaneous sarcoidosis with chloroquine. Review of the literature. Arch Dermatol. 1991;127(7):1034–40.
7. Nathan SD. Lung transplantation: disease-specific considerations for referral. Chest. 2005;127(3):1006–16.
8. Jalisi S, et al. Sarcoidosis masquerading as carotid body tumor. Arch Otolaryngol Head Neck Surg. 2010;136(11):1132–5.
9. Laudien M. Orphan diseases of the nose and paranasal sinuses: pathogenesis – clinic – therapy. GMS Curr Top Otorhinolaryngol Head Neck Surg. 2015;14:Doc04. https://doi.org/10.3205/cto000119
10. Plaschke CC, et al. Clinically isolated laryngeal sarcoidosis. Eur Arch Otorhinolaryngol. 2011;268(4):575–80. https://doi.org/10.1007/s00405-010-1449-y.
11. Hybels RL, Rice DH. Neuro-otologic manifestations of sarcoidosis. Laryngoscope. 1976;86(12):1873–8. https://doi.org/10.1002/lary.5540861214.
12. Ozdogan A, et al. A difficult case: sarcoidosis of the middle ear. Am J Otolaryngol. 2009;30(4):281–4.
13. Vairaktaris E, et al. Salivary gland manifestations of sarcoidosis: report of three cases. J Oral Maxillofac Surg. 2005;63(7):1016–21.
14. Takase H, et al. Validation of international criteria for the diagnosis of ocular sarcoidosis proposed by the first international workshop on ocular sarcoidosis. Jpn J Ophthalmol. 2010;54(6):529–36.
15. Bihan H, et al. Sarcoidosis: clinical, hormonal, and magnetic resonance imaging (MRI) manifestations of hypothalamic-pituitary disease in 9 patients and review of the literature. Medicine (Baltimore). 2007;86(5):259–68.
16. Rao DA, Dellaripa PF. Extrapulmonary manifestations of sarcoidosis. Rheum Dis Clin North Am. 2013;39(2):277–97. https://doi.org/10.1016/j.rdc.2013.02.007
17. Miyoshi S, et al. Comparative evaluation of serum markers in pulmonary sarcoidosis. Chest. 2010;137(6):1391–7.
18. Stanton KM, et al. The utility of cardiac magnetic resonance imaging in the diagnosis of cardiac sarcoidosis. Heart Lung Circ. 2017;26(11):1191–9.
19. Davies CW, et al. Air trapping in sarcoidosis on computed tomography: correlation with lung function. Clin Radiol. 2000;55(3):217–21.
20. Palmucci S, et al. Clinical and radiological features of extra-pulmonary sarcoidosis: a pictorial essay. Insights Imaging. 2016;7(4):571–87. https://doi.org/10.1007/s13244-016-0495-4
21. Diamantopoulos PT, et al. An unusual case report of unilateral parotid gland sarcoidosis with spontaneous remission. Medicine (Baltimore). 2019;98(49):e18172. https://doi.org/10.1097/MD.0000000000018172
22. Mostard RL, et al. Inflammatory activity assessment by F18 FDG-PET/CT in persistent symptomatic sarcoidosis. Respir Med. 2011;105(12):1917–24.
23. Teirstein AS, et al. Results of 188 whole-body fluorodeoxyglucose positron emission tomography scans in 137 patients with sarcoidosis. Chest. 2007;132(6):1949–53.

24. Ahmadian A, et al. The response of FDG uptake to immunosuppressive treatment on FDG PET/CT imaging for cardiac sarcoidosis. J Nucl Cardiol. 2017;24(2):413–24.
25. Oki M, et al. Prospective study of endobronchial ultrasound-guided transbronchial needle aspiration of lymph nodes versus transbronchial lung biopsy of lung tissue for diagnosis of sarcoidosis. J Thorac Cardiovasc Surg. 2012;143(6):1324–9.
26. Rawala MS, et al. An atypical presentation of extrapulmonary sarcoidosis. Case Rep Rheumatol. 2020;8840245:6 p. https://doi.org/10.1155/2020/8840245
27. Silverman KJ, Hutchins GM, Bulkley BH. Cardiac sarcoid: a clinicopathologic study of 84 unselected patients with systemic sarcoidosis. Circulation. 1978;58:1204–11.
28. Nunes H, et al. Sarcoidosis. Orphanet J Rare Dis. 2007;2:46. https://doi.org/10.1186/1750-1172-2-46
29. Lower EE, Baughman RP. Prolonged use of methotrexate for sarcoidosis. Arch Intern Med. 1995;155(8):846–51.
30. Doty JD, et al. Treatment of corticosteroid-resistant neurosarcoidosis with a short-course cyclophosphamide regimen. Chest. 2003;124(5):2023–6.
31. Timmermans WMC, et al. Immunopathogenesis of granulomas in chronic autoinflammatory diseases. Clin Transl Immunol. 2016;5(12):e118. https://doi.org/10.1038/cti.2016.75
32. Kataria YP. Chlorambucil in sarcoidosis. Chest. 1980;78(1):36–43.
33. York EL, et al. Cyclosporine and chronic sarcoidosis. Chest. 1990;98(4):1026–9.
34. Doty JD, et al. Treatment of sarcoidosis with infliximab. Chest. 2005;127(3):1064–71.
35. Callejas-Rubio JL, et al. Tumor necrosis factor-alpha inhibitor treatment for sarcoidosis. Ther Clin Risk Manag. 2008;4(6):1305–13.

23 Crohn's Disease

Abstract

Crohn's disease is chronic granulomatous transmural inflammatory disease of the gastrointestinal tract. Typically, Crohn's lesions attain segmental and asynchronous distribution, although the sites most frequently involved are the terminal ileum and the proximal colon. Transmural inflammation of the gut results in fissures, abscess, fistula, thickening of the bowel wall, and limited distensibility and causes abdominal pain, anemia, arthralgia, repeated bouts of diarrhea, and weight loss. In the oral cavity, itmanifests as diffuse nodular swelling, cobblestone appearance, ulcers, hyperplasia, granulomatous gingivitis, and angular cheilitis. CD may trigger pyostomatitis vegetans. Persistent cervical lymphadenopathy is often associated. Diagnosis of CD is confirmed by clinical evaluation and a combination of endoscopic, histological, radiological, and/or biochemical investigations. In recent years, many studies have been performed to investigate the diagnostic potential of less invasive and more patient-friendly imaging modalities in the evaluation of Crohn's disease, including conventional enteroclysis, ultrasonography, color-power Doppler, contrast-enhanced ultrasonography, multidetector CT enteroclysis, MRI enteroclysis, and 99mTc-HMPAO-labeled leukocyte scintigraphy. Elevated C-reactive protein levels, anti-Saccharomyces cerevisiae antibodies (ASCA) and serum p-anti-neutrophil cytoplasmic antibodies (p-ANCA) aid the diagnosis. Anti-inflammatory and immunosuppressive medications such Sulfasalazine, Prednisone, Azathioprine, and 6-Mercaptopurine are recommended. Surgery is required in case of obstructive bowel disease or oral granulomas.

Synonyms

Crohn's syndrome; granulomatous enteritis; regional enteritis; Lesniowski–Crohn's disease [1, 2].

23.1 Background

Crohn's disease (CD) is a granulomatous inflammatory bowel disorder that mainly affects the gastrointestinal tract, including the oral cavity. Crohn's disease was first described in 1932 by three doctors—Burrill Crohn, Leon Ginzberg, and Gordon D. Oppenheimer. At the time, any disease in the small intestine was thought to be intestinal tuberculosis. Crohn's disease is named after the famous gastroenterologist Dr. Burrill Crohn. It first became regarded as a medical condition when it was described by Crohn and colleagues in 1932 [2]. Extraintestinal manifestations and other immune disorders are also prevalent in CD patients [1, 2].

S. V. Nemade, K. J. Shinde, *Granulomatous diseases in Otorhinolaryngology, Head and Neck*,
https://doi.org/10.1007/978-981-16-4047-6_23

23.2 Epidemiology

CD can develop at any age, but most patients develop the disease by the age of 40 years [3]. CD is much more prevalent in whites than in other races. It is prevalent in western countries. In the developed countries, the prevalence is 3.2/100,000 population. It is more common in whites (HLA-DR1/DQw5), Jews, smokers; monozygotic twins have 30–50% concordance. Overall, there is no sex predilection, but the younger the age of onset, the greater the likelihood that the disease will affect males. It peaks in the tens or twenties and at ages 50–70. Recent epidemiologic studies suggest increasing incidence rates worldwide, including within pediatric populations [1–3].

23.3 Etiopathogenesis

Like sarcoidosis, CD is a multifactorial disease with genetic and environmental factors, including diet, psychological stress and smoking, playing important roles in disease pathogenesis and/or exacerbation. The disease affects any part of the gastrointestinal tract, with terminal ileum being most common [2, 4, 5].

Inappropriate acquired T-cell immune response to commensal enteric bacteria developing in genetically susceptible host T-cells is the primary pathogenesis in CD. Autophagy plays an integral role in the innate immune response to intracellular microorganisms. Autophagy-associated genes, including ATG16L1, CARD9, IRGM, and LRRK2, have also been identified in subsets of CD patients [1, 5].

Other genes, including those implicated in the regulation of intestinal barrier function, lymphocyte differentiation, leukocyte migration, adaptive immunity and apoptosis, have also been linked to CD; most still require detailed investigations. However, irrespective of which protein may be implicated in disease pathogenesis, none of these currently explain the appearance of granulomatous inflammation within affected tissues [1, 2].

23.4 Clinical Features

Constitutional signs and symptoms include abdominal pain, anemia, arthralgia, repeated bouts of diarrhea, and weight loss. In addition 20% have abrupt onset of symptoms resembling acute appendicitis or bowel perforation [1, 2].

Intestinal Manifestations: Transmural inflammation of gut results in fissures, abscess, fistula, thickening of the bowel wall, and limited distensibility. Aphthous like superficial ulceration, cobblestone appearance of bowel mucosa are the typical presentations. Usually involves the small intestine; 40% of patients have colon involvement [1, 6, 7].

23.4.1 Extraintestinal Manifestations

Oral cavity and neck—Oral Manifestation occurs at any time during the course of the disease.

- Diffuse mucosal erythema (Fig. 23.1) or nodular swelling of oral and perioral tissues (Fig. 23.2)
- Cobblestone appearance of the oral mucosa
- Deep linear ulcers involving vestibule, aphthous ulcers
- Fibro epithelial hyperplasia

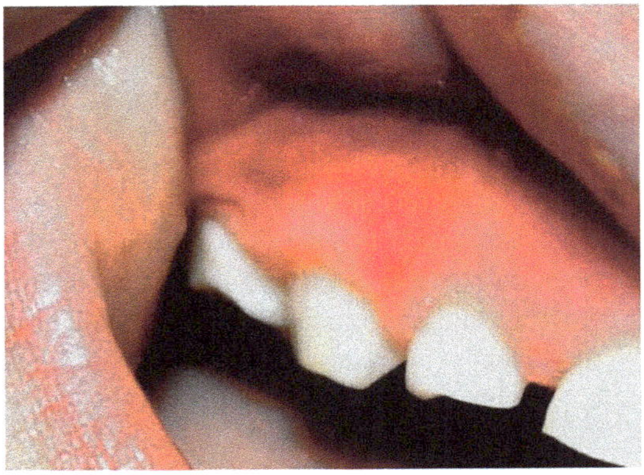

Fig. 23.1 Mild mucosal erythema of the right anterior maxillary gingiva [8]

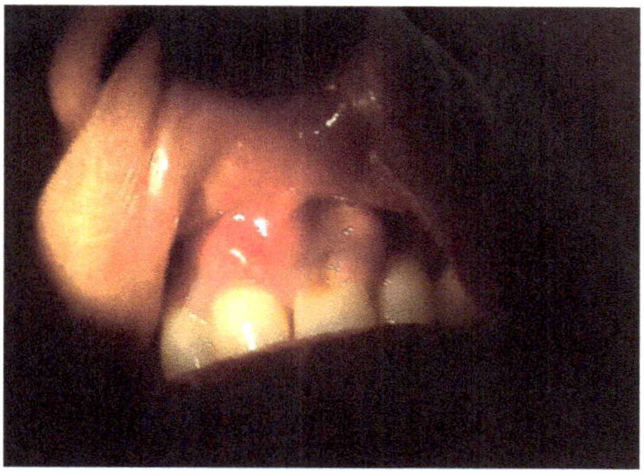

Fig. 23.3 Granulomatous gingivitis

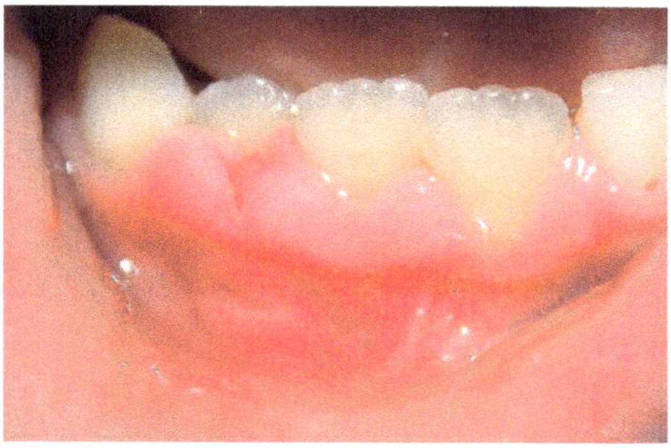

Fig. 23.2 Nodular swellings of the interdental papillae between the right permanent mandibular central and lateral incisors and primary canine. Ulceration of the free gingival margin between the incisors is seen. Also, note a linear ulceration with hyperplastic margins involving the alveolar mucosa [8]

- Granulomatous gingivitis (Fig. 23.3), angular cheilitis, metallic dysgusia
- Persistent submandibular and superficial cervical lymphadenopathy [6, 7]

Similar to the intestinal manifestations, oral lesions of CD may wax and wane over extended periods of time. In rare cases, CD may trigger pyostomatitis vegetans, which is characterized by pustular mucosal lesions and superficial erosions, oftentimes with concomitant peripheral eosinophilia [7].

- Skin—Erythema nodosum, pyoderma gangrenosum, pyodermatitis vegetans, and neutrophilic dermatoses are common manifestations [7, 9].
- Eyes—CD may cause conjunctivitis, anterior uveitis and episcleritis [7].

23.5 Diagnosis

It is confirmed by clinical evaluation and a combination of endoscopic, histopathological, radiographic and biochemical investigation [7].

23.5.1 Histopathology

It is an important diagnostic test that typically reveals non-caseating granulomatous inflammation (Fig. 23.4). However, only about 50% of CD biopsies reveal granulomas. In the intestine, the CD is characterized by the appearance of "skip lesions" and gross and histologic evidence of transmural inflammation that helps to differentiate CD from ulcerative colitis [8, 9].

23.5.2 Blood Tests [10]

- A complete blood count may reveal anemia, which commonly is caused by blood loss leading to iron deficiency or by vitamin B12 deficiency, usually caused by ileal disease impairing vitamin B12 absorption. Rarely autoimmune hemolysis may occur—anemia of chronic disease results in normocytic anemia.
- Serum iron, total iron-binding capacity and transferrin saturation may be more easily interpreted in inflammation.
- Erythrocyte sedimentation rate (ESR) and C-reactive protein help assess the degree of inflammation, which is important as ferritin can also be raised in inflammation.

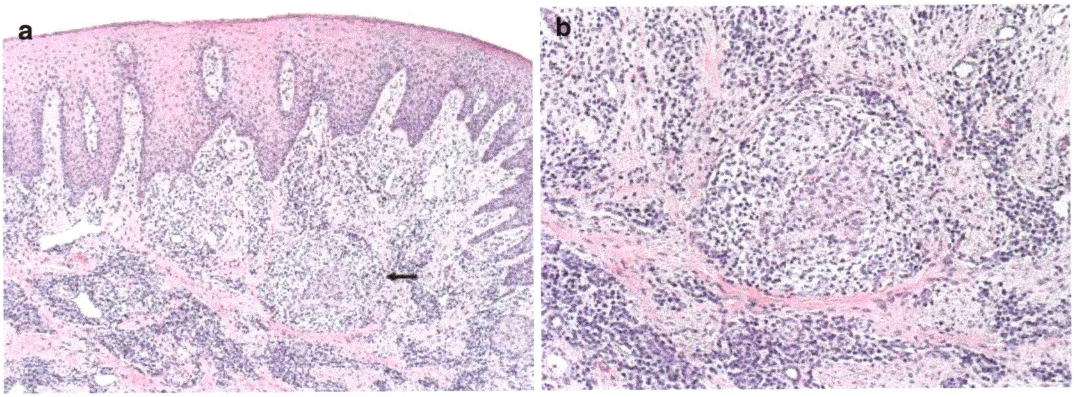

Fig. 23.4 Histopathologic images of the right mandibular gingiva. (**a**) Low-power view showing stratified squamous epithelium with scattered intraepithelial lymphocytes (exocytosis). The underlying fibrous connective tissues are characterized by a patchy chronic inflammatory cell infiltrate and an isolated granuloma (arrow) (hematoxylin and eosin, 40×). (**b**) High-power view showing a well-defined, non-caseating granuloma composed predominantly of epithelioid histiocytes and lymphocytes (hematoxylin and eosin, 100×) [8]

23.5.3 Serology

Elevated C-reactive protein levels and anti-Saccharomyces cerevisiae antibodies (ASCA) are frequently observed in CD patients [9, 11].

Calprotectin is a fecal granulocyte protein that is a promising marker of gastrointestinal inflammation. Fecal calprotectin levels are significantly increased in CD and may have predictive value in identifying active CD in adults and children [1].

Serum p-anti-neutrophil cytoplasmic antibodies (p-ANCA) may be elevated in inflammatory bowel diseases, including CD and ulcerative colitis [9].

23.5.4 Molecular Assay

In tissues affected by IBDs such as Crohn's disease and ulcerative colitis, several genes are differentially expressed, such as—the expression of mRNA for interleukin (IL)-1 and IL-1 receptor antagonist differs in colonic biopsy specimens from patients with IBD and in patients with acute colitis; IL-12 is expressed and actively released by intestinal lamina propria mononuclear cells from Crohn's disease specimens in contrast with ulcerative colitis specimens; tumour necrosis factor α, IL-1β, and IL-6 are also overexpressed in the inflamed areas of Crohn's disease tissue specimens.

To date, RNA fingerprinting such as differential display and RNA arbitrarily primed-polymerase chain reaction (RAP-PCR) using reverse transcriptase coupled to the PCR appears to be the most promising approach for the identification of such molecular markers [12].

23.5.5 Imaging

Advanced imaging technology has enabled the prompt and accurate diagnosis of Crohn's disease.

- Conventional Enteroclysis (CE)
  Crohn's disease has been traditionally investigated with the use of small-bowel barium enteroclysis, which detects early mucosal disease (sensitivity 69.6%, specificity 95.8%) as well as complications such as strictures, fistulae, and abscesses (diagnostic accuracy 80.3%) [10].
- Ultrasonography (US)
  Ultrasonography is an accurate, noninvasive, painless diagnostic tool with the capability of being used extensively in the clinical setting [10].
- Color-Power Doppler (PD)

Color and power Doppler US permits the measurement of arterial and venous flows in the upper mesenteric vessels, the evaluation of the increase of the relevant loop, determination of alterations in the vascular and microvascular nature of the inflammatory process and association with neoangiogenesis in the intestinal wall [13].

- Contrast-Enhanced Ultrasonography (CEUS)
It helps assess bowel wall vascularization and the differentiation between thickening due to active inflammation or fibrosis that cannot be reliably made with ultrasound [14].
- Multidetector CT Enteroclysis (MDCT-E)
MDCT-E is highly accurate in revealing mural and extraluminal manifestations of disease, including abscesses, while conventional enteroclysis is superior for luminal abnormalities and ulceration (Fig. 23.5) [15]
- MRI Enteroclysis (MR-E)
MRI enteroclysis is a noninvasive, nonionizing radiation diagnostic technique able to obtain multiplanar diagnostic information about intra- and extraintestinal lesions and evaluate disease activity [12]. The high soft-tissue contrast, multiplanar capabilities, and possibility of obtaining functional information make MR imaging the ideal technique for evaluating small-bowel inflammatory disease.

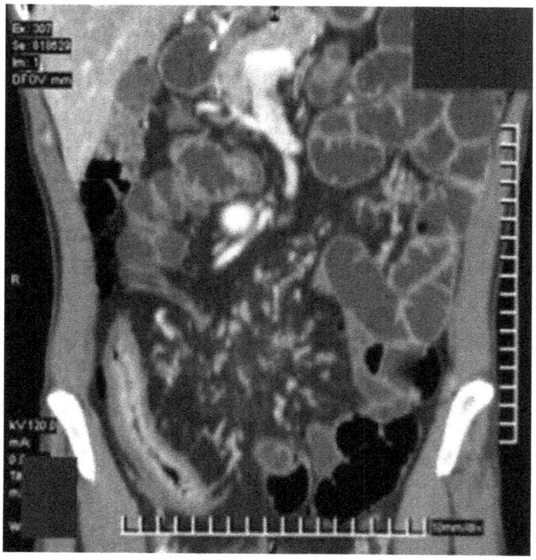

Fig. 23.5 Intramural wall thickening revealed on MDCT-E [15]

23.6 Treatment

An assessment of disease severity is necessary to design an appropriate treatment plan. A patient with a mildly to moderately active Crohn's disease may benefit from oral budesonide, but it is inappropriate in oral intolerance and severely active disease with systemic symptoms as fever in which parenteral corticosteroids should be necessary.

Crohn's Disease Activity Index (CDAI) is widely used disease assessment scores:

1. Clinical remission (CDAI <150): spontaneous or post-treatment remission.
2. Mild to moderate Crohn's disease (CD I 150–220): good oral intake, absence of dehydration, abdominal tenderness/mass, obstruction, or weight loss of >10%. Ambulatory follow-up is sufficient.
3. Moderate to severe Crohn's disease (CDAI 220–450): patients with mild to moderate Crohn's disease irresponsive to first-line therapy; the presence of two or more of the following systemic symptoms: fever, weight loss, abdominal pain, nausea and vomiting, and anemia.
4. Severe-fulminant Crohn's disease (CD I >450): ambulatory patients with persisting symptoms despite optimal therapy, presence of high fever, or obstruction symptoms as refractory nausea/vomiting, peritoneal signs, cachexia, or intraabdominal abscess [16].

Management aims to suppress the inflammation, promote mucosal healing, and interrupt disease progression to obviate disease morbidity (Figs. 23.6 and 23.7) [1, 3].

- Anti-inflammatory and immunosuppressive medications such as Budesonide Prednisone, Azathioprine and 6-Mercaptopurine are recommended (Table 23.1). Patients show variable responses to topical and systemic corticosteroid therapy [1, 16].

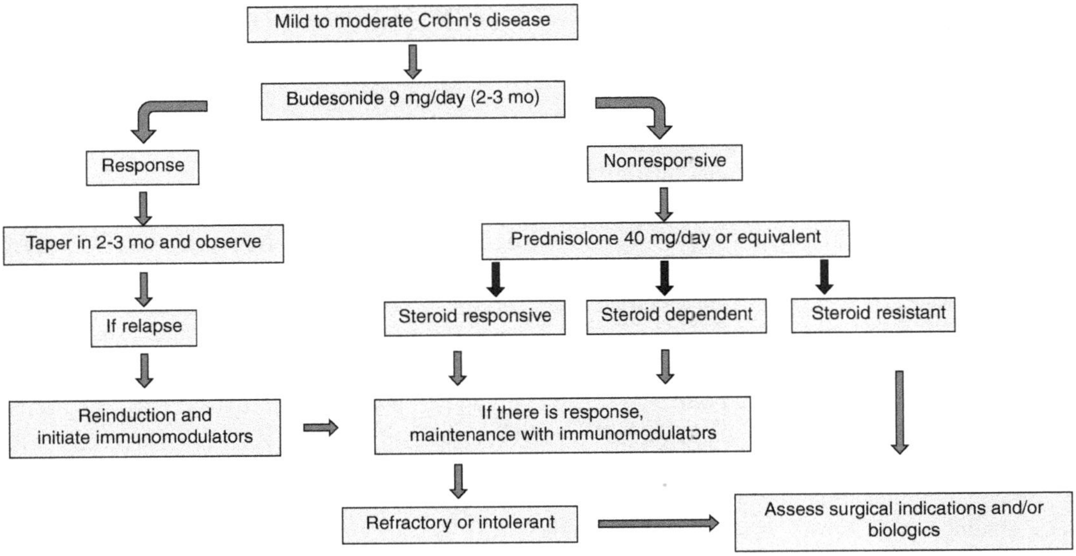

Fig. 23.6 Algorithm for management of mild to moderate Crohn's disease [16]

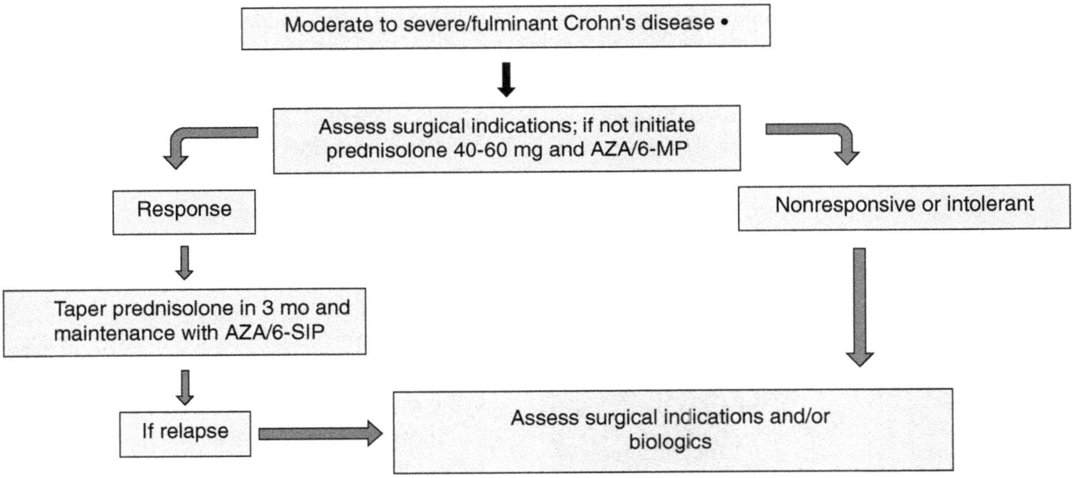

Fig. 23.7 Algorithm for management of moderate to severe/fulminant Crohn's disease. *Top-down strategy with biologics may be more appropriate in selected patients with risk factors [16]

- Anti TNF antibodies such as infliximab block the TNF—key inflammatory cytokine and mediator of intestinal inflammation (Table 23.1) [1, 3, 16].
- Antibiotics, including Metronidaloze or Ciprofloxacin, may be necessary for patients with abscess or fistula [2].
- Surgery is required for 50–80% of patients—in case of obstructive bowel disease or oral granulomas [4].

23.7 Essential Features

- Crohn disease (CD) is a transmural granulomatous enteritis. It mainly affects the gastrointestinal (GI) tract, including the oral cavity, but discontinuous.
- Transmural inflammation of gut results in fissures, abscess, fistula, thickening of bowel wall and limited distensibility. Causes abdom-

Table 23.1 Dose and duration of medications in Crohn's disease [16]

Drug	Severity of disease	Dose	Duration
Budesonide	Mild-moderate	9 mg/day	3–6 months
Prednisolone	All	40–60 mg/day	3–4 months
Azathioprine	All	2–2.5 mg/kg	Indefinite
6-Mercaptopurine	All	1–1.5 mg/kg	Indefinite
Methotrexate	All	25 mg/week	Indefinite
Infliximab	Moderate to severe with fistula/abscess	5 mg/kg/dose	Indefinite
Adalimumab	Moderate to severe with fistula/abscess	40 mg/dose	Indefinite

inal pain, anemia, arthralgia, repeated bouts of diarrhea, and weight loss.

- In the oral cavity, it manifests as diffuse nodular swelling, cobblestone appearance, ulcers, hyperplasia, granulomatous gingivitis and angular cheilitis. CD may trigger pyostomatitis vegetans. Persistent cervical lymphadenopathy is often associated.
- Clinical diagnosis is aided with endoscopy and biopsy. Appearance of "skip lesions" on endoscopy and typical non-caseating granulomatous inflammation on histopathology makes the diagnosis.
- Less invasive and more patient-friendly imaging modalities in the evaluation of Crohn's disease include conventional enteroclysis, ultrasonography, color-power Doppler, contrast-enhanced ultrasonography, multidetector CT enteroclysis, MRI enteroclysis, and 99mTc-HMPAO-labeled leukocyte scintigraphy.
- C-reactive protein levels, anti-Saccharomyces cerevisiae antibodies (ASCA) and serum p-anti-neutrophil cytoplasmic antibodies (p-ANCA) are often elevated.
- Anti-inflammatory and immunosuppressive medications such Sulfasalazine, Prednisone, Azathioprine and 6-Mercaptopurine are recommended.
- Surgery is required for 50–80% of patients—in case of obstructive bowel disease or oral granulomas.

References

1. Baumgart DC, Sandborn WJ. Crohn's disease. Lancet. 2012;380(9853):1590–605.
2. Crohn BB, et al. Regional ileitis: a pathologic and clinical entity. 1932. Mt Sinai J Med NY. 2000;67(3):263–8.
3. Miheller P, et al. Recommendations for identifying Crohn's disease patients with poor prognosis. Expert Rev Clin Immunol. 2013;9:65–75.
4. Ananthakrishnan AN. Environmental triggers for inflammatory bowel disease. Curr Gastroenterol Rep. 2013;15:302.
5. Tsianos EV, et al. Role of genetics in the diagnosis and prognosis of Crohn's disease. World J Gastroenterol. 2012;18:105–18.
6. Fritz T, et al. Crohn's disease: NOD2, autophagy and ER stress converge. Gut. 2011;60:1580–8.
7. Hegarty AM, et al. Pyostomatitis vegetans. Clin Exp Dermatol. 2004;29:1–7.
8. Woo VL. Oral manifestations of Crohn's disease: a case report and review of the literature. Case Rep Dent. 2015;2015:830472. https://doi.org/10.1155/2015/830472
9. Lewis JD. The utility of biomarkers in the diagnosis and therapy of inflammatory bowel disease. Gastroenterology. 2011;140:1817–26.
10. Fraser GM, Findlay JM. The double contrast enema in ulcerative and Crohn's colitis. Clin Radiol. 1976;27(1):103–12.
11. Glas J, et al. Anti-saccharomyces cerevisiae antibodies in patients with inflammatory bowel disease and their first-degree relatives: potential clinical value. Digestion. 2002;66:173–7.
12. Lafontaine D, et al. Identification of a Crohn's disease specific transcript with potential as a diagnostic marker. Gut. 1998;42:878–82.

13. Maconi G, et al. Factors affecting splanchnic haemodynamics in Crohn's disease: a prospective controlled study using Doppler ultrasound. Gut. 1998;43(5):645–50.
14. Serra C, et al. Ultrasound assessment of vascularization of the thickened terminal ileum wall in Crohn's disease patients using a low-mechanical index real-time scanning technique with a second generation ultrasound contrast agent. Eur J Radiol. 2007;62(1):114–21.
15. Gatta G, et al. Crohn's disease imaging: review. Gastroenterol Res Pract. 2012;816920:15 p. https://doi.org/10.1155/2012/816920.
16. Baran B, Karaca C. Practical medical management of Crohn's disease. Int Scholar Res Notices. 2013; 208073:12 p. https://doi.org/10.1155/2013/208073

24 Orofacial Granulomatosis

Abstract

Orofacial granulomatosis (OFG) is a chronic inflammatory disorder characterized by persistent or recurrent soft tissue swelling, oral ulceration, and a variety of orofacial features. Focal granulomas may occur anywhere in the oral mucosa or in the subcutaneous tissue of the skin, where they present as the localized firm mass that is occasionally multinodular. The diagnosis of OFG is made by the clinical presentation of recurring orofacial swellings that histologically consist of non-caseating granulomas. The patient should be evaluated for several systemic diseases such as Crohn's disease, sarcoidosis, and tuberculosis. When it presents in a triad encompassing facial nerve palsy, lip swelling, and fissured or furrowed tongue it is called Melkersson–Rosenthal syndrome, while monosymptomatic or oligosymptomatic forms are referred to as granulomatous cheilitis. Corticosteroids have been shown to be effective in reducing facial swelling and preventing recurrences and are considered the mainstay of therapy. Reduction cheiloplasty with intralesional triamcinolone and systemic tetracycline offers the best results in cheilitis granulomatosis. Facial nerve decompression may be required in the treatment of recurrent facial nerve palsy.

Synonyms

Melkersson–Rosenthal syndrome (MRS), Granulomatous cheilitis, cheilitis granulomatosa, Miescher–MRS [1, 2].

24.1 Background

Orofacial Granulomatosis (OFG) is a group of conditions affecting oral and maxillofacial regions and characterized microscopically by non-caseating granulomatous inflammation. Melkerson–Rosenthal syndrome is a type of orofacial granulomatosis as it includes one of the features as cheilitis granulomatosis. The term orofacial granulomatosis was proposed by Wiesenfield et al. in 1985 [1]. The onset of OFG during childhood may predict the future development of Crohn's disease. Thus, there is still no consensus as to whether OFG is a distinct clinical disorder or simply the initial manifestation of Crohn's disease or possibly sarcoidosis [1–3]. Melkersson described an association between facial edema and facial paralysis. Rosenthal added the features of lingua plicata or scrotal tongue. Other clinical features include granulomatous cheilitis, edema of the gums and scalp, salivary gland dysfunction, granulomatous blepharitis, trigeminal neuralgia, Raynaud's phe-

S. V. Nemade, K. J. Shinde, *Granulomatous diseases in Otorhinolaryngology, Head and Neck*,
https://doi.org/10.1007/978-981-16-4047-6_24

nomenon, and even chronic hypertrophic granulomatous vulvitis [4, 5]. Patients with this disorder do not have chest radiography changes, nor uveitis, and the Kveim–Siltzbach skin test is negative [1, 2].

24.2 Etiopathogenesis

The suggested etiology is the abnormal immune reaction. A delayed-type allergic reaction to foods, dental materials or some other environmental agent has been suggested. It primarily involves the mouth and adjacent tissues, involving the oral mucosa, gum, lips, tongue, pharynx, eyelids, and skin of the face [1, 2].

Although various etiological agents such as food substances, food additives, dental materials, and various microbiological agents have been implicated in the disease process, its precise pathogenesis is yet to be elucidated. The delayed type of hypersensitivity reaction appears to play a significant role, although the exact antigen inducing the immunological reaction varies in individual patients. However, evidence for the role of genetic predisposition to the disease is sparse. Cytokine production by monoclonal lymphocytic proliferation can stimulate granuloma formation. This is evident in oral mucosal lymphocytes, and it is associated with a local T-cell clonal expansion [1, 2].

24.3 Clinical Features

Lip edema: Painless, persistent diffuse swelling involving one or both lips (macrocheilia) [6, 7]. In the initial phase, swelling is soft intermittent and recurrent. It may be associated with angular cheilitis and gingival edema (Figs. 24.1, 24.2, and 24.3). Later it is permanent and fibrotic or granulomatous (Chelitis granulomatosis) [3, 4, 6].

Generalized edema, erythema, and nonspecific erosions or ulcerations are seen in the mouth. Gingivitis, facial edema with or without lip involvement is common. Other manifestations include fissures of the tongue, taste alteration, decreased salivary production and cobblestone appearance of buccal mucosa (Fig. 24.4). Lateral aspects of the dorsum of the tongue are usually fissured (Fig. 24.5) [3, 8].

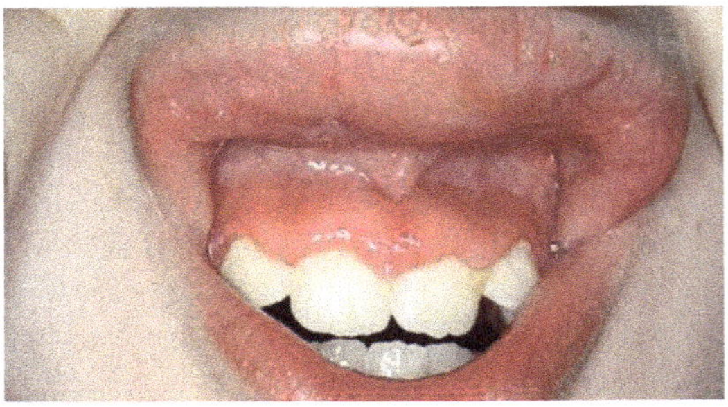

Fig. 24.2 Chronic swelling of the upper lip. Redness, swelling, and hypertrophy of the gingivae [6]

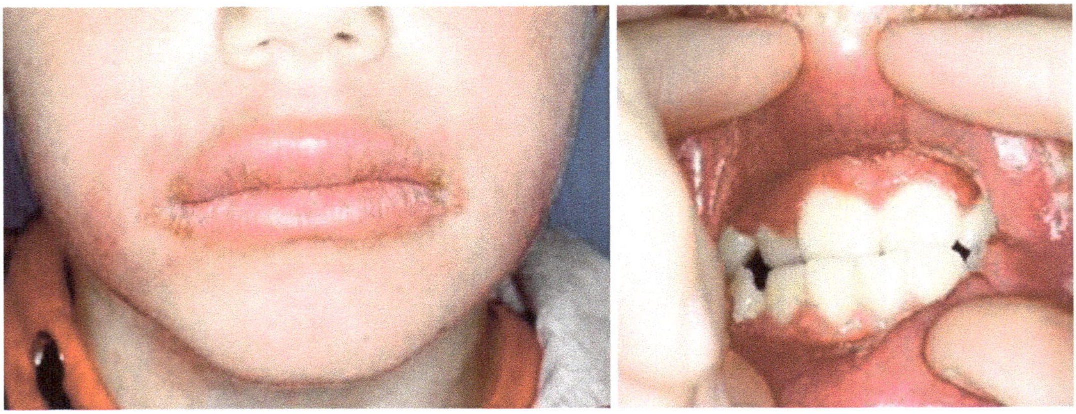

Fig. 24.1 Perioral edema, severe fissuring of the lips, angular cheilitis and gingival edema [6]

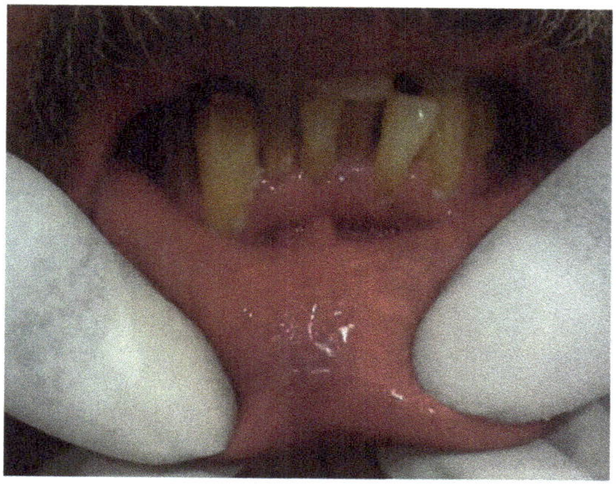

Fig. 24.3 Diffuse swelling of the lower lip [7]

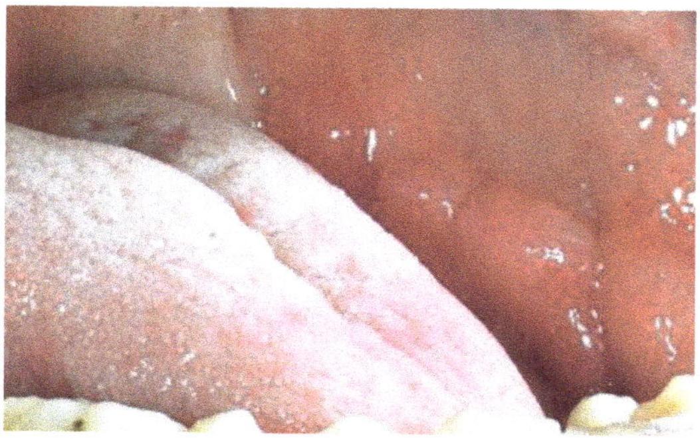

Fig. 24.4 Cobblestone appearance of buccal mucosa

Cheilitis granulomatosa associated with fissured tongue and recurrent facial paralysis is a well-known entity as Melkerson Rosenthal syndrome (Fig. 24.6) [9]. Sometimes cheilitis Granulomatosa is considered to be a monosymptomatic form of Melkersson–Rosenthal syndrome [4, 5, 10]. Painless recurrent orofacial edema, also called Miescher MRS or cheilitis granulomatosa of Miescher, is the most common monosymptomatic presentation of MRS, and diagnosis is suggested by the identification of a non-caseating granuloma on a mucocutaneous biopsy of the subjects [11, 12].

In few cases, it may be associated with granulomatous blepharitis, trigeminal neuralgia, Raynaud's phenomenon, and even chronic hypertrophic granulomatous vulvitis [5, 10].

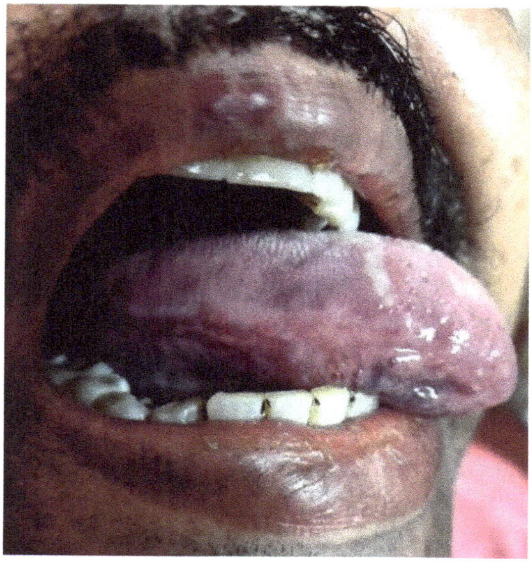

Fig. 24.5 Fissured lateral border of the tongue with granulomatous swelling

24.4 Diagnosis

Systemic workup such as clinical, laboratory, and radiographic investigations is mandatory to rule out underlying local or systemic disease.

24.4.1 Culture

Culture of the oral swabs and staining with PAS stain, Grocott–Methamine silver stain, Ziehl–Neelsen stain and Gram stain may enable to show fungal or specific bacterial organisms but is usually negative [9, 11].

24.4.2 Histopathology

Histopathology of oral granulomatous lesion reveals non-necrotizing granulomas with dilation of lymphatic vessels and perivascular lymphocytic infiltration. Fibrosis may also be present in long-term lesions (Fig. 24.7) [12, 13].

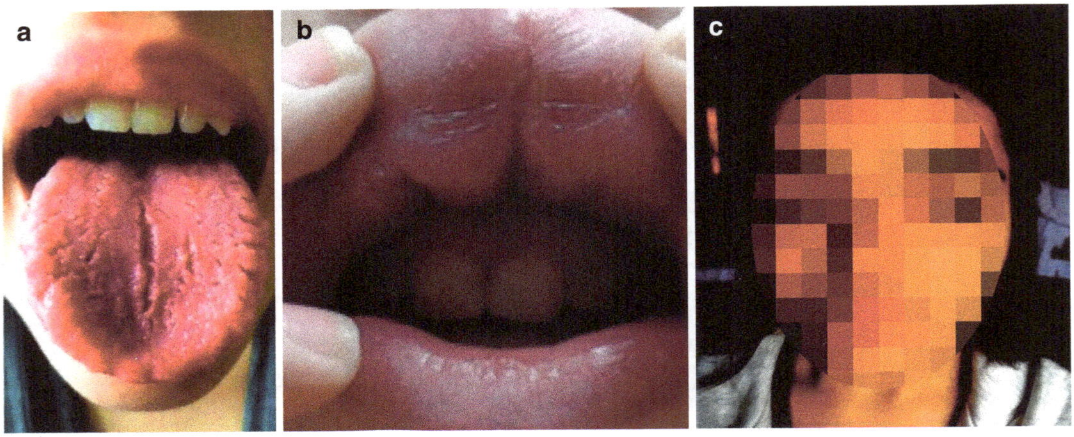

Fig. 24.6 (**a**) Fissured tongue, (**b**) Cheilitis granulomatosis and (**c**) facial paralysis [9]

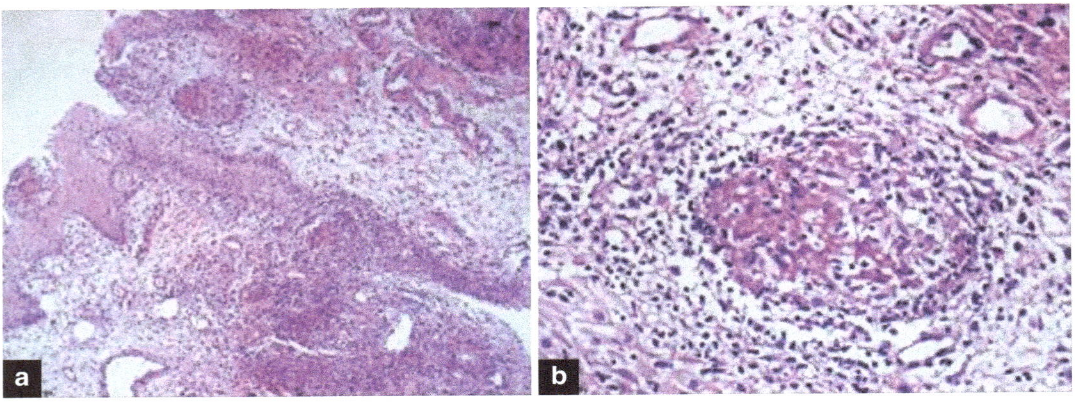

Fig. 24.7 Well-demarcated granulomas in an edematous stroma under the hyperplastic stratified squamous epithelium (hematoxylin-eosin stain, original magnification: ×100). (**b**) Granuloma formation consisting of epithelioid cells surrounded by lymphocytes in an edematous stroma (hematoxylin-eosin stain, original magnification: ×400) [13]

Complete blood count, ESR and serum levels of folic acid, vit B12, and iron is useful in patients with unusual gastrointestinal manifestation. Specialized gastrointestinal examination to assess for Crohn's disease is important. Tuberculin test and chest radiograph should be done to rule out tuberculosis [3, 8].

24.5 Treatment

- Although a spontaneous recovery is possible, currently, the initial therapeutic approach is based on intralesional or systemic corticosteroids administration. In particular, a short course of systemic corticosteroids (prednisolone1–1.5 mg/kg/day), tapered over 3–6 weeks, depending on the severity of the manifestations, improves symptoms in 50–80% of the patients, with a recurrence rate decrease of 60–75% [14, 15].
- Combined use of steroids with minocycline (200 mg/day) and metronidazole (1.5 gm/day) in patients with MRS has reported promising results [14, 16, 17].
- Other measures are Hydroxychloroquines, Methotrexate, Clofazimine, Metronidazole, or Minocycline alone or in combination with oral

Prednisolone, Thalidomide, and Dapsone [4, 18, 19].
- For lipedema and granulomatosis, simple compression for several hours daily may produce sustained improvement. Compression devices can be worn overnight to reduce lipedema. Extensive labial swelling can be disfiguring and can have serious social consequences; hence patient's psychology should be taken into consideration when choosing treatment options. Furthermore, comorbid psychiatric diseases and other affective phenomena may be linked to relapse frequency of Miescher–Melkersson–Rosenthal syndrome [20].
- As HSV is a rare but potentially devastating cause of facial palsy, it is common practice to add antiviral agents (acyclovir) to steroid therapy, at least until exclusion of a viral etiology [14].
- Intravenous immunoglobulins are tried successfully in patients unresponsive to standard treatment. Elimination diets to identify and exclude dietary allergens have been advocated in a number of case studies. Granulomatous cheilitis or OFG may improve with the implementation of a cinnamon- and benzoate-free diet. Benefit has been reported in 54–78% of patients [14].

24.5.1 Surgical Management

Surgery and radiation have been used in treating cheilitis granulomatosa. Surgery alone is relatively unsuccessful. Reduction cheiloplasty with intralesional triamcinolone and systemic tetracycline offers the best results. Medical therapy is necessary to maintain the results of reductive cheiloplasty during the postoperative period. Intralesional corticosteroid injections are periodically given after surgery to avoid an exaggerated recurrence [21].

Facial nerve decompression has been successful in the treatment of recurrent facial nerve palsy [14, 22].

24.6 Essential Features

- Rare neurological disorder characterized by orofacial swelling (usually of upper lip), peripheral facial nerve paralysis and fissured tongue.
- Manifests as perioral edema, severe fissuring of the lips, angular cheilitis and gingival edema.
- Onset is in childhood or early adolescence.
- After recurrent episodes, lip swelling may persist and eventually become permanent.
- Lips become hard, cracked, and fissured with a reddish brown discoloration.
- Cheilitis granulomatosis: Lips become fibrotic and nodular. Sometimes considered to be a monosymptomatic form of Melkersson–Rosenthal syndrome.
- May be associated with granulomatous blepharitis, trigeminal neuralgia, Raynaud's phenomenon.
- Culture of oral swabs and biopsy of oral lesions: Staining with PAS stain, Grocott–Methamine silver stain.
- Histopathology of oral granulomatous lesion reveals non-necrotizing granulomas with dilation of lymphatic vessels and perivascular lymphocytic infiltration.
- Gastrointestinal endoscopic examination to assess for Crohn's disease is important.
- Intralesional corticosteroids are the gold standard treatment. In severe cases, oral steroids combined with metronidazole, dapsone, or hydroxychlroroquine are preferred.
- Compression devices are used to reduce lipedema. Reduction cheiloplasty with intralesional triamcinolone and systemic tetracycline offers the best results in cheilitis granulomatosa.

References

1. Wiesenfeld D, et al. Oro-facial granulomatosis—a clinical and pathological analysis. Q J Med. 1985;54(213):101–13.

2. Yadav S, et al. Orofacial granulomatosis responding to weekly azithromycin pulse therapy. JAMA Dermatol. 2015;151(2):219–20.
3. Grave B, et al. Orofacial granulomatosis—a 20-year review. Oral Dis. 2009;15(1):46–51.
4. Mignogna MD, et al. The multiform and variable patterns of onset of orofacial granulomatosis. J Oral Pathol Med. 2003;32(4):200–5.
5. Lloyd DA, et al. Melkersson-Rosenthal syndrome and Crohn's disease. J Clin Gastroenterol. 1994;18(3):213–7.
6. Simonsen AB, Deleuran M. Orofacial granulomatosis in children can be the initial manifestation of systemic disease: a presentation of two cases. Dermatol Rep. 2014;6(1):5039. https://doi.org/10.4081/dr.2014.5039.
7. Ravindran R, Karunakaran A. Idiopathic orofacial granulomatosis with varied clinical presentation. Case Rep Dentistry. 2013;701749:3 p. https://doi.org/10.1155/2013/701749
8. El-Hakim M, Chauvin P. Orofacial granulomatosis presenting as persistent lip swelling: review of 6 new cases. J Oral Maxillofac Surg. 2004;62(9):1114–7.
9. Savasta S, et al. Melkersson-Rosenthal syndrome in childhood: report of three paediatric cases and a review of the literature. Int J Environ Res Public Health. 2019;16(7):1289. https://doi.org/10.3390/ijerph16071289
10. Greene RM, Rogers RS. Melkersson-Rosenthal syndrome: a review of 36 patients. J Am Acad Dermatol. 1989;21(6):1263–70.
11. Bohra S, et al. Clinicopathological significance of Melkersson-Rosenthal syndrome. BMJ Case Rep. 2015;2015:3–6. https://doi.org/10.1136/bcr-2015-210138.
12. Lalosevic J, et al. Orofacial granulomatosis in a 12-year-old girl successfully treated with intravenous pulse corticosteroid therapy and chloroquine. Pediatr Dermatol. 2017;34:e324–7. https://doi.org/10.1111/pde.13279.
13. Afsar FS, et al. Clinicopathological diagnosis of orofacial granulomatosis. Indian Dermatol Online J. 2017;8(1):32–4. https://doi.org/10.4103/2229-5178.198768.
14. Pryce DW, King CM. Orofacial granulomatosis associated with delayed hypersensitivity to cobalt. Clin Exp Dermatol. 1990;15:384–6.
15. Leao JC, et al. Review article – orofacial granulomatosis. Ailment Pharmacol Ther. 2004;20:1019–27.
16. Kano Y, et al. Treatment of recalcitrant cheilitis granulomatosa with metronidazole. J Am Acad Dermatol. 1992;27(4):629–30.
17. Coskun B, et al. Treatment and follow-up of persistent granulomatous cheilitis with intralesional steroid and metronidazole. J Dermatolog Treat. 2004;15(5):333–5.
18. Campbell HE, et al. Review article: cinnamon- and benzoate-free diet as a primary treatment for orofacial granulomatosis. Aliment Pharmacol Ther. 2011;34(7):687–701.
19. Ziem PE, et al. Melkersson-Rosenthal syndrome in childhood: a challenge in differential diagnosis and treatment. Br J Dermatol. 2000;143(4):860–3.
20. Alves P, et al. Melkersson-Rosenthal syndrome: a case report with a psychosomatic perspective. Adv Mind Body Med. 2017 Winter;31(1):14–7.
21. Kruse-Losler B, et al. Surgical treatment of persistent macrocheilia in patients with Melkersson-Rosenthal syndrome and cheilitis granulomatosa. Arch Dermatol. 2005;141(9):1085–91.
22. Tan Z, et al. Recurrent facial palsy in Melkersson Rosenthal syndrome: total facial nerve decompression is effective to prevent further recurrence. Am J Otolaryngol. 2015;36(3):334–7.

Part IV

Hereditary Granulomatous Diseases

Chronic Granulomatous Disease (CGD)

25

Abstract

Chronic granulomatous disease (CGD) is a primary immunodeficiency caused by defects in any of the five subunits of the NADPH oxidase complex responsible for the respiratory burst in phagocytic leukocytes. Patients with CGD are at increased risk of life-threatening infections with catalase-positive bacteria and fungi and inflammatory complications such as CGD colitis. CGD is characterized by granuloma and abscess formation in the skin, liver, lungs, spleen, and lymph nodes. These granuloma and abscess are caused by the inability of macrophages to kill ingested organisms. Inflammatory complications are a significant contributor to morbidity in CGD, and they are often refractory to standard therapies. Life expectancy for patients with CGD has increased, largely due to universal antibacterial and antifungal prophylaxis and increased awareness of infectious complications. At present, hematopoietic stem cell transplantation (HCT) is the only curative treatment, and transplantation outcomes have improved over the last few decades, with overall survival rates now >90% in children less than 14 years of age. In recent years, gene therapy has been proposed as an alternative to HCT for patients without an HLA-matched donor. However, results to date have not been encouraging.

Synonyms
CGD; chronic dysphagocytosis; congenital dysphagocytosis; septic progressive granulomatosis [1, 2].

25.1 Background

Chronic Granulomatous Disease (CGD), firstly described in 1957 [3, 4], is a primary inherited immunodeficiency leading the body vulnerable to chronic inflammation and frequent bacterial and fungal infections. The features of this condition usually develop in infancy or early childhood; however, milder forms may be diagnosed in the teen years or even in adulthood. It is caused by changes (mutations) in any one of five different genes and is usually inherited in an autosomal recessive or X-linked recessive manner. Treatment consists of continuous therapy with antibiotic and antifungal medications to treat and prevent infections. The only cure for the disease is allogeneic hematopoietic stem cell transplantation (HSCT) [2–4].

25.2 Epidemiology

The prevalence of CGD varies among the population, with studies reporting variations from 1 case per 1 million individuals to 1 case per 160,000 individuals. It is a genetically heterogeneous disease with all ethnic groups equally affected.

S. V. Nemade, K. J. Shinde, *Granulomatous diseases in Otorhinolaryngology, Head and Neck*,
https://doi.org/10.1007/978-981-16-4047-6_25

Approximately 80% of patients with CGD are male, because the main cause of the disease is a mutation in an X-chromosome-linked gene. However, defects in autosomal genes may also underlie the disease and cause CGD in both males and females. Symptoms onset typically occurs at a young age, although the diagnosis may be done at an older age in some patients [3–5].

25.3 Etiopathogenesis

Chronic granulomatous disease (CGD) is a rare disease caused by mutations in any one of the five components of the nicotinamide adenine dinucleotide phosphate (NADPH) oxidase in phagocytes. This enzyme generates superoxide and is essential for the intracellular killing of pathogens by phagocytes.

CGD is a primary immunodeficiency that affects phagocytes of the innate immune system and leads to recurrent or persistent intracellular bacterial and fungal infections. Leukocytes ingest bacteria but do not kill them because of a defect in the production of the superoxide anion. Most infections in CGD are caused by *Staphylococcus aureus*. Infections are also caused by unusual opportunistic organisms such as *Chromobacterium violaceum*, *Serratia marcescens*, and Nocardia, Legionella, and atypical Mycobacteria species. The most common fungal infections in these patients are caused by Aspergillus species.

The most common infecting organisms, on the basis of the type and site of infection, include the following [3, 4]:

- Pneumonia—Aspergillus species, Staphylococcus aureus, Nocardia, and Serratia species and *Burkholderia cepacia* (formerly *Pseudomonas cepacia*).
- Subcutaneous, liver, or perirectal abscess—Staphylococcus, Serratia, and Aspergillus species.
- Lung abscess—Aspergillus species.
- Brain abscess—Aspergillus species.
- Suppurative adenitis—Staphylococcus and Serratia species.
- Osteomyelitis—Due to hematogenous spread of organisms (*S. aureus*, Salmonella species, *S marcescens*) or contiguous invasion of bone, seen typically with non-*Aspergillus fumigatus* pneumonia, such as *Aspergillus nidulans* spreading to the ribs or vertebral bodies.
- Bacteremia and/or fungemia—Salmonella and Candida species and *B. cepacia.*
- Other frequently encountered catalase-positive microbial agents—*Escherichia coli* species, Listeria species, Klebsiella species, and Nocardia.

The intracellular survival of ingested bacteria and fungi leads to the development of granulomata in the lymph nodes, skin, lungs, liver, gastrointestinal tract, and/or bones.

25.3.1 Genetics and Inheritance

CGD is usually inherited in an X-linked recessive fashion. Most patients (approximately 80%) are males, who have hemizygous mutations on the X-linked gene coding for gp91phox. The gene responsible for this form of the disease has been mapped to the p21.1 region of the X chromosome [6, 7].

25.4 Clinical Features

Patients with CGD usually present with recurrent bacterial and fungal infections in infancy and early childhood, however, presentation in old age is also reported.

The manifestations are as follows:

1. Ear Nose Throat Manifestations—Ear, nose, and throat (ENT) infections occur in 12% of CGD patients. Among them, the most common infection is otitis media and otitis externa, which accounts for 33% of ENT infections, while parotitis takes up 5% [7]. In particular, necrotizing otitis externa, an infection that occurs in the cartilage and bones of the external auditory canal, develops mainly in immunocompromised patients. Parotitis is

accompanied by inflammatory change in subcutaneous soft tissues [8]. Nasal septal abscess (Fig. 25.1), recurrent multiple gingival abscesses due to *S. aureus* infection may be seen (Fig. 25.2).

2. Pulmonary Manifestations—Pneumonia is the most common infectious disease among CGD patients and is detected in about 80% of CGD patients [4]. The most common causative organism is Aspergillus spp. (41%), followed by staphylococci (11%) and Nocardia spp. (6%) [9]. Severe pneumonia may progress to a lung abscess, while inflammation in the adjacent chest wall may propagate to the ribs and vertebral bodies to cause osteomyelitis [4, 9].

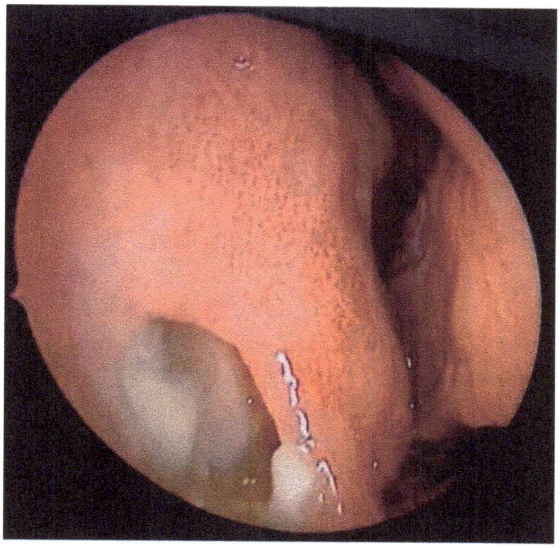

Fig. 25.1 Nasal endoscopy showing nasal septal abscess and perforation

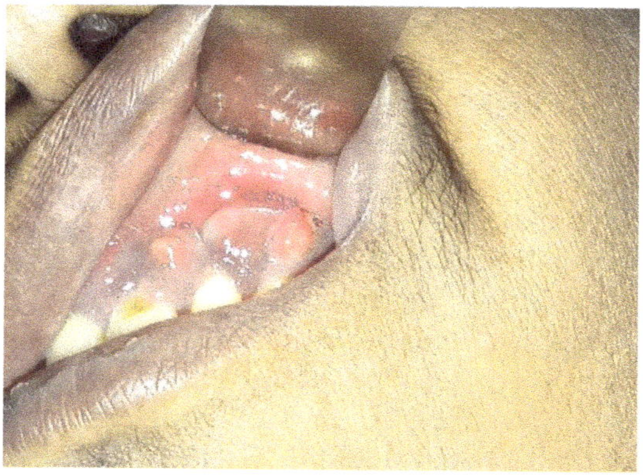

Fig. 25.2 Multiple granulomatous gingival abscesses in patient with CGD

3. Lymphadenopathy: Lymphadenopathy is fairly common in patients with CGD. (Suppurative lymphadenitis is found in 60% of CGD patients, having the second-highest rate next to lung infection, while *Staphylococcus aureus* is the most common pathogen for this infection. With respect to lesions, cervical lymphadenitis is the most common affliction [3].
4. CNS Manifestations—The central nervous system (CNS) infection is rather rare in CGD patients, showing a prevalence rate of 5% or less. Brain abscess may occur as a secondary infection caused by pathogens like Aspergillus spp. or *S. aureus* through hematogenous transmission [3].
5. Gastrointestinal Manifestations—Gastrointestinal infection in CGD patients may be caused by granulomatous inflammations in the entire gastrointestinal system from the mouth to anus. The pathogens that cause granulomatous inflammation include mostly Gram-positive *S. aureus* and Gram-negative organisms such as *Escherichia coli*, and Salmonella and Klebsiella spp. [4] Granulomatous inflammation of the upper gastrointestinal tract leads to diffuse edematous wall thickening of the esophagus and the stomach. This, in turn, causes malabsorption, perianal abscesses and fistulae and characteristic obstructive lesions associated with granulomatous infiltration.
6. Hepatosplenic Manifestations—More than 90% of CGD patients are afflicted with hepatosplenomegaly. Liver and splenic abscesses are found in 25–50% of CGD patients. Since a liver abscess is generally very rare among children, its presence should give rise to suspicion of CGD. Patients usually present with fever, malaise, and weight loss [4].
7. Musculoskeletal Manifestations—Soft tissue abscess is the third most common infection among CGD patients, caused most commonly by staphylococci. An abscess may occur even in the subcutaneous layer, which is usually

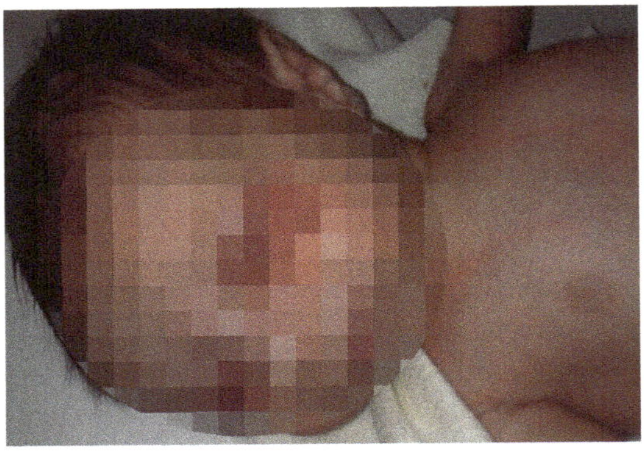

Fig. 25.3 Vesiculopustular lesions in a 24 days old neonate with CGD [10]

accompanied by inflammation in the adjacent skin (Fig. 25.3).

Osteomyelitis occurs in 25% of all CGD patients [3].

8. Genitourinary Manifestation—Infection of the urinary system is relatively rare in CGD patients, but repeated urinary tract infections, cystitis, renal, and perinephric abscesses may occur. Granulomatous cystitis leads to diffuse nodular bladder wall thickening [4].

25.5 Diagnosis

25.5.1 Histopathology

Biopsy obtained from lymph node, skin lesions, mucosal lesions or visceral granulomas is important in correctly diagnosing chronic granulomatous disease.

It is characterized by a mixed suppurative and granulomatous inflammation. A typical feature of visceral granulomas is the presence of golden-brown-pigmented histiocytes along with neutrophils and diffuse areas of necrosis [11]. Histochemical stains show that this material is composed of unsaturated fatty acids, phospholipids, and glycoproteins. Electron microscopic findings suggest that the pigment represents lipofuscin bodies and appears to be derived from lysosomes (Fig. 25.4).

Periodic acid-Schiff (PAS) staining demonstrates the presence of polysaccharides such as mucoproteins. These substances stain reddish purple with the PAS reaction.

25.5.2 Culture

Culture and sensitivity studies may be helpful. Bacteria isolated from lesions in patients with the chronic granulomatous disease are usually catalase positive.

Histopathology and culture are complimentary and allow accurate identification of the infecting organism and antifungal susceptibility testing. Fungal elements seen in pathology specimens may assist in the identification of the infecting organism; however, different fungal species can appear morphologically very similar, and identification should not rely on histopathology alone [11].

25.5.3 Specialized Blood Tests

Blood tests such as the nitroblue tetrazolium test and/or flow cytometry with dihydrorhodamine help to confirm the diagnosis. Both of these tests can be used to determine whether or not the immune cells are making toxic substances that the body uses to fight infections.

- The Nitroblue Tetrazolium (NBT) Dye TestLaboratory diagnosis of chronic granulomatous disease (CGD) can be made using the NBT test, stimulated with substances such as phorbol myristate acetate or *Escherichia coli* lipopolysaccharide, which promote an oxidative response in 90–100% of normal neutrophils. Neutrophils in patients with the chronic granulomatous disease are unable to reduce oxidized NBT to insoluble blue formazan; this principle forms the basis of the standard diagnostic screening test for the chronic granulomatous disease. This test is best used to identify gene carriers, and it has been used for the prenatal diagnosis of chronic granulomatous disease [12, 13].
- Flow Cytometric Reduction of Dihydrorhodamine (DHR):This test can also

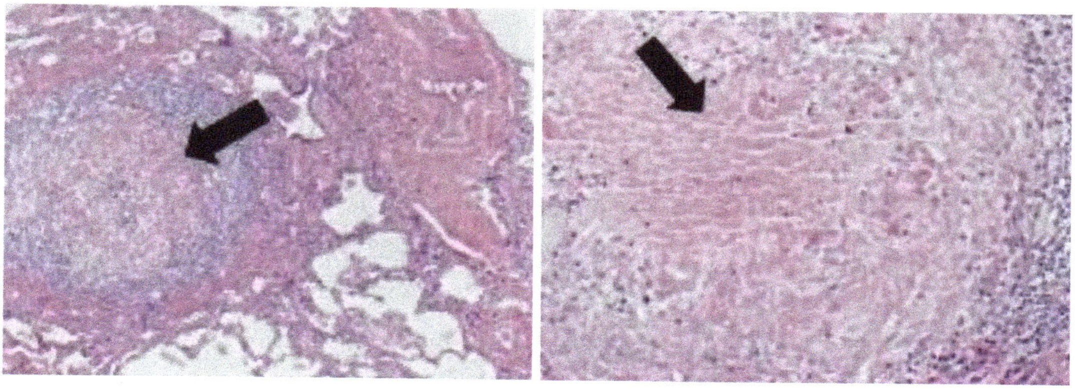

Fig. 25.4 Histopathological examination (hematoxylin and eosin stain) shows granulomas as indicated by arrows in the lung tissue obtained by surgical biopsy [11]

be used to diagnose chronic granulomatous disease. The principles are the same as for the NBT dye test, but a different dye is used. Additionally, X-linked carrier status can also be detected [12, 13].

25.5.4 Complete Blood Cell Counts

Peripheral blood leukocytosis (>8.5 × $10^3/\mu L$) is a characteristic finding that reflects increased numbers of circulating neutrophils. Most patients are anemic (hemoglobin <11 gm%), usually with a microcytic hypochromic picture [14–16].

25.5.5 Serology

Levels of the three major classes of immunoglobulins- IgG, IgM, and IgA, are increased. IgE levels are increased or in the reference range [12, 14].

25.5.6 Molecular Assay [10–13, 17]

- Polymerase chain reaction.
- Gene Sequencing and mutational analysis for subtypes.
  The diagnosis of CGD is established with the identification of the mutation(s) in one of five genes:
  1. CYBA, NCF1, NCF2, and NCF4 (the genes related to autosomal recessive chronic granulomatous disease).
  2. CYBB is the gene related to the X-linked chronic granulomatous disease.
- Allele-specific restriction enzyme analysis [11].

25.5.7 Imaging

25.5.7.1 Radiography and CT Imaging

The radiologic studies for acute pneumonia show findings of consolidation, ground-glass attenuation, empyema, nodules, and lung abscess (Figs. 25.5, 25.6 and 25.7). Less specific reticulonodular shadowing and hilar lymphadenopathy are also commonly observed [10].

Radiologic findings of external and middle ear diseases in CGD patients are similar to those of patients with normal immunity. On the CT scan, the skin of the external auditory canal and the auricle are thick with contrast enhancement. Cases accompanied by bony destruction of the tympanic bone and mastoid bone especially suggest a grave prospect of life-threatening necrotizing external otitis [8].

On CT scan, suppurative lymphadenitis presents with enlarged and contrast-enhanced lymph nodes with a necrosis-induced central low-density area. Ultrasonography shows internal

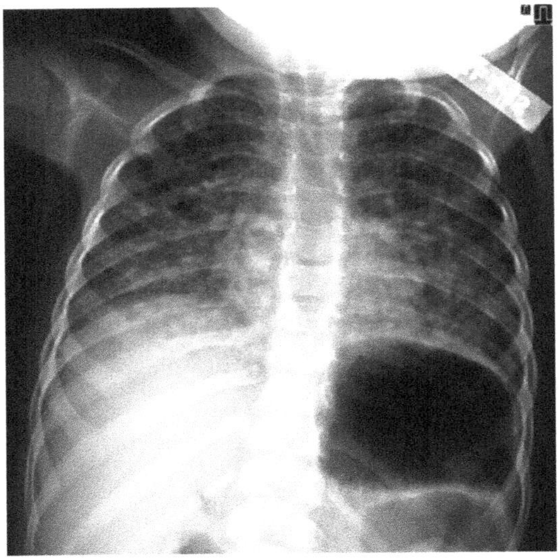

Fig. 25.5 Chest radiograph demonstrating focal opacities extensive diffuse nodularity [18]

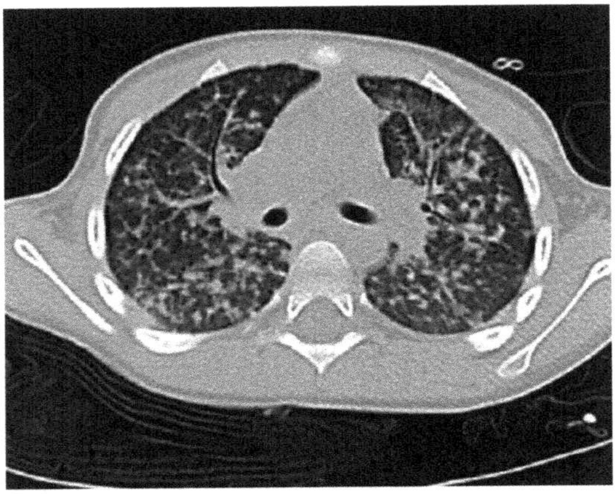

Fig. 25.6 Chest CT showing diffuse nodular pattern involving different areas of the lungs [18]

debris in volute shapes, and some cases reveal a thick septation as well as increased color flow signals within the septation.

25.5.7.2 MRI

It is particularly useful in CNS infection, which usually occurs in the gray matter-white matter junction. Contrast-enhanced MRI may show typical ring-enhancing lesions with peripheral vasogenic edema (Fig. 25.8) [9].

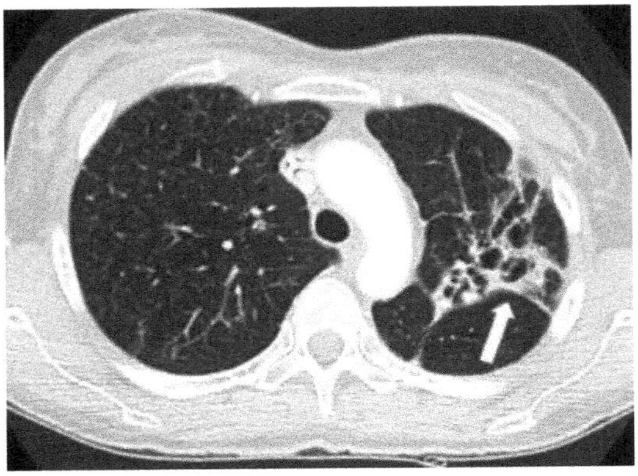

Fig. 25.7 Chest CT showing patchy areas of consolidation and cavitation primary in the left upper lung lobe (arrow) [11]

Osteomyelitis can be better assessed in Tc99m whole-body scan (Fig. 25.9) [10, 16].

25.5.7.3 Other Diagnostic Tests Include the Following

1. Chemiluminescence immunoassay (CLIA) test to detect the degree of light generated by activated phagocytic cells. Chemiluminescence immunoassay (CLIA) is an assay that combines the chemiluminescence technique with immunochemical reactions. Similar with other labeled immunoassays (RIA, FIA, ELISA), CLIA utilize chemical probes which could generate light emission through chemical reaction to label the antibody [13, 17, 19].
2. Direct measurements of oxygen consumption: Optical methods for the measurement of oxygen consumption rates (OCRs) have become both widely used and accessible in the last several years. While palladium and ruthenium-based phosphores are used for oxygen sensing, Pt-phosphores have become the most relied upon oxygen sensor dye and have been used routinely in research and industry for over 20 years [5, 19].
3. Direct measurements of superoxide anion production: The capacity of human phagocytes to generate superoxide anion (O_2-), a free radical of oxygen, and a possible role for this radical or its derivatives in the killing of

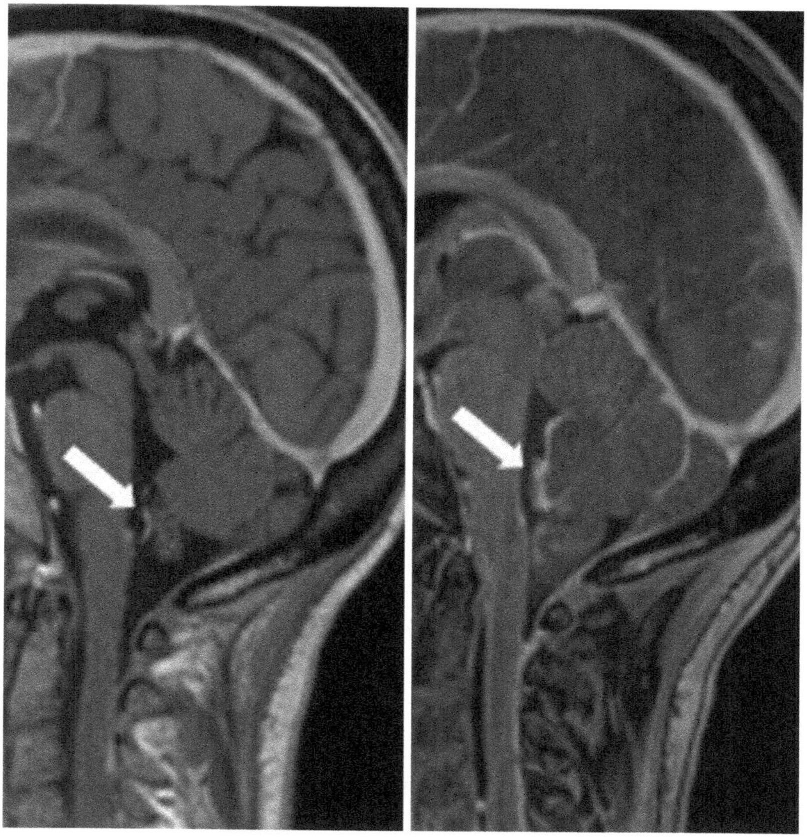

Fig. 25.8 Magnetic resonance imaging demonstrating multiple contrast-enhanced nodular masses along the leptomeninges (arrow). Left- minimal disease at the time of the first visit. Right- disease progression in 3 weeks [11]

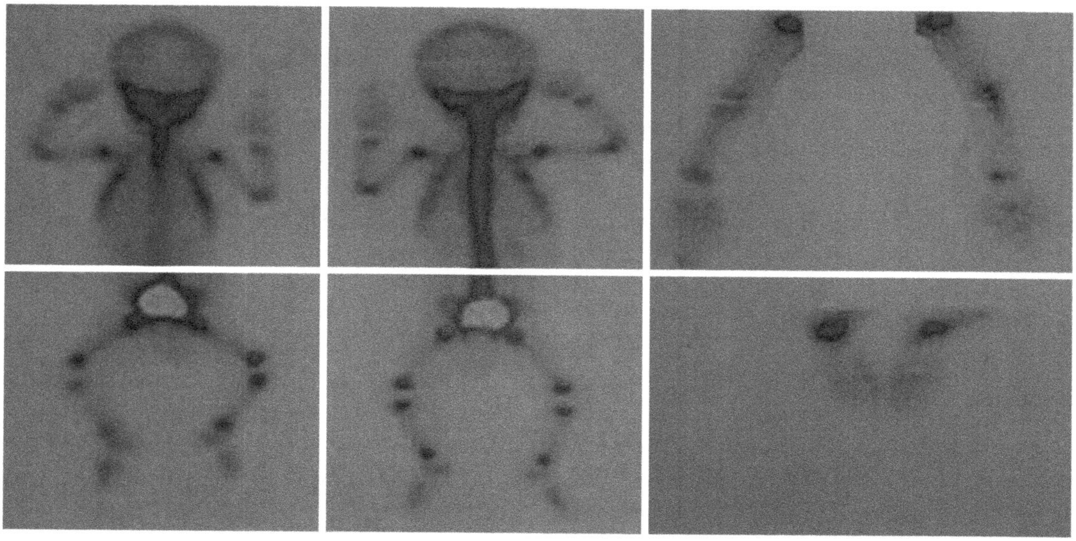

Fig. 25.9 Osteomyelitis of the left ankle, right elbow, and right wrist [10]

phagocytized bacteria are explored using leukocytes from patients with the chronic granulomatous disease (CGD) [5, 20].

25.6 Treatment

Early diagnosis and treatment can significantly improve the prognosis. Modern therapy for chronic granulomatous disease (CGD) includes aggressive and prolonged administration of antibiotics and Prednisolone [5, 11, 21].

- Sulfasalazine and Azathioprine are useful steroid-sparing agents. Tumor necrosis factor-α (TNF-α) inhibitors such as Infliximab are effective anti-inflammatory agents but might significantly increase the risk of severe and even fatal infections [5].
- Methotrexate and Hydroxychloroquine (Plaquenil) can be effective in those with arthritides or lupus-like problems.

25.6.1 Lifelong Anti-Infectious Prophylaxis Includes

A. Antibiotics such as Trimethoprim-Sulfamethoxazole (TMP-SMZ-5 mg/kg/day (maximum 320 mg P.O in two divided daily doses) [22].
B. Antimycotics such as Itraconazole (Itraconazole 5 mg/kg (maximum dose 200 mg orally daily) [23].
C. And/or Interferon (INF)-gamma (50 μg/m^2 (subcutaneous) three times a week 15 μg/kg (subcutaneous) three times a week for children <0.5 m^2) [10–12].

If a fungal invasive infection is identified or strongly suspected, intravenous voriconazole is recommended as initial treatment. Voriconazole has been the recommended first-line antifungal agent for invasive aspergillosis. This triazole antifungal agent is active against both *A. fumigatus* and *A. nidulans*, the most frequent fungal pathogens observed in CGD, and has good central nervous system (CNS) penetration making it the first line of treatment as well in CNS aspergillosis [24].

Another promising azole antifungal, isavuconazole, has recently been shown to be non-inferior to voriconazole in the invasive mold infections in adult allogeneic hematopoietic stem-cell transplantation (HSCT) patients and adult patients with hematological malignancies [22, 24].

When infections are refractory to voriconazole or when there is intolerance, intravenous liposomal Amphotericin B and Caspofungin have been shown effective. Posaconazole, an orally well-tolerated broad-spectrum triazole antifungal agent, has proven efficacy as prevention of and salvage therapy for invasive fungal infection [12, 22].

Immunomodulatory Therapy: INF-gamma 1b (Actimmune) therapy (50 μg/m^2 subcutaneous three times a week OR 15 μg/kg subcutaneous three times a week for children <0.5 m) appears to be a promising way of improving neutrophil and monocyte function and may prove to be of particular value in the prevention or treatment of deep fungal infections. INF-gamma possesses antiviral, immunomodulatory, and antiproliferative activity also [14, 22].

Stem cell Transplant: In the case of multidrug resistance, life-threatening infections (e.g., aspergillosis), hematopoietic stem cell transplantation (HSCT) with reduced-intensity conditioning represents a valid curative option [18]. HLA identical sibling umbilical cord stem cell transplantation (UCSCT) after myeloablative conditioning (Stem cell transplantation from an HLA-identical donor) may, at present, be the only proven curative approach to CGD [25].

Present HSCT indication criteria in children are one or more life-threatening infections, non-compliance with antimicrobial prophylaxis, or steroid-dependent autoinflammation. Indication criteria in adolescents and young adults are more difficult to apply because organ dysfunction is frequent and transplant-related mortality after HSCT has been high [9, 15, 18].

Gene therapy for CGD: Gene therapy for hematopoietic cells (GT-HSC) represents an attractive alternative to HSCT as therapy for CGD patients without a matched donor [8, 16, 25].

25.6.2 Surgical Treatment

In addition to systemic antifungal treatment, surgical debridement or excision of consolidated infection is advised when possible [19], including surgical drainage of abscesses and resection (when possible) of granulomas.

25.7 Essential Features

- CGD is a rare immunodeficiency disease characterized by repeated infections that invade multiple organs. CGD patients are prone to catalase-positive bacterial or fungal infections.
- Pneumonia is the most common presentation. It often gets complicated with lung abscess, which is an unlikely prospect for children with normal immunologic functions.
- Persistent suppurative adenitis is the second common presentation.
- Fulminant infections such as liver abscess, brain abscess, osteomyelitis unresponsive to treatments, repeated infections, unusual location of the infection, or a severe infection that propagates to adjacent tissues are the characteristic presentation.
- Ear, nose, and throat (ENT) infections occur in 12% of CGD patients. It includes otitis media and otitis externa, parotitis, nasal septal abscess and recurrent multiple gingival abscesses due to *S. aureus* infection.
- Histopathology is characterized by a mixed suppurative and granulomatous inflammation.
- Culture helps to isolate the causative organism.
- Blood tests such as the nitroblue tetrazolium test and/or flow cytometry with dihydrorhodamine help to confirm the diagnosis.
- Chemiluminescence immunoassay, Direct measurements of oxygen consumption, and superoxide anion production may aid in diagnosis.
- Treatment includes aggressive and prolonged administration of antibiotics and Prednisolone.
- Lifelong prophylaxis with Trimethoprim-Sulfamethoxazole, itraconazole, and/or Interferon in required
- Hematopoietic stem cell transplantation (HSCT) is the only curative approach.
- Surgical management is limited to drainage of abscess and excision of granuloma.

References

1. Lun A, et al. Unusual late onset of X-linked chronic granulomatous disease in an adult woman after unsuspicious childhood. Clin Chem. 2002;48(5):780–1.
2. Wolach B, et al. Unusual late presentation of X-linked chronic granulomatous disease in an adult female with a somatic mosaic for a novel mutation in CYBB. Blood. 2005;105(1):61–6.
3. Winkelstein JA, et al. Chronic granulomatous disease. Report on a national registry of 368 patients. Medicine (Baltimore). 2000;79:155–69.
4. Khanna G, et al. Imaging of chronic granulomatous disease in children. Radiographics. 2005;25:1183–95.
5. Song E, et al. Chronic granulomatous disease: a review of the infectious and inflammatory complications. Clin Mol Allergy. 2011;9:10. https://doi.org/10.1186/1476-7961-9-10
6. Roos D, de Boer M. Molecular diagnosis of chronic granulomatous disease. Clin Exp Immunol. 2014;175(2):139–49.
7. Liese J, et al. Long-term follow-up and outcome of 39 patients with chronic granulomatous disease. J Pediatr. 2000;137:687–93.
8. Trojanowska A, et al. External and middle ear diseases: radiological diagnosis based on clinical signs and symptoms. Insights Imaging. 2012;3:33–48.
9. Towbin AJ, Chaves I. Chronic granulomatous disease. Pediatr Radiol. 2010;40:657–68.
10. Afrough R, et al. An uncommon feature of chronic granulomatous disease in a neonate. Case Rep Infect Dis. 2016;5943783:4 p.
11. Schwenkenbecher P, et al. Chronic granulomatous disease first diagnosed in adulthood presenting with spinal cord infection. Front Immunol. 2018;9:1258. https://doi.org/10.3389/fimmu.2018.01258
12. Tafti SF, et al. Chronic granulomatous disease with unusual clinical manifestation, outcome, and pattern of inheritance in an Iranian family. J Clin Immunol. 2006;26(3):291–6.
13. Martire B, et al. Clinical features, long-term follow-up and outcome of a large cohort of patients with chronic granulomatous disease: n Italian multicenter study. Clin Immunol. 2008;126(2):155–64.
14. Arnold DE, Heimall JR. A review of chronic granulomatous disease. Adv Ther. 2017;34(12):2543–57.

15. Jurkowska M, et al. Genetic and biochemical background of chronic granulomatous disease. Arch Immunol Ther Exp. 2004;52(2):113–20.
16. Kliegman S, St Geme S. Nelson textbook of pediatrics, 2-volume set, chapter 128, 20th ed. Elsevier; 2015.
17. Chiriaco M, et al. Chronic granulomatous disease: clinical, molecular, and therapeutic aspects. Pediatr Allergy Immunol. 2016;27(3):242–53.
18. Gutierrez MJ, et al. Residual NADPH oxidase activity and isolated lung involvement in X-linked chronic granulomatous disease. Case Rep Pediatr 2012;974561:6 p.
19. Strovas TJ, et al. Direct measurement of oxygen consumption rates from attached and unattached cells in a reversibly sealed, diffusionally isolated sample chamber. Adv Biosci Biotechnol. 2010;5(5):398–408.
20. Johnston RB, et al. The role of superoxide anion generation in phagocytic bactericidal activity. Studies with normal and chronic granulomatous disease leukocytes. J Clin Invest. 1975;55(6):1357–2. https://doi.org/10.1172/JCI108055
21. Yamazaki-Nakashimada MA, et al. Corticosteroid therapy for refractory infections in chronic granulomatous disease: case reports and review of the literature. Ann Allergy Asthma Immunol. 2006;97(2):257–61.
22. King J, et al. Aspergillosis in chronic granulomatous disease. J Fungi (Basel). 2016;2(2):15.
23. Gallin JI, et al. Itraconazole to prevent fungal infections in chronic granulomatous disease. N Engl J Med. 2003;348(24):2416–22.
24. Herbrecht R, et al. Voriconazole vs. amphotericin b for primary therapy of invasive aspergillosis. N Engl J Med. 2002;347:408–15. https://doi.org/10.1056/NEJMoa020191.
25. Seger RA. Modern management of chronic granulomatous disease. Br J Haematol. 2008;140(3):255–66.

Part V

Neoplastic Granulomatous Diseases

NK/T-Cell Lymphoma (Midline Lethal Granuloma)

26

Abstract

Lethal midline granuloma is a midfacial necrotizing lesion that is characterized by destructive mucosal lesions of the upper aerodigestive tract. The patients complain of rhinorrhea, epistaxis, nasal stuffiness, obstruction, and pain. The underlying mucosa is thickened and the patient usually develops extensive midfacial destructive lesions, perforated nasal septum and erosion of the nasal bone. The disease is localized to the upper aerodigestive tract at presentation but dissemination to distant sites may occur. Constitutional symptoms may develop. Also referred to as polymorphic reticulosis, midline malignant reticulosis, Stewart's granuloma most of the lethal midline granulomas are NK/T-cell lymphomas. Untreated, this disease has a very high mortality reaching almost 100% due to septicemia, perforation into blood vessels or penetration into brain leading to abscess. Clinical diagnosis is aided by histopathology that typically reveals granulomatous lesion with a mixed cellular infiltrate of eosinophils, lymphocytes, plasma cells and histiocytes. Angiocentric and angiodestructive pattern is usually seen. Immunohistochemistry (IHC) is positive for T-cell markers. Combined chemotherapy followed by involved field external radiation beam to be beneficial in patients and prolonged progression-free survival rates.

Synonyms

Stewart's granuloma, Polymorphic reticulosis, Nasal NK/T-cell lymphomas, midline malignant reticulosis, Non-Hoghkins T-cell lymphoma [1, 2].

26.1 Background

Nasal NK/T-cell lymphomas are aggressive, locally destructive, midfacial, necrotizing lesions. Most of them were initially diagnosed as lethal midline granuloma, a term that is slowly being phased out. The term "lethal midline granuloma" was first described by "McBride" in 1897 [3, 4] LMG was thought to be a manifestation of three or four different diseases: the well-characterized disease of Granulomatosis with polyangiitis (GPA), the ill-defined disorders of polymorphic reticulosis or midline malignant reticulosis, and an incompletely defined form of non-Hodgkins lymphoma [1, 2]. Subsequent studies found that the cells infiltrating the midline tissues in cases of lethal midline granuloma that were not clearly diagnosed as Granulomatosis with polyangiitis were: (a) infected by the Epstein–Barr virus and (b) malignant lymphocytes, usually NK cells or, rarely, cytotoxic T-cells. The disease is therefore now regarded as an NK/T-cell malignancy, is grouped with other Epstein–Barr virus-associated lymphoproliferative disease and is classified by the World Health Organization (2017 update) as a

S. V. Nemade, K. J. Shinde, *Granulomatous diseases in Otorhinolaryngology, Head and Neck*,
https://doi.org/10.1007/978-981-16-4047-6_26

manifestation of the well-defined disease, extra-nodal NK/T-cell lymphoma, nasal type (ENKTCL-NT) [1, 2, 5].

Macroscopically the lesions usually look like necrotic granulomas and are characterized by ulceration and destruction of the nose and para-nasal sinus es with the erosion of soft tissues, bone, and cartilage of the region. The patients show an aggressive and lethal course with rapid destruction of the nose and face (midline); therefore the term "lethal midline granuloma" [3, 4].

26.2 Epidemiology

This disease occurs around the fourth decade, and the male to female ratio is 8:1 to 2:1 [2]. It is more prevalent in the Asians and Native American populations of Mexico, Central America and South America. Low frequency of HLA-A*0201 alleles is reported in patients with EBV+ nasal NKTL. T-/NK cell sinonasal lymphoma is most commonly seen in Asia, and an increased incidence has also been described in Latin American countries such as Mexico, Guatemala, and Peru [1, 2].

26.3 Etiopathogenesis

This entity is associated with the Epstein–Barr virus, and the presence of EBV-encoded RNA-1, EBV-encoded RNA-2, and, less commonly, LMP-1 has been identified in the neoplastic lymphoid cells [3–5]. Morphologically it is characterized by extensive ulceration of mucosal sites with a lymphomatous infiltrate that is diffuse but has an angiocentric and angiodestructive growth pattern. These tumors have specific characteristics of NK cells. NK cells are active against tumor cells and cells infected with bacteria or viruses without prior sensitization. These develop from precursor cells that can differentiate into NK/T--cells, and this explains why some of the NK cells can also express T-cell markers. The most common immunophenotype is CD56+, CD3+, and surface CD20. Nasal NK/T-cell lymphoma is an aggressive disease with a rapid downhill course.

Untreated, this disease has a very high mortality reaching almost 100% due to septicemia, angioinvasion, or intracranial extention leading to brain abscess [4, 6, 7].

26.4 Clinical Features

26.4.1 ENT and Head Neck Manifestations

It commonly involves the nasal cavity, oral cavity, and/or pharynx and may extend to the eyes [4, 7]. The patients complain of rhinorrhea, epistaxis, nasal stuffiness, obstruction, and pain. There is often a history of longstanding sinusitis with purulent and foul-smelling nasal discharge. There may or may not be a tumor mass. The underlying mucosa is thickened, and the patient usually develops extensive midfacial destructive lesions (Figs. 26.1 and 26.2), perforated nasal septum and erosion of the nasal bone. Nasal septal perforation has been reported in 40% of cases. Systemic symptoms such as fever, weight loss, night sweats and anemia are not typically noted except in advanced cases. The disease is local-

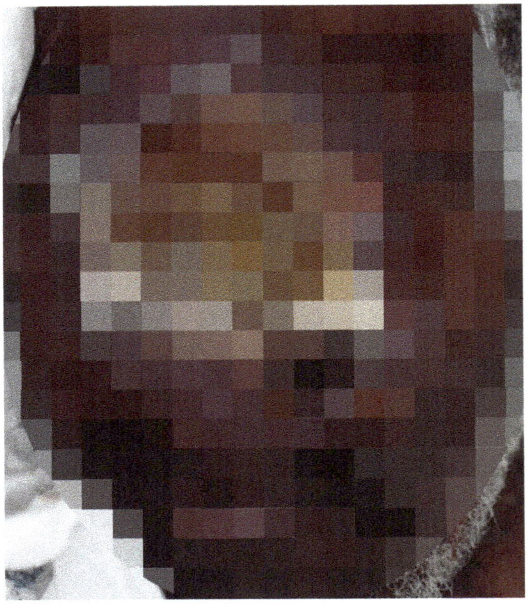

Fig. 26.1 Destruction of the midface with swelling of surrounding facial tissues and lower part of the nose [8]

Fig. 26.2 NK/T-cell lymphoma involving nasal cavity extending to right nare [9]

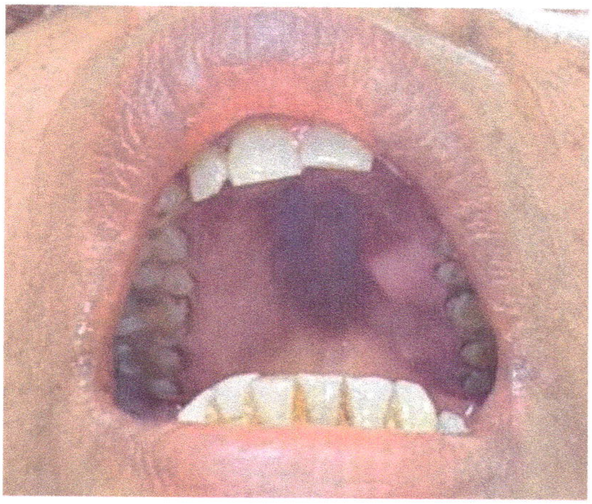

Fig. 26.3 Bulge on the left posterior hard palate extending to soft palate

ized to the upper aerodigestive tract at presentation, but dissemination to distant sites may occur [7–9].

Swelling of the soft palate or posterior hard palate (Fig. 26.3) may precede the formation of a deep, necrotic ulceration, which usually occupies a midline position. This ulceration may progress to destroy the palate, which typically creates an oronasal fistula.

The clinical course of NK-cell lymphoma varies with the clinical stage. Patients with limited stage disease (usually nasal disease) typically have an indolent course with tumor restriction to the original site, but others with advanced stage suffer rapid progression to systemic dissemination and may involve the lung, gastrointestinal tract, skin, and various other tissues. It is often accompanied by hemophagocytosis or disseminated intravascular coagulation [4, 9].

26.5 Diagnosis

Hematological investigations are usually normal except raised ESR and absolute eosinophil count.

26.5.1 Histopathology

Biopsy of granulomatous lesion typically shows a mixed cellular infiltrate of eosinophils, lymphocytes, plasma cells and histiocytes. A diffuse dense infiltrate of atypical small and large lymphocytes with pleomorphism may be present. A diffuse lymphomatous infiltrate having an angiocentric and angiodestructive pattern is usually seen (Figs. 26.4 and 26.5) [4, 7, 9].

Immunohistochemistry (IHC) is positive for T-cell markers, such as CD3 (Fig. 26.1) and CD45RO but is negative for a B-cell marker, i.e., CD20. IHC for an NK cell marker, i.e., CD56 is

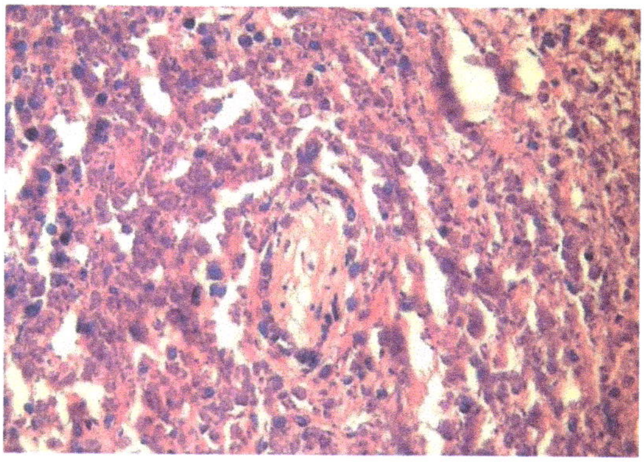

Fig. 26.4 Photomicrograph showing angiocentric (around the blood vessels) distribution of atypical lymphoid cells with hyperchromatic nuclei infiltrating the wall and filling the lumen of a blood vessel (H and E 40×) [4]

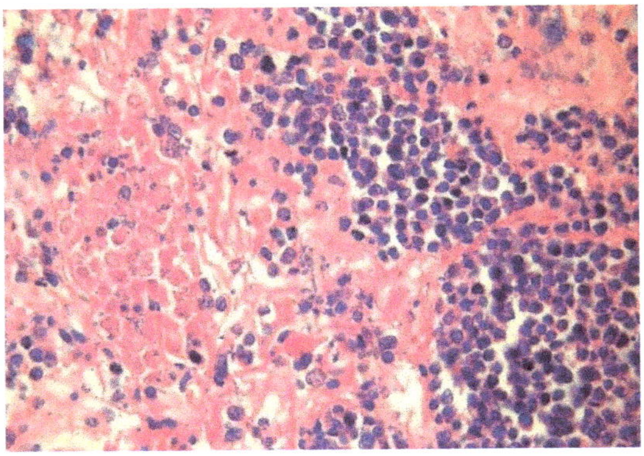

Fig. 26.5 Photomicrograph showing areas of necrosis and atypical lymphoid cells with hyperchromatic nuclei (H and E stain 40×) [4]

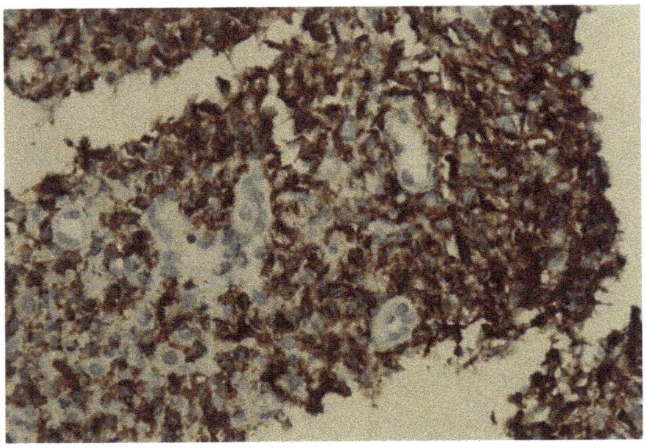

Fig. 26.6 Immunohistochemistry showing atypical lymphocytes positive for CD56 (original magnification ×40) [8]

most sensitive (Figs. 26.6 and 26.7). Fungal strains, Periodic Acid Schiff (PAS) should be done to exclude fungal disease [3, 4, 8, 10].

26.5.2 Imaging

CT paranasal sinuses show destruction of midline structures, especially nasal septum (bony and cartilaginous both) and hard palate with bony sequestration (Fig. 26.8). It may be associated with sinusitis. MRI better delineates the soft tissue involvement with intraorbital or intracranial extension (Fig. 26.9) [4, 5, 8].

26.5.3 Serology

The active involvement of EBV in the pathogenesis of extranodal NK/T-cell lymphoma, nasal type, is further supported by the direct positive correlation between EBV load in the tumor and the extent of the disease, and by the high titers of IgG antibodies to EBV in persons with the disease. Plasma titer of EBV DNA serves as a marker of tumor viral burden and fluctuates with the status of the disease and the response to treatment because EBV DNA fragments are released from apoptotic tumor cells and escape into the circulation [11].

26.5.4 Molecular Assay

High levels of serum or plasma cell-free EBV DNA by quantitative PCR is considered to be a negative prognostic marker.

26.6 Treatment

26.6.1 Therapy for Localized Extranodal NK-Cell Lymphoma

Chemotherapy and external beam irradiation is beneficial in patients and prolong the progression-free survival rates to 70% [7]. Injection methotrexate 50 mg I.V. for 12 weeks along with external beam irradiation (total 34 Gy units) is the preferred regimen [4, 12].

26.6.2 Therapy for Advanced Extranodal NK-Cell Lymphoma

Four cycles of multidrug chemotherapy regimen and third-generation anthracycline-containing regimen followed by external beam irradiation

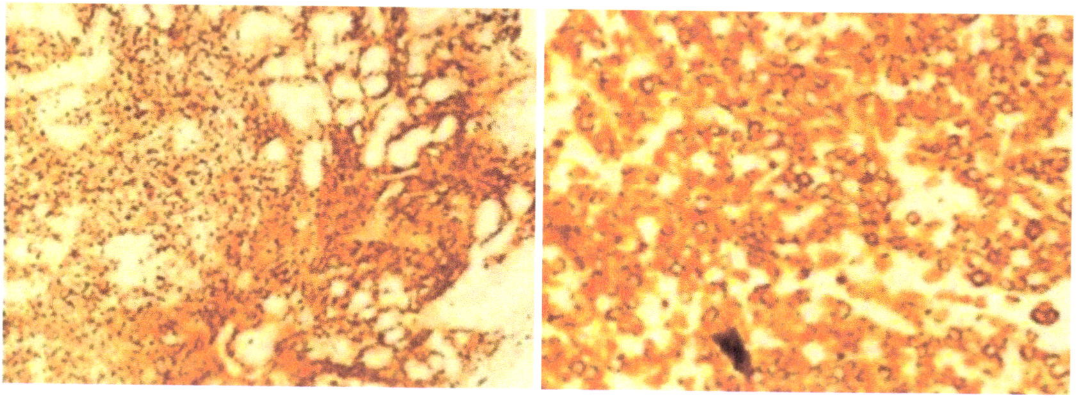

Fig. 26.7 Immunohistochemistry showing atypical lymphocytes positive for CD3+MP ×10 and HP ×40 [9]

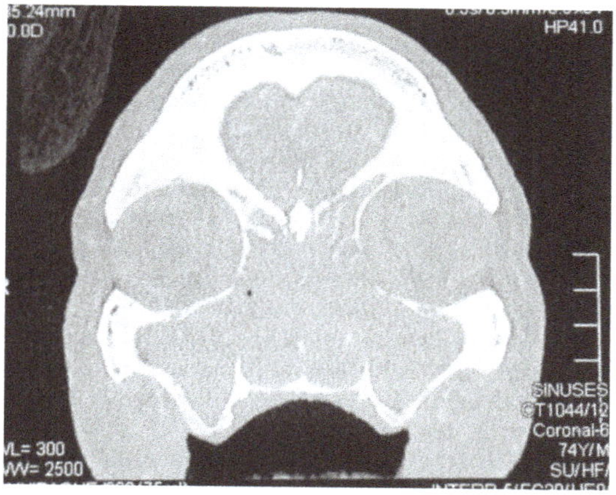

Fig. 26.8 Destruction of the medial walls of the maxillary sinuses and veiling of maxillary sinuses, ethmoidal sinus, frontal sinus and the nasal cavity [8]

(36 Gy) is the choice of therapy, but most patients respond poorly and mortality is high [4, 12, 13].

Treatment Regimens [14]:

- SMILE
  - S (steroid), M (methotrexate), I (ifosfamide), L (L-asparaginase) and E (etoposide)
  - Frontline therapy in fit patients
  - Improved response rates in relapsed or advanced-stage disease

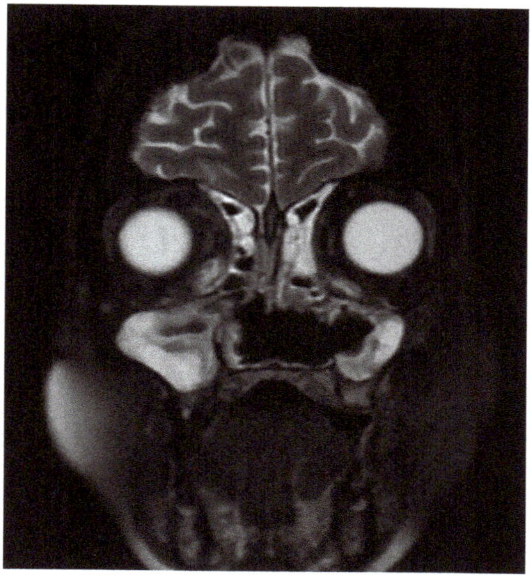

Fig. 26.9 MRI showing midline destruction involving nasal septum and the medial wall of maxillary sinuses. Extension of granuloma to inferomedial aspect of the orbits

- CHOP
  - C (cyclophosphamide), H (hydrxydaunorubicin), O (vincristin), P (prednisone)
- ESHAP
  - Etoposide, methylprednisolone, cytarabine, and cisplatin

- DeVIC
  - D (dexamethasone), E (etoposide), VI (ifosfamide) and C (carboplatin)
  - Overall response rate (ORR) of 81% and complete remission in 77% of patients when associated with concurrent radiation therapy.

    Hematopoietic stem cell transplantation (HSCT)-Several reports demonstrated successful treatment using hematopoietic stem cell transplantation (HSCT) for these diseases. Currently, HSCT is the only therapy expected to be curative in advanced cases. However, the results of transplants during relapse are poor, and this requires the development of more effective chemotherapeutic regimens for NK-cell neoplasms [4, 12].

26.7 Essential Features

- Lethal midline granuloma is also known as Nasal NK/T-cell lymphoma, is an aggressive, locally destructive, midfacial, necrotizing lesion.
- Known to be associated with the Epstein–Barr virus.
- Ulceration and destruction of the nose and paranasal sinuses with erosion of soft tissues, bone, and cartilage of the region.
- The disease is localized to the upper aerodigestive tract at presentation, but mat spread fast, leading to septicemia, angioinvasion, or intracranial extension leading to brain abscess.
- Histopathology: Granulomatous lesion typically shows a mixed cellular infiltrate of eosinophils, lymphocytes, plasma cells and histiocytes. Angiocentric and angiodestructive pattern is usually seen.
- Immunohistochemistry (IHC) is positive for T-cell markers, such as CD3, CD45RO, and NK cell marker CD56
- Computed Tomography helps to delineate bone, cartilage destruction along with the extent of disease.
- Chemotherapy with CHOP (cyclophosphamide, doxorubicin, vincristine, prednisone) regimen followed by external beam irradiation (36Gy) is the choice of therapy.
- The SMILE regimen (steroid hormone, methotrexate, ifosfamide, L-asparaginase, and etoposide) is found to be effective with Improved response rates in advanced-stage disease.

References

1. Aozasa K, et al. Nation-wide study of lethal midline granuloma in Japan: frequencies of Wegener's granulomatosis, polymorphic reticulosis, malignant lymphoma and other related conditions. Int J Cancer. 1989;44(1):63–6.
2. Hartig G, et al. Nasal T-cell lymphoma and the lethal midline granuloma syndrome. Otolaryngol Head Neck Surg. 1996;114(4):653–6.
3. Ghosh SN, et al. Lethal midline granuloma. Indian J Dermatol. 1995;40:53–4.
4. Metgud RS, et al. Extranodal NK/T-cell lymphoma, nasal type (angiocentric T-cell lymphoma): a review about the terminology. J Oral Maxillofac Pathol. 2011;15:96–100.
5. Rezk SA, et al. Epstein—Barr virus—associated lymphoid proliferations, a 2018 update. Hum Pathol. 2018;79:18–41.
6. Mehta V, et al. D. Nasal NK/T cell lymphoma presenting as a lethal midline granuloma. Indian J Dermatol Venereol Leprol. 2008;74:145–7.
7. Patel V, et al. Nasal extranodal NK/T-cell lymphoma presenting as a perforating palatal ulcer: a diagnostic challenge. Indian J Dermatol Venereol Leprol. 2006;72:218–21.
8. Tlholoe MM, et al. Extranodal natural killer/T-cell lymphoma, nasal type: 'midline lethal granulomá' case report. Head Face Med. 2013;9:4. https://doi.org/10.1186/1746-160X-9-4.
9. Schwarz ER, et al. Extranodal NK/T-cell lymphoma, nasal type, presenting as refractory *Pseudomonas aeruginosa* facial cellulitis. J Investig Med High Impact Case Rep. 2017;5(3):2324709617716471. https://doi.org/10.1177/2324709617716471
10. Wang B, et al. Combined chemotherapy and external beam radiation for stage IE and IIE natural killer cell T-cell lymphoma of nasal cavity. Leuk Lymphoma. 2007;48:396–402.
11. Al-Hakeem DA, et al. Extranodal NK/T-cell lymphoma, nasal type. Oral Oncol. 2007;43:4–14. https://doi.org/10.1016/j.oraloncology.2006.03.011.
12. Suzuki R. Leukemia and lymphoma of natural killer cells: review. Hema. 2005;45:51–70.
13. Yamaguchi M, et al. Extranodal NK/T-cell lymphoma: updates in biology and management strategies. Best Pract Res Clin Haematol. 2018;31(3):315–21.
14. Marques-Piubelli ML, et al. Extranodal NK/T cell lymphoma, nasal type. PathologyOutlines.com website. https://www.pathologyoutlines.com/topic/lymphomanonBnasal.html

Part VI

Reactive Granulomatous Diseases

27 Reparative Giant Cell Granuloma

Abstract

Giant cell reparative granuloma (GCRG) is an uncommon benign non-neoplastic osteolytic lesion that occurs mainly within the mandible and maxilla and occasionally in the skull, spine and small bones of the hands and feet. The term "giant cell granuloma" is now more frequently used as this lesion has been found in patients without a history of trauma. In addition, several cases with a destructive nature, in contrast to a reparative one, have been observed. Depending on the origin, these are known as central if intraosseous and peripheral if extraosseous. Central giant cell granuloma (CGCG) usually results from an inflammatory response to intraosseous hemorrhage following trauma, while peripheral giant cell granuloma (PGCG) is reactive gingival mass resembling pyogenic granuloma, it pushes teeth aside and may erode alveolar bone or involve periodontal membrane. It arises from periodontal ligament enclosing the root of tooth. Imaging modalities such as CT scan, Orthopantomogram are helpful in the diagnosis. Radiology in CGCG typically reveals radiolucent mass with honeycomb/ soap bubble appearance (multilocular lesion that helps to differentiate it from PGCG). Surgical excision of the granulomatous mass and thorough curettage is the gold standard treatment. Repeat curettage may be necessary to prevent a recurrence. In extensive granuloma, reconstructive surgery is necessary.

Synonyms

Giant cell granuloma (GCG)

27.1 Background

The term "giant cell reparative granuloma" (GCRG) was introduced by "Jaffe" in 1953 as a benign lesion originating from an inflammatory response due to intraosseous hemorrhage following trauma [1, 2]. It is a non-neoplastic fibro-osseous lesion, mostly found in the mandible and maxilla [3, 4]. Initially referred to as a "giant cell reparative granuloma," due to the previously accepted notion of its nature in attempting to repair areas of injury, the term "giant cell granuloma" is now more frequently used as this lesion has been found in patients without a history of trauma. In addition, several cases with a destructive nature, in contrast to a reparative one, have been observed [5]. Giant cell granulomas occurring within the bone (intraosseous) are called central giant cell granuloma (CGCG) and those occurring on edentulous alveolar processes or gingivae (extraosseous) are called peripheral giant cell granuloma (PGCG). "Bernier Cahn" suggested that these lesions should be called

S. V. Nemade, K. J. Shinde, *Granulomatous diseases in Otorhinolaryngology, Head and Neck*,
https://doi.org/10.1007/978-981-16-4047-6_27

either a peripheral or central giant cell reparative granuloma [6]. Although the CGCG is rare in nature, making up 7% of total benign lesions of the jaws it is at times uncompromising in nature, especially in young patients [5, 7]. Contrary to that, PGCG is a more common giant cell lesion of the jaw and can arise either in response to local irritation or from the connective tissue of the gingiva, periodontal membrane, or from the periosteum of the alveolar ridge. Temporal bone location is less frequent and was first described in 1974 by "Hirschl and Katz" [8].

27.2 Epidemiology

CGCG is seen twice more common in females than males. It usually occurs before 30 years of age, but can occur from infants to the seventh decade of life. Multiple CGCGs are seen in people with Noonan syndrome. Mutations in PTPN 11 or RAS pathway genes are seen [2].

PGCG mainly affects female patients (60% of cases) and, although it can occur at any age, has a peak incidence between 40 and 60 years [2, 9]. Peripheral type is four times more common than central type [2].

27.3 Etiopathogenesis

CGCG—Central giant cell granuloma is a non-neoplastic proliferative lesion of an unknown etiology. The former theory suggests that it usually results from an inflammatory response to intraosseous hemorrhage following trauma [9].

PGCG—Peripheral giant cell granuloma is one of the reactive hyperplastic lesions of the oral cavity, which originates from the periosteum or periodontal membrane following local irritation or chronic trauma [10].

The predisposing factors include trauma (tooth extraction), badly finished restorations/dentures, plaque, calculus, chronic infections, and impacted food. Furthermore, marked female predilection of PGCG suggests a possible hormonal influence, especially ovarian and thyroid hormones influence the growth of this lesion; however, the effect is secondary. Bodner et al. suggested that irritation, infection, or trauma leads to an abnormal proliferative response in the periodontal membrane and causes aggregation and granuloma formation. The lesion simulates pyogenic granuloma [11, 12].

27.4 Clinical Features

CGCG: It is common in the anterior mandible often crossing the midline. It is the most common giant cell lesion of the jaw. It may involve the nasal cavity, paranasal sinuses, or the orbit along with the invasion of cranium. It has been reported in other parts of the body including small bones, skull, spine, clavicle, tibia, humerus, and ribs [13]. Giant cell reparative granuloma of the ethmoid sinuses is exceedingly rare, but is reported [14, 15].

It is a localized fibrous tissue tumor presenting as a painless swelling that grows and expands rapidly. It erodes through the alveolar ridge and presents as soft tissue swelling typically purple in color (Fig. 27.1). It may be associated with lip paresthesia and loosening of teeth [2, 13].

PGCG: The most common site is the mucosa over the mandible followed by the maxilla. It presents as painless, soft, nodular mass, usually red to reddish-blue in color. It may be mistaken as a fibroma or pyogenic granuloma that closely resembles PGCG, the PGCG seems to arise from deeper tissues and presents as a sessile or pedunculated lesion (Fig. 27.2). PGCG has a typical bluish—red hue and is painless (Fig. 27.3), in contrast to pyogenic granuloma that has a characteristic bright red color and is painful. The lesion is usually asymptomatic; however, repeated trauma due to occlusion can lead to its growth with eventual ulceration and secondary infection [9, 11, 12, 16].

Temporal bone giant cell granuloma is more common in males than females and tends to present at a slightly older age (mean ~30 years) than its gnathic counterpart. Aside from temporal bone involvement, there can also be an extension into the TMJ joint and involvement of the sphenoid bone. Symptoms vary but can include hearing loss, otalgia, and dizziness [17].

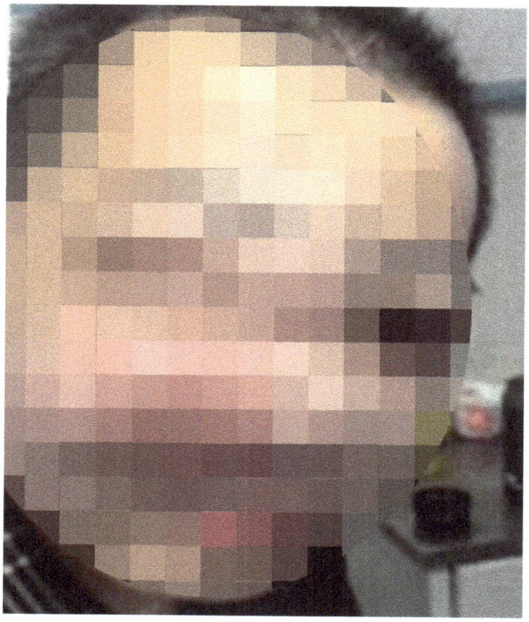

Fig. 27.1 Central giant cell granuloma involving right maxilla [15]

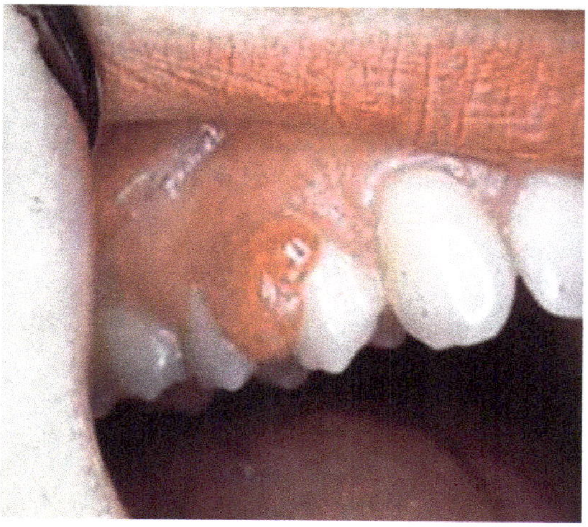

Fig. 27.2 Peripheral giant cell granuloma of right maxilla [10]

27.5 Diagnosis

27.5.1 Imaging

As PGCG is a soft tissue lesion that presents on gingival and alveolar mucosa; X-ray features

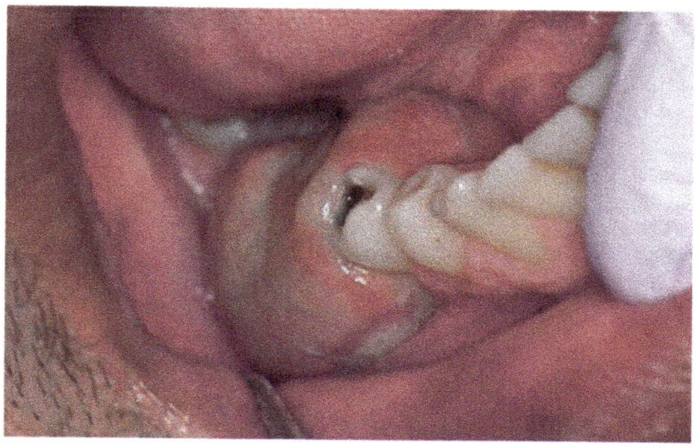

Fig. 27.3 Clinical photograph of intraoral gingival soft tissue swelling in the area of the right lower mandibular molar teeth [16]

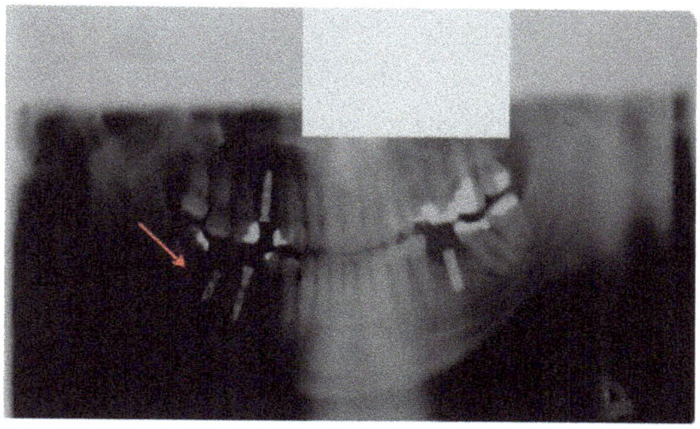

Fig. 27.4 Panoramic radiograph of a patient with PGCG showing no evidence of intra-bony pathology in association with the soft tissue lesion (arrow) [16]

are thereby nonspecific. Occasionally, bone involvement beneath the lesion is evident that presents as superficial bone resorption (Fig. 27.4) [16, 18].

On Computed tomography, giant cell granulomas usually show an expansile lesion with thinning of the surrounding bone and bone remodeling (Fig. 27.5). Foci of mineralization can be seen. On MRI, there can be a thick low T1-weighted and T2-weighted signal with a variable central signal [17]. CGCG shows a rounded, cyst-like radiolucent mass with well-defined margins or in few cases, scalloped margins. The mass may have multilocular (honeycomb or soap bubble) appearance (Figs. 27.5 and 27.6). This typical appearance helps to differentiate it from PGCG [13, 15, 19, 20].

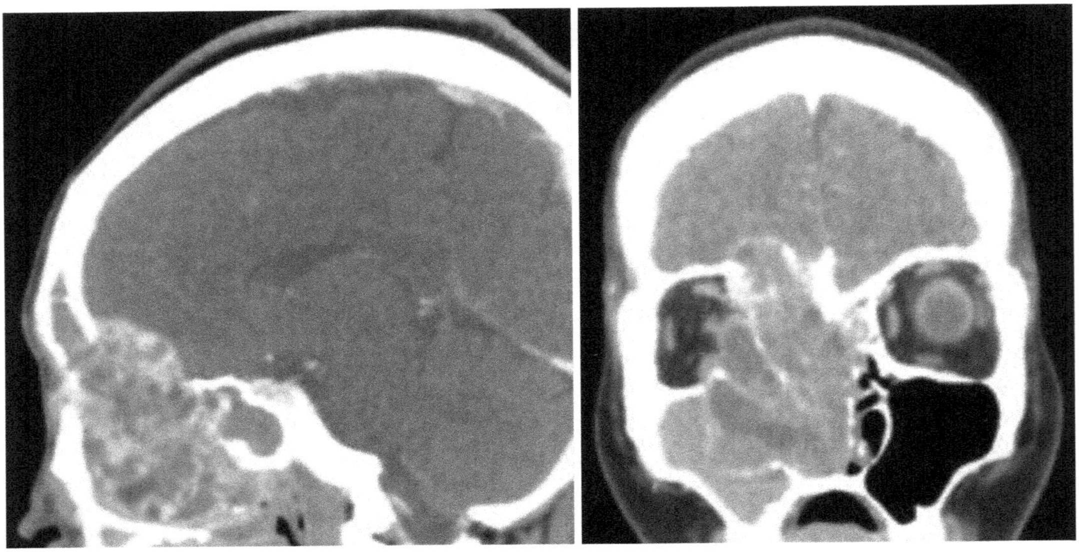

Fig. 27.5 CT scan (contrast-enhanced) demonstrates the mass occupied right nasal cavity with intracranial invasion and extension into the orbit [19]

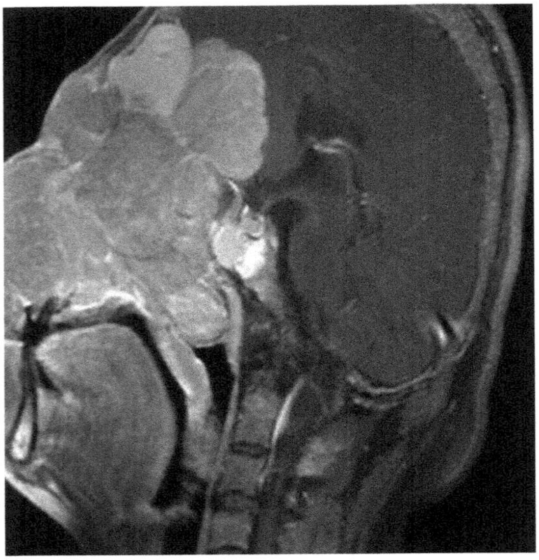

Fig. 27.6 MRI showing the lesion involved in the right nasal cavity, maxillary sinus, right frontal lobe, right eye, and skull base bone [15]

27.5.2 Histopathology

CGCG—It typically shows a lobulated mass composed of vascular connective tissue and multinucleated giant cells (osteoclasts). The giant cells may be diffusely located throughout the lesion or focally aggregate in the lesion, often clustered around hemorrhagic areas hemosiderin deposits. Lobules of the lesion can be separated by fibrous tissue or even a thin layer of bone or osteoid (Fig. 27.7) [13, 15, 21].

PGCG—Microscopic examination of the section shows the presence of hyperplastic parakeratinized stratified squamous epithelium [10, 18, 21].

Histopathology of PGCG centers around three main features:

- Presence of numerous young proliferating fibroblasts.
- Vascularized fibrocellular stroma with numerous capillaries.
- Abundant multinucleated giant cells (Fig. 27.8) [18].

27.5.3 Immunohistochemistry

It is particularly helpful in PGCG.

Serum Ki67 (proliferative marker) is expressed through G1, S, G2, and M phases of the cell cycle and its demonstration indicates the proliferative stage of the cell. Ki67 positive cells were more in PGCG. Although CGCG is more aggressive;

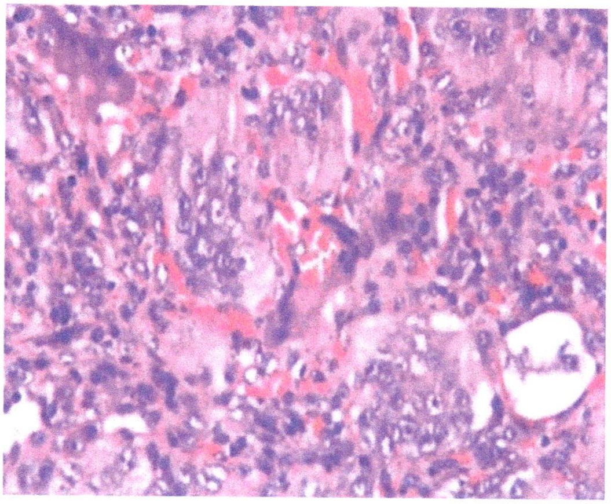

Fig. 27.7 Histopathological features of CGCG—hypertrophic shuttle fibroblasts scattered in the distribution of multicore giant cells; cells of different sizes; cells with small nuclei; no overtly mitotic cells and visible interstitial bleeding [15]

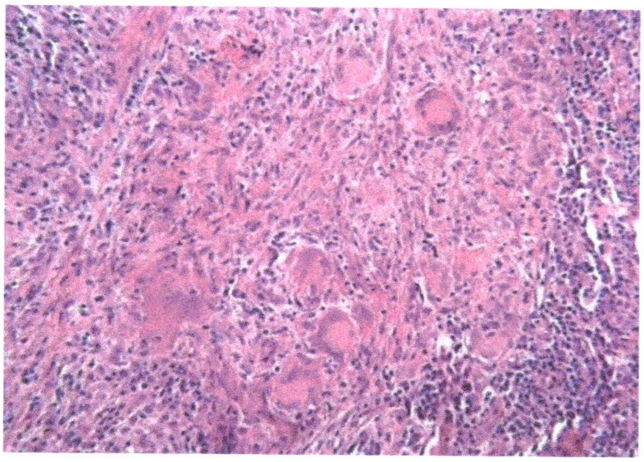

Fig. 27.8 Histological appearance of peripheral giant cell granuloma. Fibrillar and reticular connective tissue stroma with abundant young connective tissue cells of fusiform shape, and multinucleated giant cells (H&E stain, magnification ×400) [10]

however, PGCG is more proliferative than CGCG [10, 21].

Expression of α-SMA which is a cytoskeletal marker is highly correlated with myofibroblasts in the granulation tissue of PGCG. This denotes increased fibroblastic activity of the lesion [21].

27.6 Treatment

27.6.1 CGCG and PGCG

- Correction of underlying etiological factors.
- Surgery: It is the gold standard treatment that includes thorough curettage of the granuloma. Curettage is done using various methods ranging from the conventional blade, an electric scalpel to cryosurgery using liquid nitrogen or cryoprobe and lasers [17, 18].

Recurrence ranges from 15% to 20%, second curettage is sufficient to prevent further recurrence. Rapidly growing tumors are more likely to recur and can sometimes require full excision with the surrounding bone. Large lesions can require en-bloc resections. Reconstruction with full-thickness skin graft may be required.

Alternatives or adjuncts to surgery [22]:

- Intralesional corticosteroids which convert lesions into fibrous tissue
- Calcitonin which slows the growth of lesion
- Interferon α-2a which slows the growth of lesion
- Biphosphonates which slows the growth of lesion
- Thermal sterilization using laser or cryoprobe
- More recently, denosumab, a monoclonal antibody has been used in gnathic giant cell granulomas [17, 23]

These therapeutic approaches provide possible alternatives for small, slow-growing lesions, or in children where facial growth following surgery might be affected [2, 7, 14]. Radiation therapy is contraindicated. There have been cases reported in which radiation-treated lesions have undergone malignant transformation [22].

27.6.2 Essential Features

- "Giant cell reparative granuloma" (GCRG) originates from an inflammatory response due to intraosseous hemorrhage following trauma. Intraosseous form is called central giant cell granuloma (CGCG) and extraosseous form (alveolar process and gingiva) is called peripheral giant cell granuloma (PGCG).
- CGCG is the most common giant cell tumor of the jaw. Presents as a painless, rapidly growing mass that erodes the alveolus causing soft tissue swelling.
- PGCG usually presents as reddish, painless, soft nodular mass and may be mistaken with pyogenic granuloma.
- Imaging modalities such as CT scan, Orthopantomogram are helpful in the diagnosis. Radiology in CGCG typically reveals radiolucent mass with honey-comb/soap bubble appearance (multilocular lesion that helps to differentiate it from PGCG)
- Histopathology shows vascular connective tissue and multinucleated giant cells (osteoclasts).
- Immunohistochemistry is particularly helpful in PGCG. Serum Ki67 (proliferative marker) is expressed. Although CGCG is more aggressive, however, PGCG is more proliferative than CGCG.
- Surgical excision of the granulomatous mass and thorough curettage is the gold standard treatment. Repeat curettage may be necessary to prevent a recurrence. In extensive granuloma, reconstructive surgery is necessary.
- Corticosteroids, Calcitonin, Interferon α-2a, and Biphosphonates are adjuncts to surgery which slows the growth of lesion.

References

1. Boedeker CC, et al. Giant cell reparative granuloma of the temporal bone: a case report and review of the literature. Ear Nose Throat J. 2003;82:926–9.
2. Chaparro Avendaño AV, et al. Peripheral giant cell granuloma. A report of five cases and review of the literature. Medicina Oral Patologia Oral Cirugia Bucal. 2005;10(1):48–57.
3. Morris JM, et al. Giant cell reparative granuloma of the nasal cavity. AJNR Am J Neuroradiol. 2004;25:1263–5.
4. Montero EH, et al. Giant-cell reparative granuloma in temporal bone. Am J Otolaryngol. 2003;24:191–3.
5. Maerki J, et al. Giant cell granuloma of the temporal bone in a mixed martial arts fighter. J Neurol Surg Rep. 2012;73(1):60–3. https://doi.org/10.1055/s--0032-1323158. Published online 2012 Aug 8.
6. Bernier JL, Cahn LR. The peripheral giant cell reparative granuloma. J Am Dent Assoc. 1954;49:141–8.
7. Kruse-Lösler B, et al. Central giant cell granuloma of the jaws: a clinical, radiologic, and histopathologic study of 26 cases. Oral Surg Oral Med Oral Pathol Oral Radiol Endod. 2006;101:346–54.
8. Hirschl S, Katz A. Giant cell reparative granuloma outside the jaw bone: diagnostic criteria and review of the literature with the first case described in the temporal bone. Hum Pathol. 1974;5:171–81.
9. Amaral FR. Clonality analysis of giant cell lesions of the jaws. Braz Dent J. 2010;21(4):361–4. https://doi.org/10.1590/S0103-64402010000400013.
10. Shadman N, et al. Peripheral giant cell granuloma: a review of 123 cases. Dent Res J (Isfahan). 2009;6(1):47–50.
11. Bodner L, et al. Growth potential of peripheral giant cell granuloma. Oral Surg Oral Med Oral Pathol Oral Radiol Endod. 1997;83:548–51.
12. Shirani G, Arshad M. Relationship between circulating levels of sex hormones and peripheral giant cell granuloma. Acta Med Iran. 2008;46:429–33.
13. Shah UA, et al. Giant cell reparative granuloma of the jaw: a case report. Indian J Radiol Imag. 2006;16(4):677–8. https://doi.org/10.4103/0971-3026.32297.
14. Bhalodiya NH, Singh N. Giant cell reparative granuloma of posterior ethmoid: a case report. Indian J Otolaryngol Head Neck Surg. 2005;57(4):325–7. https://doi.org/10.1007/BF02907701.
15. Zhang Q, et al. Radiotherapy for recurrent central giant cell granuloma: a case report. Radiat Oncol. 2019;14:130. https://doi.org/10.1186/s13014-019-1336-7. Published online 2019 Jul 19.
16. Ogbureke EI, et al. A peripheral giant cell granuloma with extensive osseous metaplasia or a hybrid peripheral giant cell granuloma-peripheral ossifying fibroma: a case report. J Med Case Rep. 2015;9:14. https://doi.org/10.1186/1752-1947-9-14. Published online 2015 Feb 4.
17. Martinez AP, Torres-Mora J. Selected giant cell rich lesions of the temporal bone. Head Neck Pathol. 2018;12(3):367–77. https://doi.org/10.1007/s12105-018-0906-6. Published online 2018 Aug 1.
18. Goyal R, et al. Peripheral giant cell granuloma: a case report. Guident. 2011;5:76–7.
19. Ishinaga H, et al. Aggressive giant cell reparative granuloma of the nasal cavity. Case Rep Otolaryngol. 2013;2013:690194, 3 pages. https://doi.org/10.1155/2013/690194.

20. Nemoto Y, et al. Central giant cell granuloma of the temporal bone. AJNR Am J Neuroradiol. 1995;16:982–5.
21. Souza PE, et al. Evaluation of p53, PCNA, Ki-67, MDM2 and AgNOR in oral peripheral and central giant cell lesions. Oral Dis. 2000;6:35–9.
22. Jeevan Kumar KA, et al. Reparative giant cell granuloma of the maxilla. Ann Maxillofac Surg. 2011;1(2): 181–6. https://doi.org/10.4103/2231-0746.92791.
23. Bredell M, et al. Denosumab as a treatment alternative for central giant cell granuloma: a long-term retrospective cohort study. J Oral Maxillofac Surg. 2017.

28 Cholesterol Granuloma

Abstract

Cholesterol granuloma (CG) also known as cholesterol cyst is rare and expansile, round, or ovoid cyst containing cholesterol crystals surrounded by foreign body giant cells and chronic inflammation, all contained within a thick fibrous capsule. Cholesterol granuloma was first described in 1894. It is commonly encountered in the petrous apex, middle ear, and mastoid air cells. It occurs after the obstruction of the normally aerated spaces due to associated diseases such as otitis media. CG at the petrous apex presents with sensorineural hearing loss, tinnitus, vertigo, or cranial nerve impairment. CG of the mastoid and middle ear is mistaken as cholesteatoma. Blue bulging eardrum is the typical finding of CG involving the middle ear. HRCT temporal bone and MRI are diagnostic. The extent of the lesion and bone destruction is evident. MRI is useful to know the soft tissue integrity especially in lesions extending to the middle cranial fossa or posterior cranial fossa. Histopathology examination shows typical foreign body giant cells surrounding cholesterol crystals.CG of the petrous apex is treated with complete surgical excision along with the capsule. In CG of the mastoid, simple mastoidectomy with insertion of a ventilation tube is preferred.

Synonyms Cholesterol cyst [1, 2]

28.1 Background

Cholesterol granuloma (CG) is a rare condition consisting of a foreign body reaction to cholesterol crystals and hemosiderin derived from the ruptured erythrocytes. Cholesterol is an unusual endogenous substance; in that, it is relatively resistant to absorption by giant cells [1, 2]. This condition involves diverse temporal bone sites: petrous apex, middle ear, mastoid. Rarely it may involve other facial bones such as the maxilla and frontal bone. The lesion is secondary to chronic obstruction of air cells within the petrous pyramid. Cholesterol granuloma was first described in 1894. Tympanomastoid disease occurs after the obstruction of the normally aerated spaces due to associated diseases such as otitis media [3]. In the literature, it is considered the most common benign pathological lesion of the petrous apex, involving about 40% of the lesions in that area [4].

28.2 Etiopathogenesis

"Nager" described the pathogenesis of cholesterol granulomas as being dependent upon three factors: hemorrhage, obstruction of drainage, and impair-

S. V. Nemade, K. J. Shinde, *Granulomatous diseases in Otorhinolaryngology, Head and Neck*,
https://doi.org/10.1007/978-981-16-4047-6_28

ment of ventilation. The source of blood may be infection, trauma, or inflammation, and obstruction to drainage coupled with lack of ventilation leads to stasis of erythrocytes and other tissue elements that break down to deposit cholesterol and other lipids. These irritants stimulate a foreign body reaction that leads to the formation of granuloma [3].

These are predominantly found incidentally during surgical treatment of chronic otitis media and can also occur in the context of post-traumatic hemorrhage of the temporal bones. In each case, internal hemorrhage is thought to be the cause of the formation of cholesterol granuloma [2, 4].

"Beegun and Bottrill" suggested that aggressive extension of cholesterol granuloma into the middle ear and mastoid is because of intense bleeding which is an essential component for both the initiation and maintenance of aggressive cholesterol granuloma [5]. Three theories have been hypothesized for the processes that may contribute to such intensive bleeding:

1. Vacuum Hypothesis—Obstruction of the drainage pathway leads to the reabsorption of gas, promoting the development of a vacuum with resultant seepage of blood from mucosal vessels [5, 6].
2. Exposed bone marrow—The exposed bone marrow hypothesis put forth by "Jackler" and "Cho" suggests that exuberant pneumatization of the temporal bone exposes marrow-filled spaces of the petrous apex. The resulting coaptation of the marrow and mucosa results in a proclivity toward hemorrhage. Sustained hemorrhage from exposed marrow elements is responsible for the progressive expansion of granuloma [5, 6].
3. Robust Blood Supply—This theory suggests that a robust blood supply, such as that of the sigmoid sinus, carotid artery, or large epidural vein, is essential for the maintenance and promotion of bony destruction [5].

Martin et al. suggested that benign and aggressive cholesterol granulomas are often macroscopically distinct. The commonly encountered cholesterol granulomas are fluid-like expanding masses that contain lipids and cholesterol crystals surrounded by a thin fibrous lining. The second type is the rare aggressive cholesterol granuloma surrounded by a thickened wall of fibrous tissue that is capable of eroding bone [7].

28.3 Clinical Features

Cholesterol granuloma at the petrous apex presents with symptoms related to bony erosion (e.g., sensorineural hearing loss, tinnitus, vertigo, or cranial nerve impairment) [4].

Cholesterol granulomas of the petrous apex can cause:

- Sensorineural hearing loss (Fig. 28.1)
- Tinnitus, vertigo
- Cranial nerve impairment (V, VI, VII) [4, 7]

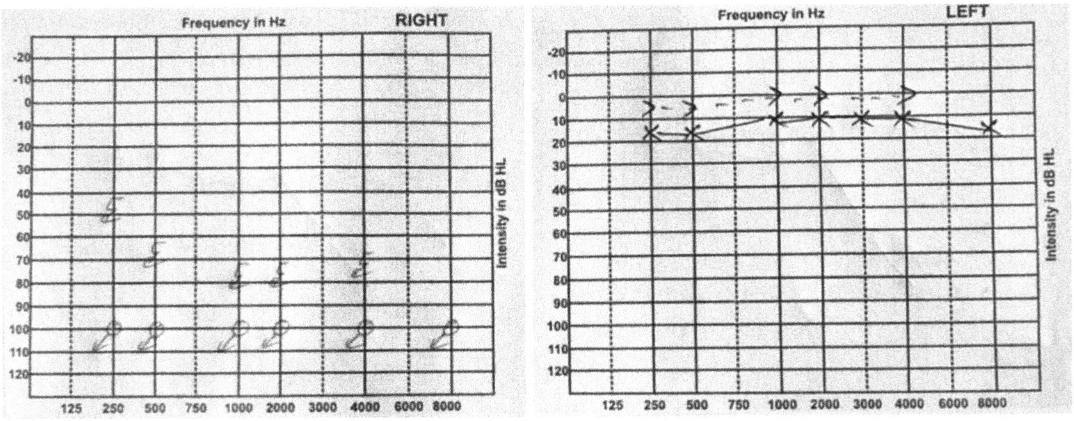

Fig. 28.1 Audiogram of the patient with cholesterol granuloma demonstrating right side sensorineural hearing loss

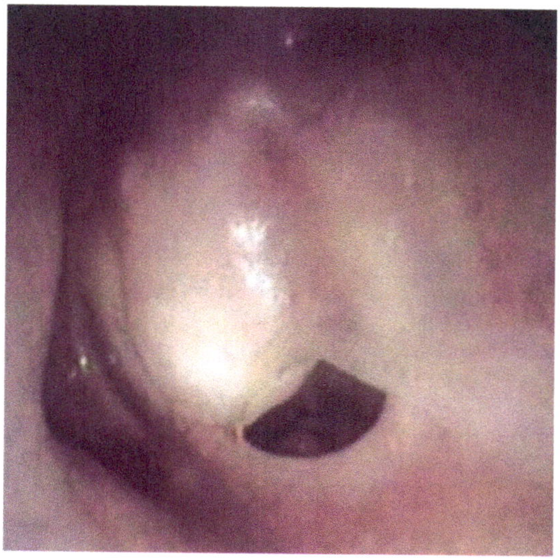

Fig. 28.2 The left tympanic membrane is thick and white. A left tympanic membrane perforation is evident, but with no discharge [8]

Cholesterol granuloma of the mastoid and middle ear may present as ear discharge, Tympanic membrane perforation (Fig. 28.2), conductive hearing loss, and facial paralysis and is mistaken as cholesteatoma. It may cause various complications, such as destruction of the inner ear, inner ear fistula, cerebrospinal fistula, and intracranial extension. Hence, early detection and treatment are crucial [7–9].

28.4 Diagnosis

Cholesterol granuloma of the middle ear typically presents with conductive hearing loss and a blue eardrum, diagnosis is easy when these findings are present [10, 11].

28.4.1 Imaging

Temporal bone HRCT: It shows a large, expansile, heterogeneous mass with bone destruction. The bone destruction may extend to the posterior and middle cranial fossa (Figs. 28.3 and 28.4) [8, 12–14].

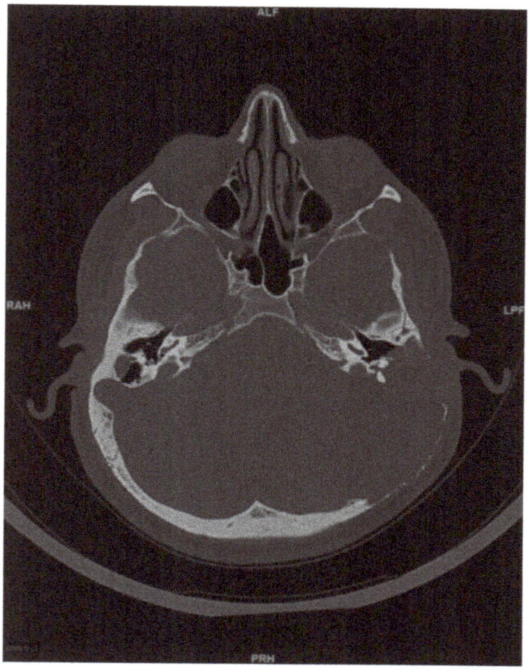

Fig. 28.3 Computed tomography (CT) scan of the temporal bone showing a mass in the left tympanomastoid region. The mass is bulging into the external auditory canal, middle ear cavity, and extending posteriorly to temporal and occipital region. A smaller lesion is seen on the right side within the mastoid cavity [12]

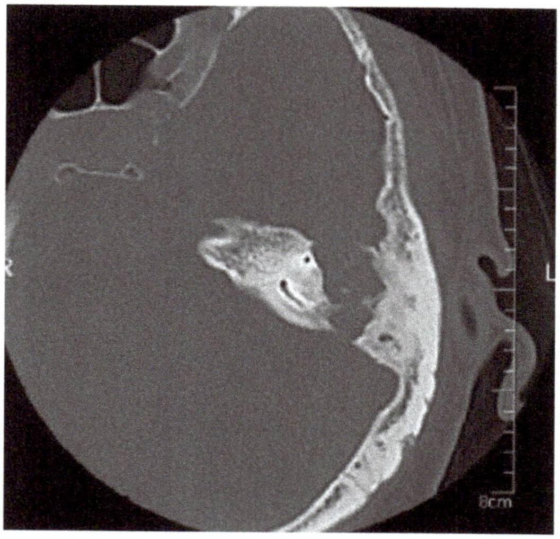

Fig. 28.4 Cholesterol granuloma of tympanomastoid region demonstrating destruction of sinus plate, dural plate and labyrinth [8]

CT scan of paranasal sinuses helps to delineate the lesions involving sinuses and soft tissue (Fig. 28.5 and 28.6) [13, 14].

MRI with gadolinium enhancement: It helps to diagnose cholesterol granuloma and differentiate between the various possible diagnoses (e.g., dermoid cyst, cholesteatoma, other tumors, and carotid aneurysm) [7]. Cholesterol granuloma is characterized by high signal intensity on both T1- and T2-weighted images, due to the paramagnetic effects of protein content and cholesterol [9] and because of the presence of areas of the void. In contrast, cholesteatomas appear to be iso- or hypodense on T1-weighted imaging and display high signal intensity on T2-weighted imaging (Fig. 28.7) [8, 13].

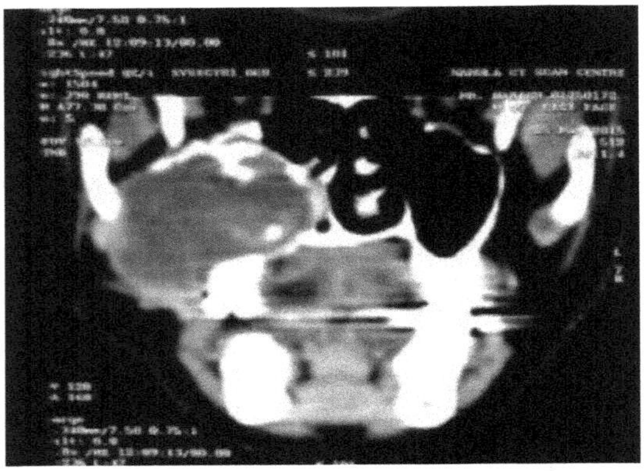

Fig. 28.5 CT scan image showing huge expansile, well-demarcated, and osteolytic mass extending from maxilla into the maxillary sinus on the right side [13]

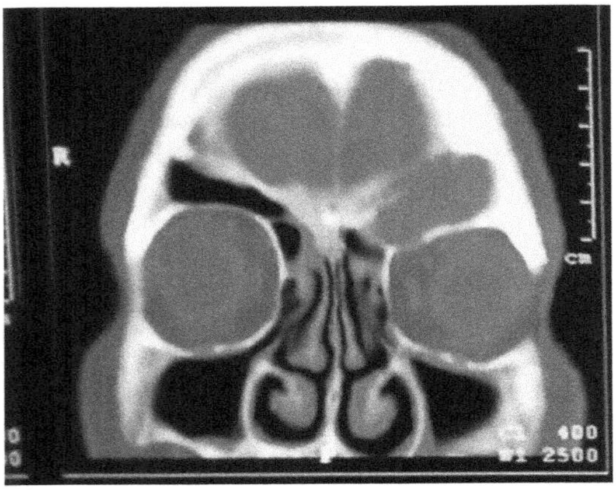

Fig. 28.6 Computed tomography (CT scan) of the orbits shows complete opacity of the left frontal sinus with anterior and inferior breach of the sinus [14]

28.4.2 Histopathology

Microscopic examination showing typical foreign body giant cells, foamy macrophages, and surrounding cholesterol crystals (Hematoxylin & Eosin stain, ×100) (Fig. 28.10) [12].

28.5 Treatment

The suitability of surgical intervention depends on the location and size of cholesterol granuloma, the existence of symptoms, and diagnostic confirmation [15–17]. Treatment strategies for cholesterol granuloma of the petrous apex include complete surgical excision along with the capsule. In the case of cystic granuloma, drainage of the cyst with excision of the capsule is recommended. In cholesterol granuloma of the mastoid, simple mastoidectomy with insertion of a ventilation tube or with additional mastoid obliteration is preferred [14, 18, 19]. Frontal sinus cholesterol granuloma needs to be excised with exposure of frontal sinus by Lynch–Howarth procedure (Fig. 28.11) [14].

28.6 Essential Features

- Cholesterol granuloma (CG) is a foreign body reaction to cholesterol crystals and hemosiderin derived from the ruptured erythrocytes.
- Involves diverse temporal bone sites: middle ear, mastoid, and petrous apex. It presents as benign or aggressive forms. Aggressive disease erodes the bone and spreads fast.
- CG at the petrous apex presents with sensorineural hearing loss, tinnitus, vertigo, or cranial nerve impairment.
- CG of the mastoid and middle ear may present as ear discharge, conductive hearing loss, and facial paralysis and is mistaken as cholesteatoma. Blue bulging eardrum is the typical finding of CG involving the middle ear.

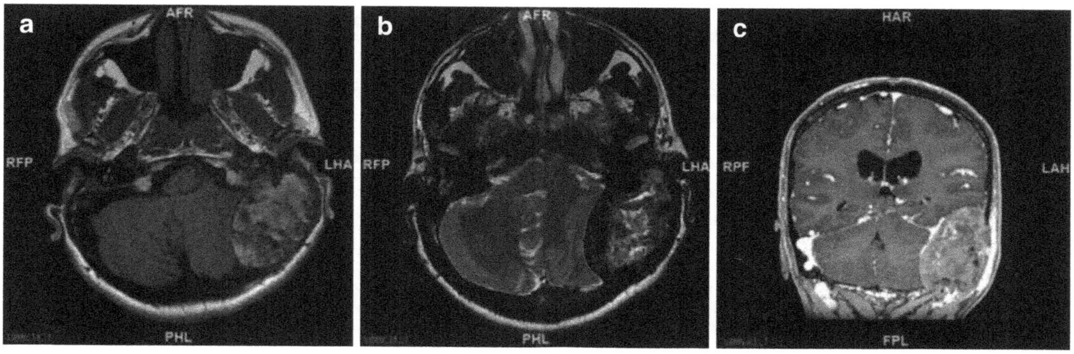

Fig. 28.7 (**a**) T1 without IV contrast. (**b**) T2-weighted image. (**c**) Coronal T1-weighted image with IV contrast. Magnetic resonance imaging (MRI) of the temporal bone showing a large, expansile, heterogenous mass in the left tympanomastoid region with involvement of the mastoid air cells, and occipital bone, and a mass effect on the cerebellum and left posterior temporal and occipital lobes. The mass shows very tiny foci of enhancement (**c**) and had intrinsic high-signal intensity on T1- and T2-weighted imaging. A similarly limited but smaller mass is seen on the right side (Figs. 28.8 and 28.9) [3, 8, 12]

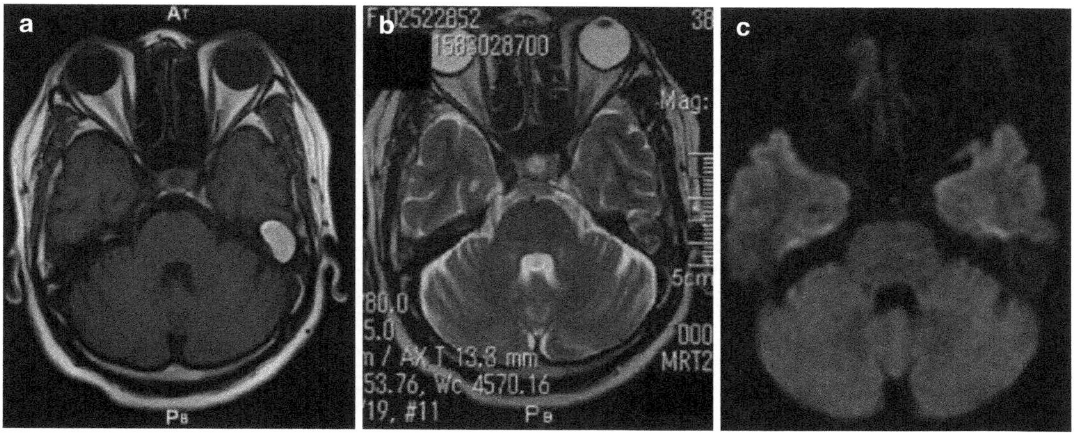

Fig. 28.8 (**a**) Axial T1-weighted temporal bone MRI showing a signal-hyperintense mass neighboring the posterior cranial fossa and extending to the middle fossa. (**b**) Axial T2-weighted imaging of the temporal bone shows a high-intensity periphery and low-intensity central mass. (**c**) DWI shows an isointense signal rather than high intensity [8]

- HRCT temporal bone is diagnostic. The extent of the lesion and bone destruction is evident. MRI is useful to know the soft tissue integrity especially in lesions extending to the middle cranial fossa or posterior cranial fossa.
- Histopathology examination shows typical foreign body giant cells surrounding cholesterol crystals.
- CG of the petrous apex is treated with complete surgical excision along with the capsule.
- In CG of the mastoid, simple mastoidectomy with insertion of a ventilation tube is preferred.

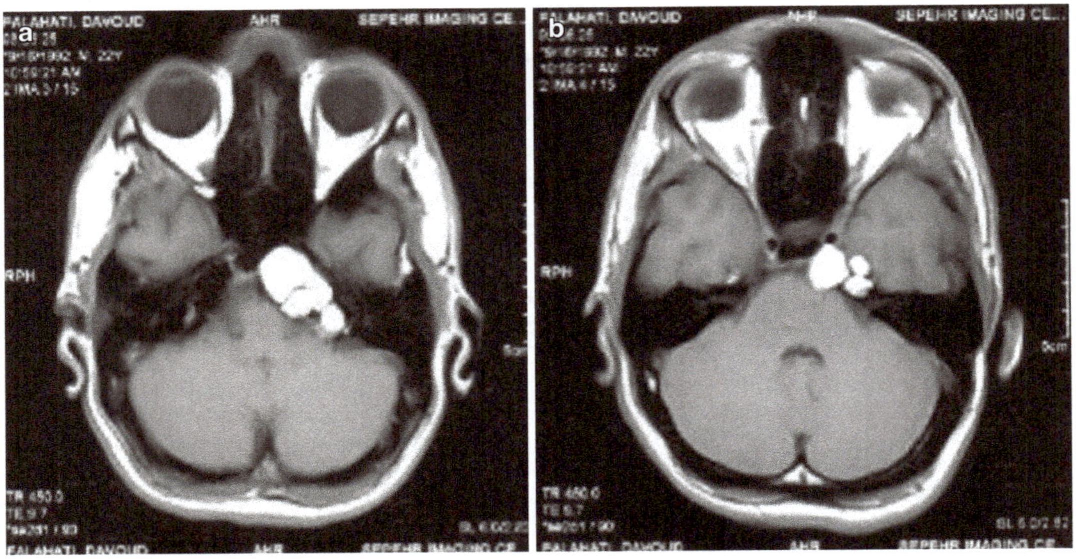

Fig. 28.9 T1-weighted MRI shows the cholesterol granuloma involving the right petrous apex [3]

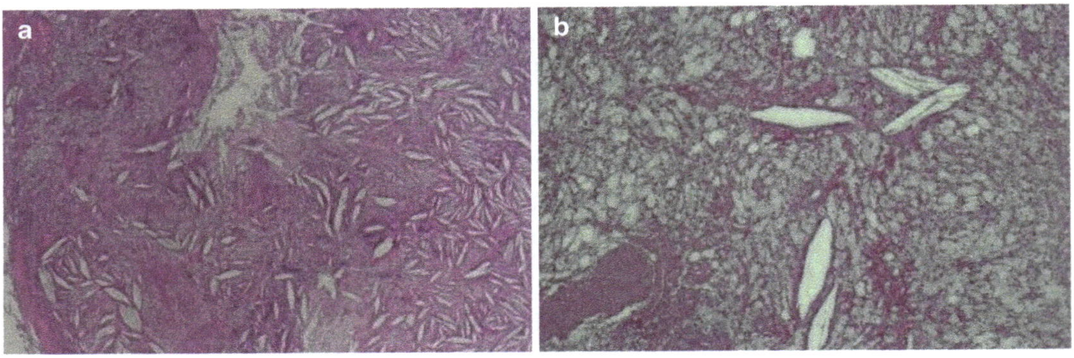

Fig. 28.10 (**a**, **b**) Cholesterol granuloma stained with hematoxylin and eosin. Histopathological evaluation with hematoxylin and eosin staining confirmed the presence of a destructive infiltrate containing foamy macrophages, foreign body giant cells, and cholesterol clefts (**b**—high power) [12]

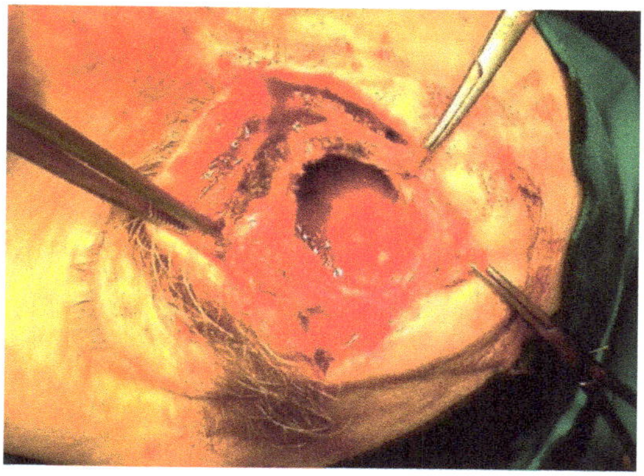

Fig. 28.11 Intraoperative photograph shows the opening of the frontal sinus with Lynch–Howarth procedure [14]

References

1. Martin TPC, et al. Large and uncharacteristically aggressive cholesterol granuloma of the middle ear. J Otol Laryngol. 2005;119:1001–3.
2. Pfister MHF, et al. Aggressiveness in cholesterol granuloma of the temporal bone may be determined by the vigor of its blood source. Otol Neurotol. 2007;28(2):232–5.
3. Samadian M, et al. Endoscopic transnasal approach for cholesterol granuloma of the petrous apex. Case Rep Neurologic Med. 2015;2015:Article ID 481231, 5 pages. https://doi.org/10.1155/2015/481231.
4. Laudien M. Orphan diseases of the nose and paranasal sinuses: pathogenesis – clinic therapy. GMS Curr Top Otorhinolaryngol Head Neck Surg. 2015;14:Doc04. https://doi.org/10.3205/cto000119. Published online 2015 Dec 22.
5. Beegun I, Bottrill ID. A large aggressive cholesterol granuloma associated with an abnormal sigmoid sinus; case report and literature review. Otorhinolaryngologist. 2009;2(3):82–4.
6. Jackler RK, Cho M. A new theory to explain the genesis of petrous apex cholesterol granuloma. Otol Neurotol. 2003;24(1):96–106. https://doi.org/10.1097/00129492-200301000-00020.
7. Martin TPC, et al. A large and uncharacteristically aggressive cholesterol granuloma of the middle ear. J Otol Laryngol. 2005;119:1001–3.
8. Kuruma T, et al. Large cholesterol granuloma of the middle ear eroding into the middle cranial fossa. Case Rep Otolaryngol. 2017;2017:3786479. https://doi.org/10.1155/2017/4793786. Published online 2017 Jun 22.
9. Brackmann DE, Toh EH. Surgical management of petrous apex cholesterol granulomas. Otol Neurotol. 2002;23(4):529–33.
10. Nager GT. Pathology of the ear and temporal bone. Baltimore, MD: Williams and Wiikins; 1993.
11. Beegun I, Bottrill ID. Large aggressive cholesterol granuloma associated with an abnormal sigmoid sinus; case report and literature review. Otorhinolaryngologist. 2009;2(3):82–4.
12. Albakheet N, et al. Familial hypercholesterolemia with bilateral cholesterol granuloma: a case series. Int J Surg Case Rep. 2019;62:135–9. https://doi.org/10.1016/j.ijscr.2019.07.018. Published online 2019 Jul 19.
13. Kamboj M, et al. Cholesterol granuloma in odontogenic cyst: an enigmatic lesion. Case Rep Dent. 2016;2016:Article ID 6105142, 5 pages. https://doi.org/10.1155/2016/6105142.
14. Marco M, et al. Cholesterol granuloma of the frontal sinus: a case report. Case Rep Otolaryngol. 2012;2012:Article ID 515986, 3 pages. https://doi.org/10.1155/2012/515986.
15. Jackler RK, Cho M. New theory to explain the genesis of petrous apex cholesterol granuloma. Otol Neurotol. 2003;24(1):96–106.
16. Goldofsky E, et al. Cholesterol cysts of the temporal bone: diagnosis and treatment. Ann Otol Rhinol Laryngol. 1991;100(3):181–7.
17. Shih TY, et al. Erosive cholesterol Granuloma. Otol Neurotol. 2013;34(4):e26–7.
18. Shihada R et al. Spontaneous regression of petrous apex cholesterol granuloma. Otol Neurotol. 2012;33(2):e10.
19. Bohra V, et al. Cholesterol granuloma of the petrous apex: benign lesion with aggressive behavior. Neurol India. 2011;59(6):927–9.

Chemical Granuloma (Cocaine, Talc, Beryllium, Tattoo)

29

Abstract

Exposure to certain harmful agents through inhalation, chronic skin exposure, or intravenous use may lead to chemical toxicity with granulomatous inflammatory reaction. The common forms of such toxicity include Cocaine abuse, Berryliosis seen in industrial workers, Talcosis (Silicosis) due to talcum powder use, and Tattooing. Cocaine snorting is associated with a peculiar type of drug-induced chronic rhinitis, which leads to inflammation of the sinonasal mucosa, slowly progressing to a destruction of nasal, palatal and pharyngeal tissues. These characteristic lesions due to cocaine abuse are commonly called cocaine-induced midline destructive lesions (CIMDL). Chronic beryllium disease (CBD) is a granulomatous lung disorder that results from beryllium exposure in a genetically susceptible host. Pulmonary talcosis, a form of pulmonary foreign body granulomatosis (PFBG), can occur in drug addicts as a result of intravenous injection of oral medications. The condition has been termed intravascular talcosis, to differentiate it from disorders arising from exposure to inhalational talc, such as simple talcosis, progressive massive fibrosis, talcosilicosis, and talcoasbestosis, often with pleural disease. Skin reactions caused by tattoo (especially red pigment) and silicon needle acupunctures vary from simple dermatitis to lichenoid, pseudolymphomatous and granulomatous reactions.

29.1 Background

Exposure to certain harmful agents through inhalation, chronic skin exposure, or intravenous use may lead to chemical toxicity with granulomatous inflammatory reaction. The common forms of such toxicity include Cocaine abuse, Berryliosis seen in industrial workers, Talcosis (Silicosis) due to talcum powder use, and Tattooing. Cocaine snorting is associated with a peculiar type of drug-induced chronic rhinitis, which leads to inflammation of the sinonasal mucosa, slowly progressing to a destruction of nasal, palatal, and pharyngeal tissues. These characteristic lesions due to cocaine abuse are commonly called cocaine-induced midline destructive lesions (CIMDL) [1–3]. A berylliosis is a form of metal poisoning caused by inhalation of beryllium dust, vapors, or its compounds or implantation of the substance in the skin. The toxic effects of beryllium most commonly occur due to occupational exposure. Acute berylliosis causes diffuse inflammation in the airway manifesting as rhinopharyngitis, laryngotracheobronchitis. Chronic berylliosis causes granulomas in the airway. Pulmonary talcosis is most commonly seen secondary to occupational exposure

S. V. Nemade, K. J. Shinde, *Granulomatous diseases in Otorhinolaryngology, Head and Neck*,
https://doi.org/10.1007/978-981-16-4047-6_29

or intravenous (IV) drug abuse and, occasionally, in excessive use of cosmetic talc. Drugs that are abused intravenously often involve contamination with cutting or bulking substances including cornstarch and talcum powder (talc). It affects the central nervous leading to intracranial talc granulomas. Tattoos are popularly used worldwide especially by the young generation. Tattoo pigments, particularly red, are the most common cause of reactions in tattoos and this can present in various clinical and histological variants with dermatitis and lichenoid being the most common. Granulomatous reactions can also occur in tattoos.

29.2 Cocaine Abuse

Cocaine, a potent CNS stimulant, is abused predominantly in Western countries. Current estimates indicate that >5.9 million Americans used this drug in 2018, and >18 million individuals have been using it worldwide [4–6].

Acute and chronic cocaine use predisposes the abuser to a wide range of local and systemic complications. Cocaine is a naturally occurring alkaloid. It is extracted from the leaves of the Erythroxylon coca plant, which is indigenous to three countries in northern South America [4, 6].

Cocaine is a psychologically disruptive and dependence-inducing drug; classified as a psychostimulant, it exhibits both local anesthetic and neurotransmitter effects [5, 7, 8]. Cocaine is commonly taken intravenously, by smoking or inhalation of the "crack" or "freebase" form, or by snorting [9, 10]. Cocaine has an acidic pH of 4.0. Its purity, sterility, and the type of adulterants it is mixed with, all directly affect its potential for local and systemic complications [11].

29.2.1 Etiopathogenesis

Cocaine is a crystalline alkaloid obtained by conversion of some subtypes of the coca leaf (Erythroxylum coca and others) into a paste and then into cocaine hydrochloride by means of catalyzing agents like ether, gasoline, and sulfuric acid. It has an indirect sympathomimetic-mediated psychoactive action increasing the norepinephrine levels and impairing its reuptake, but it is also able to induce direct vascular smooth muscle contraction. Cocaine also blocks the sodium channels and thus interferes with nerve transmission leading to an anesthetic effect. In the nineteenth century, Köller reported its use as an anesthetic agent in his ophthalmologic medical practice and for decades it has been very popular in ENT nose surgery as an excellent topical anesthetic [10, 12, 13].

Cocaine is both vasoconstricting and locally irritating to the thin respiratory epithelium of the respiratory tract. It induces a hypersensitivity reaction in the mucosa. Irritation and vasoconstriction cause ischemia, inflammation, micronecrosis, infection, and then macronecrosis leading to destruction and perforation. Long-term use may lead to chronic granulomatous inflammatory changes [11–13].

Another pathogenic route is the recently reported ANCA-associated vasculitis attributed to levamisole, an anti-helminthic agent with immunomodulatory properties that is used as a common cocaine adulterant (even 70% of its composition) as it potentiates its stimulant effects. Moreover, impaired mucociliary transport and decreased humoral and cell-mediated immunity take place leading to bacterial and fungal local colonization with recurrent nasal infections and chronic wound superinfection. Individual predisposition is also another important factor [10, 11].

29.2.2 Clinical Features

Cocaine smoking and snorting: It results in the erosion of the midfacial structures and recurrent sinus infections and granulomatous changes. It presents as oral, sinonasal, pulmonary, systemic, and behavioral problems.

The common symptoms include [12–15]:

- loss of nasal hairs
- nasal crusting
- sinusitis/halitosis
- epistaxis, anosmia/hyposmia
- nasal septal perforation is usually asymptomatic and well-tolerated but framework destruction leads to saddle nose deformity with the widening of the tip.
- palatal perforation (Fig. 29.1) leading to nasal regurgitation of liquids, solids, and rhinolalia aperta (hypernasal voice).
- Erosion of Eustachian tubes may be associated with ear pathology.
- erosion of turbinates, ethmoids, medial sinus walls, cribriform plate, and orbital walls may lead to complications such as CSF leak or loss of visual acuity/diplopia [16, 17].

The local ischemic and traumatic complication are included in the so-called cocaine-induced midline destructive lesion (CIMDL) and is based in the clinical or radiological detection of at least two of these signs: (a) septum perforation, (b) lateral nasal wall destruction of the inferior or middle turbinate in the maxillary or ethmoid sinus destruction, and (c) hard palate involvement [10, 13].

Topical application on gingiva: It may present as a non-healing ulcer causing pain and bleeding gums, granuloma formation [13, 18].

The common features include:

- mucosal ulceration
- necrotizing ulcerative gingivitis
- rapid gingival recession
- dental erosion
- possible corrosion of gold restorations [14, 15]

Ingestion or IV use: It causes potential hepatitis, endocarditis and gastroenteritis, psychotic illness, seizures followed by chronic disseminated granulomatous inflammation.

29.2.3 Diagnosis

The biopsy of soft tissue, taken from the ulcer, granulomas, or palatal margin of the oronasal fistula, may reveal a chronic inflammation with some eosinophils. The presence of eosinophils along with inflammatory infiltrate is a common histopathological finding, as reported by Schweitzer [13]. Typical histopathological picture supports the induction of hypersensitivity reaction by cocaine. Hepatic, pulmonary, or sinonasal lesion biopsy may reveal granulomatous changes with infiltration of lymphocytes, histiocytes, and plasma cells [7, 18]. Imaging modalities such as computed tomography are helpful to assess the extent of destruction (Fig. 29.2) [18].

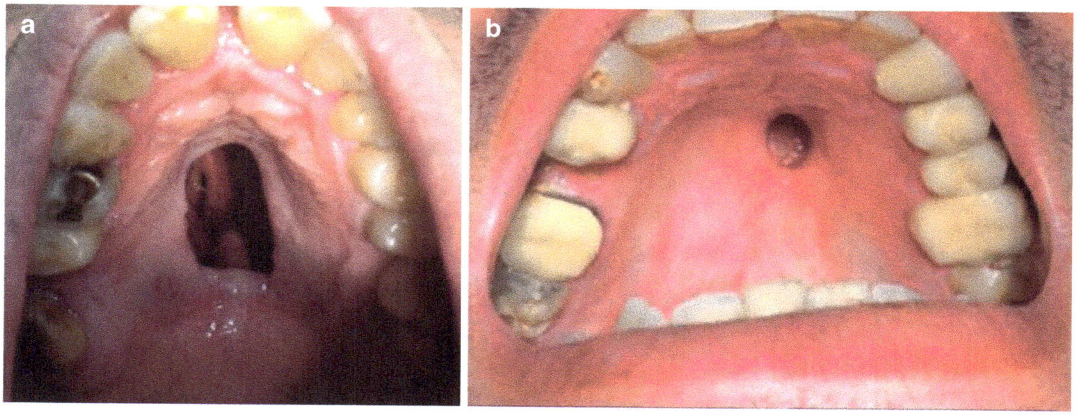

Fig. 29.1 (**a**) and (**b**) Palatal perforation due to cocaine smoking [13]

29.2.4 Treatment

Prognosis is predicated on the complete cessation of the drug. Patient counselling regarding consequences of continued cocaine use, and how to get help in quitting. The patient should avoid smoking and should use a proper filtration mask while at work.

For sinusitis, antibiotics, anti-inflammatory medications, and saline nose drops should be given. Local decongestants are to be avoided. Appropriate basic oral hygiene and restorative procedure, a removable obturator can be beneficial for the oronasal fistula (Fig. 29.3). At a later date, surgical closure of the oronasal fistula should be considered [10–13]. Regional flaps like tongue, buccinator, buccal fat pad, or temporal muscle flaps may be indicated for small to medium defects. Other pediculated flaps may be obtained from the vomer, nasolabial area, pharyngeal or nasal vestibular mucosa [13].

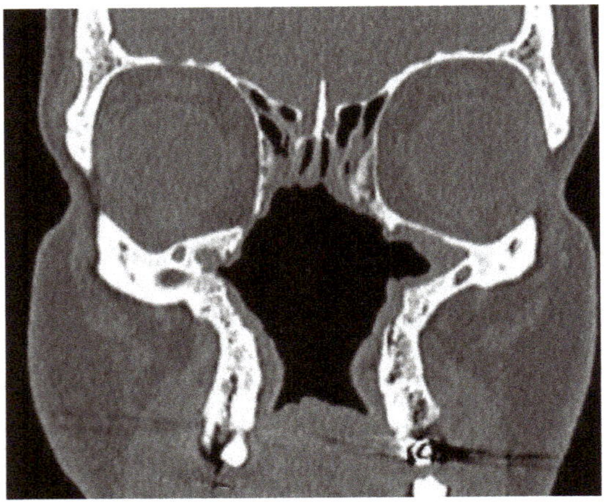

Fig. 29.2 CT scan showing massive erosion of the midline structures, with the destruction of the nasal septum, turbinates, and palate [18]

Cocaine dependence continues to be a significant public health problem in the United States. Although some cocaine-dependent patients respond well to counseling, for many standard psychological treatment is inadequate. Hence, the treatment of cocaine dependence is the research in demand. Propranolol may be helpful in promoting the initial period of stable abstinence. Potential relapse prevention medications are GABAergic medications, such as baclofen, tiagabine, and topiramate, and the glutamatergic medication, modafinil. Surprisingly, an old treatment for alcohol dependence, disulfiram, may also have efficacy for cocaine relapse prevention [19].

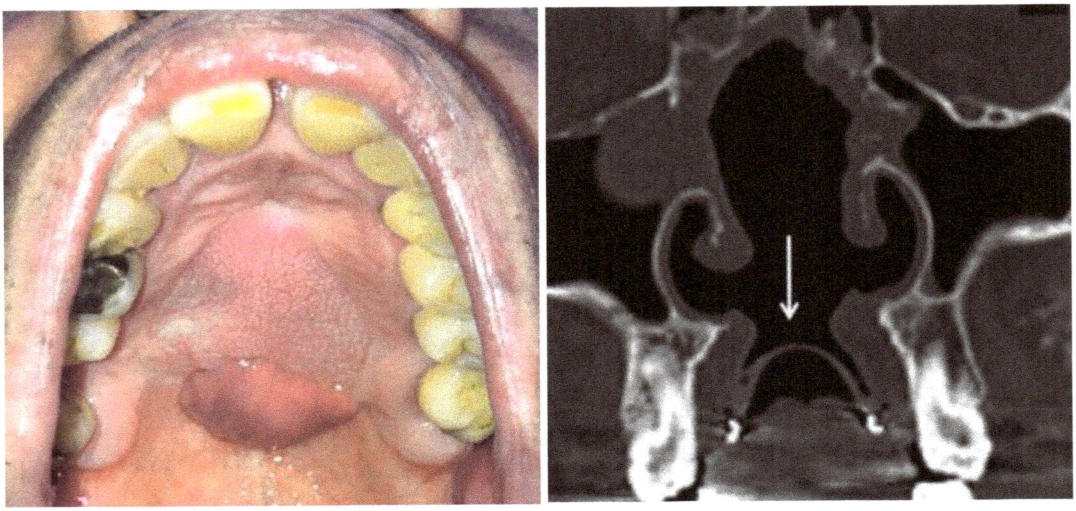

Fig. 29.3 (**a**) Obturator closing the palatal perforation. (**b**) CT scan coronal view showing septum, palate, and turbinate bone destruction. Note the presence of an obturator and its sealing effect (mark) [13]

29.3 Berylliosis

Synonyms

Acute Beryllium Disease; Beryllium Granulomatosis; Beryllium Pneumonosis; Beryllium Poisoning [20, 21].

29.3.1 Etiopathogenesis

A berylliosis is a form of metal poisoning caused by inhalation of beryllium dust, vapors, or its compounds or implantation of the substance in the skin. The toxic effects of beryllium most commonly occur due to occupational exposure. Beryllium is a metallic element used in many industries, including electronics, high-technology ceramics, metals extraction, and dental alloy preparation.

There are two forms of the beryllium-induced disease, acute and chronic.

- Acute Berylliosis (Acute Beryllium Disease)
- Chronic Berylliosis (Chronic Beryllium Disease—CBD)

Acute berylliosis: It has a sudden, rapid onset course and is characterized by severe pneumonitis causing cough, dyspnea, and other associated symptoms. It is usually associated with upper respiratory infection causing sore throat, rhinitis, and tracheobronchitis. In addition, skin or the eyes may be affected [20, 21].

Chronic berylliosis: Chronic berylliosis is a systemic disease in which there is an abnormally exaggerated immune response (hypersensitivity) to beryllium. It is a more common form that develops slowly and, in some cases, may not become apparent for many years after initial beryllium exposure. It is characterized by the abnormal formation of inflammatory nodules (granulomas) within certain tissues and organs with widespread scarring and interstitial pulmonary fibrosis. Pulmonary granulomas are often associated with hilar lymphadenopathy Although granulomas primarily affect the lungs, they may also occur within the nose and paranasal sinuses, nasopharynx, larynx, skin, liver, spleen, heart, or lymph nodes. In individuals with chronic berylliosis, associated symptoms and findings often include dry cough, fatigue, weight loss, chest pain, and increasing dyspnea [22, 23].

29.3.2 Diagnosis

Histopathology: It is helpful in chronic Berylliosis. Histopathology reveals noncaseating granulomas with infiltration of lymphocytes, histiocytes, and plasma cells [21, 24].

Pulmonary disease evaluation: It includes chest X-ray, pulmonary function tests, arterial blood gas measurements, and preferably bronchoscopy with tissue biopsy and lavage analysis for total cell count, differential cell count, and lymphocyte count [24].

Chest radiograph: findings may include diffuse infiltrates and hilar adenopathy. Infiltrates may be granular, diffuse linear, or small nodules. Hilar adenopathy is noted in 30–40% of patients, is usually mild, bilateral, and associated with parenchymal infiltrates. Severe disease may show interstitial fibrosis, honeycombing, and the formation of conglomerate masses. Pleural thickening and pneumothorax can occur but are unusual [24, 25].

Beryllium lymphocyte proliferation test (BeLPT): It is the hematological test to confirm sensitivity to beryllium. When white blood cells (lymphocytes) from affected patients are cultured in the presence of certain beryllium salts (in vitro), they begin to abnormally proliferate, demonstrating a positive immune reaction associated with beryllium sensitivity or chronic berylliosis. In some cases, the BeLPT may also be conducted on cells, bronchoalveolar lavage, and nasal secretions [26].

29.3.3 Treatment

Acute berylliosis is treated with corticosteroids, antihistaminic medicines, breathing support (oxygen support with or without the use of ventilators), and other supportive measures. With prompt, appropriate treatment, complete recovery is possible with no residual effects. However, such individuals should be regularly monitored to ensure early detection of CBD. Avoidance of further exposure to beryllium is recommended.

There is currently no cure for CBD. Symptomatic treatment with corticosteroids, mucolytics, antihistaminic medicines, and breathing support is recommended. Upper respiratory tract granulomas can be excised surgically.

Tumor necrosis factor-alpha (TNF-alpha) inhibitor: Effectiveness of the drug Infliximab (Remicade) is under trial in chronic beryllium disease (CBD). Tumor necrosis factor-alpha (TNF-a) is associated with more severe disease and inflammation in the lung. Infliximab acts by reducing TNF-alpha thus reduces pulmonary inflammation and fibrosis [22, 23].

29.4 Talcosis

Talc or magnesium silicate [Mg3Si4O10(OH)2] is a common and widely used agent in industry and daily life. Cosmetic talc is widely used as a dusting and, often, scented powder by many and is generally not considered to be a hazard when used as intended. After inhalational exposure, some talc particles are cleared by the tracheobronchial tree. However, if cleared insufficiently due to prolonged exposure or exposure to high quantities or both, pulmonary talcosis may develop. The first case of pulmonary talcosis or talc pneumoconiosis related to inhalation of talc during its extraction and processing in mines was described by Thorel in 1896 [27–29]. Pulmonary talcosis is most commonly seen secondary to occupational exposure or intravenous (IV) drug abuse and, occasionally, in excessive use of cosmetic talc. Talc has been shown to be fibrogenic due to an immunological response [27]. Inhalational talc has been associated with histological patterns of diffuse interstitial fibrosis, nodular fibrosis, and foreign body granulomatosis. It is diagnosed with radiological and histological findings when a consistent history of exposure is present [28, 29].

29.4.1 Etiopathogenesis

Talc is used in many cosmetic formulations. Reported functions of talc in cosmetics include abrasive, absorbent, anticaking agent, bulking agent, opacifying agent, skin protectant, and slip modifier [27]. Before 1976, asbestiform used to be one of the constituents of Talc. Asbestiform refers to a crystallization product of a mineral in which the crystals are thin, hair-like fibers with enhanced strength, flexibility, and durability [28]. In 1976, FDA specified that the Talc used in cosmetics should not contain asbestiform fibers, due to its proven hazardous effects. It was found to be carcinogenic for most of the sinonasal and nasopharyngeal malignancy. It induces severe inflammation with granulomatous changes in the respiratory mucosa. The mucosal absorption and hematogenous spread may induce fallopian tube inflammation leading to fibrosis, stenosis, and eventual obstruction of the fallopian tube leading to infertility in females. It is also one of the predisposing factors for ovarian cancer. Nowadays, the most common minerals associated with talc are chlorite, magnesite, dolomite, calcite, mica, quartz, and fluorapatite. Amphiboles and serpentine are associated with certain specific talc deposits.

Industrial talc can be found in paints, insecticides, roofing products, asphalt, ceramics, rubber, metal foundries, mining, and even leather. Depending on its use, talc may contain other minerals such as aluminum, iron, calcium, asbestos, and silica. High-purity talc is commonly used as a bulking agent and lubricant in oral medications. Talc is also commonly used as a sclerosing agent for the management of malignant pleural effusion. Cosmetically, talc can be found in antiperspirants or body powder [4]. Talc miners and millers are more prone to occupational exposure to talc. Talc has a threshold limit value (TLV) (respirable fraction) of 2 mg/m^3 as a 10 h time-weighted average (TWA). The National Institute for Occupational Safety and Health (NIOSH) states the immediately-dangerous-to-life-or-health (IDLH) concentration is 1000 mg/m^3 [30, 31].

29.4.2 Clinical Features

It has been recognized that talc causes disease by two routes: inhalation and intravenously.

- Inhalation

Human pulmonary effects of talc include diffuse interstitial fibrosis and progressive massive fibrosis (often called complicated pneumoconiosis), sinonasal granulomas, laryngeal granulomas, silicosis and silico-tuberculosis, malignant neoplasms of the respiratory tract, including nasopharynx, lung, bronchial and tracheal cancers.

Pulmonary disease as a result of talc exposure has been well documented and can have multiple etiologies. Inhalational talc exposure causes talc pneumoconiosis, while intravenous talc exposure causes intravascular talcosis. The disease symptoms and gross anatomic findings in these two different etiologies are essentially identical, and the histology of these two forms of talc-related lung diseases is also quite similar. Pulmonary deposition of insoluble microscopic foreign material results in a foreign body giant cell reaction within the lung parenchyma. Over time and continued exposure, this process results in pulmonary fibrosis, in some cases extensively. The differentiating feature between these two diseases is the location of the foreign material. Inhalational talc pneumoconiosis results in an alveolar distribution, and intravascular talcosis leads to a perivascular pattern of deposition [32].

Pulmonary talcosis, talcosilicosis, and talcoasbestosis may result from occupational exposures to talc dust containing pure or variable amounts of silica or asbestos, respectively.

- IV Infusion

The source of foreign material in intravascular talcosis is through the intravenous injection of drugs. Illegal street drugs commonly contain an adulterant to increase the mass, and this adulterant commonly contains microscopic insoluble material. Another common source is the injection of prescription medications meant for oral use. Pulmonary talcosis has also been reported in a wide variety of oral medications that are misused intravenously. These include methylphenidate, methadone, promethazine, diazepam, and acetaminophen [33, 34].

In these medications which are ground for intravenous injection, there are fillers and binders added to the medications. In fact, the term intravascular talcosis is a misnomer as talc is only one of several possible materials used as excipients that also include methylcellulose and crospovidone [33, 34].

With the intravenous injection of foreign material, the lungs represent the first capillary bed to serve as a filter to remove this material. Due to the size of much of this material it usually becomes lodged in the pulmonary vasculature. This results in acute small embolization of vessels. Over time the foreign material is deposited in perivascular tissues, and foreign body giant cell reaction occurs with associated fibrosis leading to the formation of perivascular granulomas. Talc particles cause disease by being entrapped in the pulmonary parenchyma also causing a granulomatous reaction resulting in fibrotic lesions [29, 35, 36].

Intranasal tissue necrosis—It can be caused by certain types of vasculitis and autoimmune diseases, infection, malignancy, and drug abuse. Drug-induced intranasal tissue necrosis (DIITN) is a well-known entity. Besides the effect of the basic drug itself, Jewers et al. hypothesized the link between necrosis and drug-concomitant substances, such as talc particles. Talc-containing substances into a peripheral artery may be the cause of ischemic necrosis of the distal extremities or other organs. Extensive necrosis may lead to septal perforation and oro-antral fistula [37].

Cerebellar talcosis—Intravenous (IV) drug abuse is a broad entity well known to perpetrate both acute and chronic insults that are deleterious to the complex physiology of the central nervous system (CNS). Psychostimulant drugs such as methamphetamines are recreationally abused through oral, inhalational, and IV routes. The latter often involves contamination with cutting or bulking substances including cornstarch and talcum powder (talc) [38]. In examination under polarized light, positively birefringent talc crystals have been demonstrated in systemic tissues of IV drug abusers, particularly in the pulmonary perivascular regions. These crystals would not be expected to traverse an intact blood–brain barrier (BBB) and have never been described in CNS tissues [38].

29.4.3 Diagnosis

Sputum and sinonasal secretions should be examined using polarized light microscopy and transmission electron microscopy [39].

29.4.3.1 Histopathology

Histopathological findings are suggestive of chronic granulomatous changes with mixed cellular infiltrate of eosinophils, lymphocytes, plasma cells, and histiocytes. Histologically, granulomas can be visualized as birefringent needle-shaped talc crystals in multinucleated giant cells under polarized light. Two patterns of inflammatory reactions have been described, either fibrosis or granulomatous formation. Histopathology can be a diffusely interstitial fibrotic reaction or irregularly nodular or as a non-caseating granulomatous reaction. Nonetheless, if a biopsy is not possible, bronchoscopy or fine-needle aspiration of pulmonary masses, coupled with an appropriate history, may provide sufficient evidence for the diagnosis [36, 39].

The finding of perivascular or intravascular polarizable foreign material in the lungs is essentially diagnostic of intravascular talcosis due to intravenous injection of illegal drugs. The most important differential to establish is between intravascular talcosis and talc pneumoconiosis due to inhalation of microscopic dust. The differentiation of these two etiologies in foreign material associated with granulomatous lung disease can be challenging as a perivascular location in some ways includes the entire lung parenchyma. The foreign material deposits of intravascular talcosis have varying morphologies such as more plate-like polarizable material, needle-like morphology, or commonly found asteroid bodies (Figs. 29.4 and 29.5) [29, 39].

29.4.3.2 Imaging

Although many of the disorders can be detected on plain radiography, high-resolution computed tomography (HRCT) is superior in delineating the upper airway and lung architecture and depicting pathology. Chest radiography, CT thorax, CT PNS may reveal pulmonary fibrosis, granulomas involving lung parenchyma or upper airway (Figs. 29.6 and 29.7) [40].

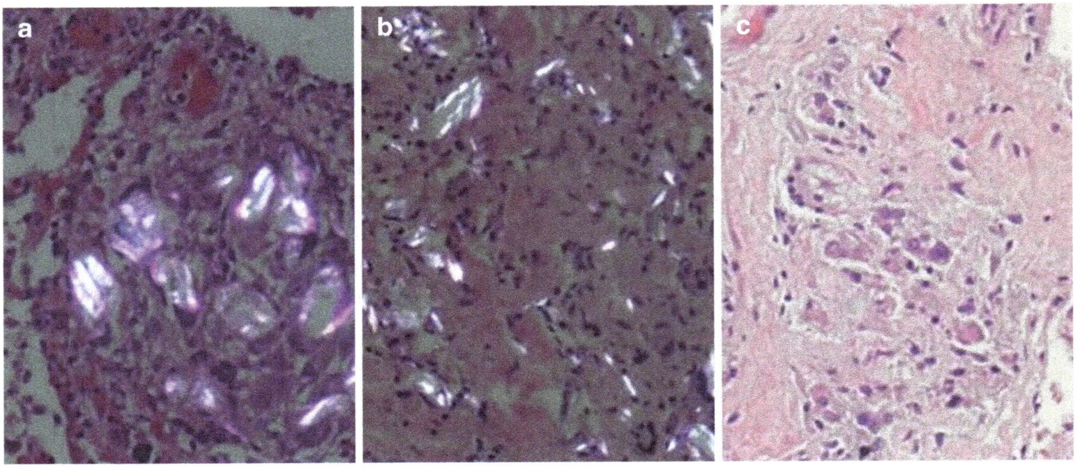

Fig. 29.4 The foreign material deposits of intravascular talcosis showing varying morphologies. (**a**) Plate-like polarizable material. (**b**) Needle-like morphology. (**c**) Asteroid bodies are a common finding in intravascular talcosis [29]

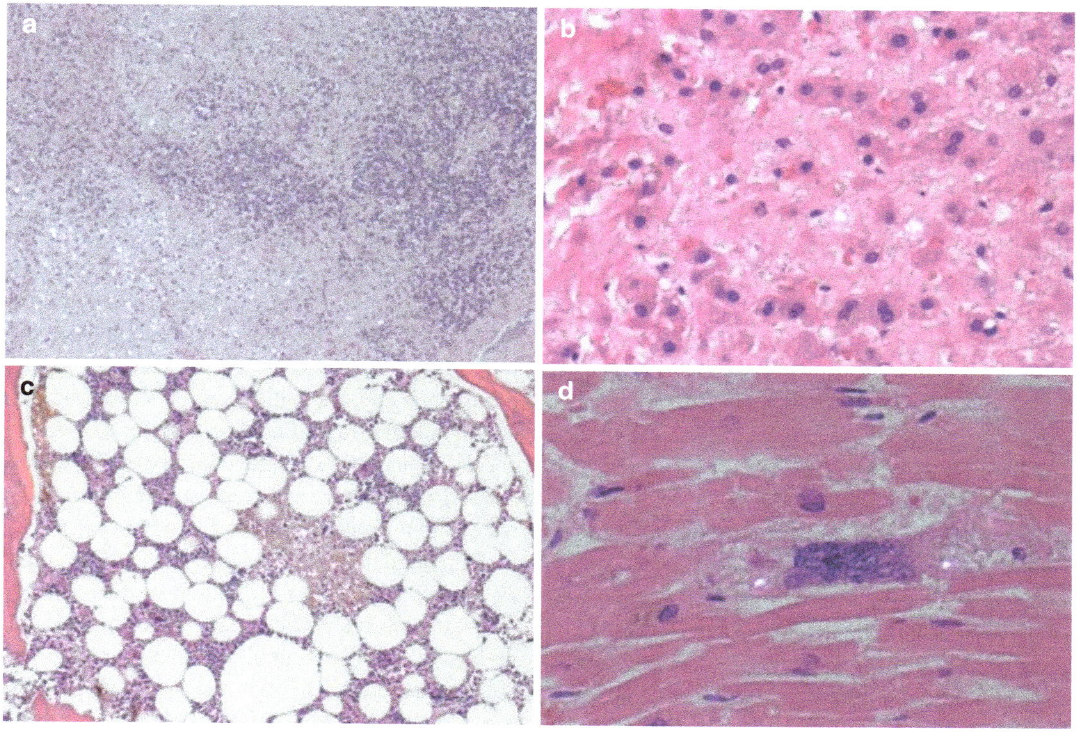

Fig. 29.5 Systemic sites of foreign material are an important feature seen in intravascular talcosis. This material is smaller than seen in the lungs and only rarely incites a foreign body giant cell reaction. Representative figures show deposition in lymph node (**a**), liver (**b**), bone marrow (**c**), and heart (**d**) [29]

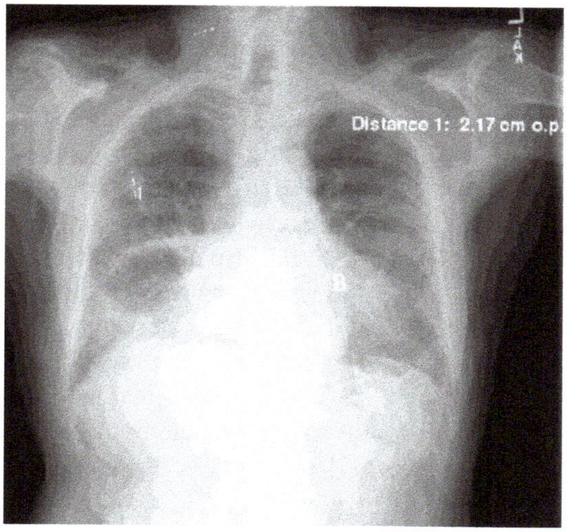

Fig. 29.6 AP chest radiograph showing extensive bilateral reticular-fibrotic pattern with honeycombing and a 217 cm nodule (talc granuloma) in the right upper lobe of his lungs [40]

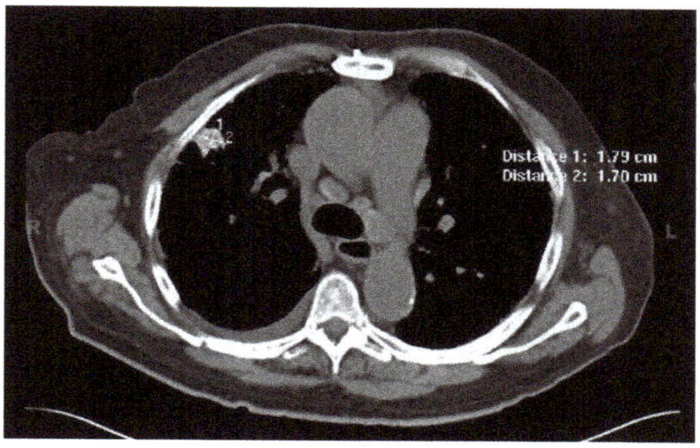

Fig. 29.7 HRCT thorax showing multiple right upper lobe pulmonary talcosis granulomatous nodules and right pleural effusion. The most prominent nodule measuring 18 × 17 cm [40]

29.4.4 Treatment

Long-term complications may include chronic respiratory failure, pulmonary hypertension, and right heart failure or corpulmonale. There is no established treatment for pulmonary talcosis, however steroids and immunosuppressants are frequently used. Transplantation is an option reserved for patients with end-stage disease. Patients are advised to stop exposure and tobacco use. However, fibrotic changes are irreversible and the disease may still continue to progress [31, 32].

29.5 Tattooing

A tattoo can be defined as the intentional insertion of pigment into the dermis using a punctate instrument. In addition to serving a broad range of decorative functions, tattooing (e.g., the procedure of tattoo placement) also includes permanent makeup and reconstructive dermatological/surgical applications. Whenever foreign material is inserted into the body, there exists an opportunity for complications, including trauma related to implantation, infection, the body's reaction to the pigment, and many other possible sequelae. Red pigment is the most common cause of reactions in tattoos and this can present in various clinical and histological variants with dermatitis and lichenoid being the most common [41–43].

29.5.1 Etiopathogenesis

Tattoos are popular and it is likely that reactions to tattoo pigment will continue to develop in various forms.

- Red pigment: cinnabar/mercuric sulfide (a most common cause of granulomatous tattoo reaction)
- Blue pigment: cobalt
- Green pigment: chromium
- Yellow pigment: cadmium
- Purple pigment: manganese
- Black pigment: carbon (India ink)
- Brown pigment: ferric oxide
- White pigment: titanium or zinc oxide [41–43].

Illegal tattooing that violated medical laws has occurred frequently. The majority of tattooists are not fully aware of the composition of the pigments they work with. This is much difficult in defining exactly which chemicals are involved. Furthermore, there are even greater challenges in recognizing the particular ingredients in a certain type of ink, especially with the creation of new mixtures. It appears that there is generally a lack of understanding regarding the risk of dangerous chemicals in tattoos. These could be carcinogenic. Several studies have reported that benign or malignant lesions could occur in tattoos [42–44].

In general, the black dye particles are the smallest, hence give a less inflammatory response. In contrast, red dye particles are bigger in size thus giving an overt inflammatory response. Mercury content in red pigment is the agent that causes reactions related to red tattoos. Modern alternatives such as sienna-ferric-hydrate, cadmium selenide, organic vegetable dyes, sandalwood, and brazilwood have largely replaced mercury. However, nowadays most reactions are not due to the traditional presence of mercury sulfides, but due to new organic pigments (e.g., Pigment Red 181 and Pigment Red 170) [45–47]. Different from a red tattoo, the blue, green, and black tattoos are a less frequent cause of tattoo reactions. Actually, allergic reactions to temporary henna tattoos due to the para-phenylenediamine are very common. Granulomas can also develop after acupuncture. Facial cosmetic acupuncture (FCA) has been widely used for antiaging, skin rejuvenation, and restoration of muscle tone. The needles used for acupuncture are silicon needles that may lead to the formation of silicon granulomas after few months to years [47].

29.5.2 Clinical Features

The various patterns of tattoo reactions are [48–51]:

- Dermatitis

Eczematous reactions to red tattoos are the most common type of reaction observed, being either allergic contact dermatitis or photo-allergic dermatitis. The exact understanding of the mechanisms behind the eczematous reactions observed in red tattoos is still lacking with type I–III hypersensitivity reactions playing a role [48, 49].

- Lichenoid

Lichenoid reaction in red organic tattoos has been shown to elicit a cytotoxic inflammatory response with lichenoid basal damage. It is produced by a delayed cellular hypersensitivity to metal particles (Fig. 29.8) [47, 48, 52].

- Pseudolymphomatous

Pseudolymphoma is a term given to a histological entity and has been reported to occur as a complication of tattoos that is histologically indistinct from malignant T or B cell lymphoma; however, the lymphoproliferative process is benign. The clinical presentation is a pruritic plaque within the tattoo, often initially mistaken for lymphoma. The distinguishing factor between pseudolymphoma and lymphoma is the polyclonal nature of the lymphocytes (Fig. 29.9) [50, 51].

- Granulomatous

Similar to lichenoid reactions, granulomatous reactions are thought to occur as a result of delayed hypersensitivity reactions to the presence of the red pigment (Fig. 29.10). Episcleral tattoo injections of various color pigments are used in western countries so as to change the color of eyes. This pigment may induce granuloma formation (Fig. 29.11) [42, 45].

Facial cosmetic acupuncture (FCA) has been touted to help with antiaging, skin rejuvenation, and restoration of muscle tone. It is commonly performed with silicon needles which may induce granuloma formation a few months to years after acupuncture (Fig. 29.12). This complication may be prevented with the use of silicone-free acupuncture needles, and early recognition by providers may prevent further disease [55].

Infection—Contaminated tattoo equipment and ink can introduce bacteria to a wound site commonest are Staphylococcus and Streptococcus. It may manifest in the form of local sepsis causing redness, swelling, and papules in the tattoo area. It may also manifest with impetigo, cellulitis to life-threatening septicemia. The skin changes that may occur can be similar to those of squamous cell carcinoma making the diagnosis more difficult.

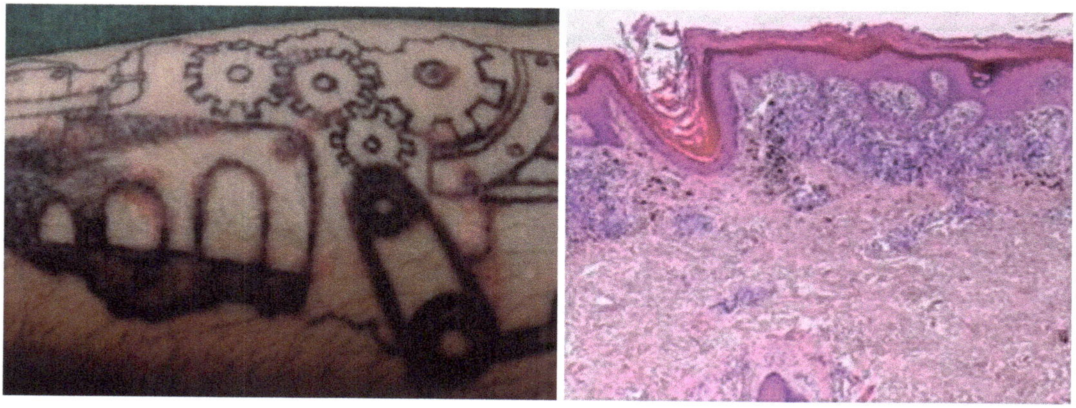

Fig. 29.8 Lichenoid reaction on a black tattoo and relative histology with a widespread vacuolar basal epidermic degeneration with a deep dermal lymphohistiocytic infiltrate into a lichenoid pattern, associated with deposition of exogenous pigment [47]

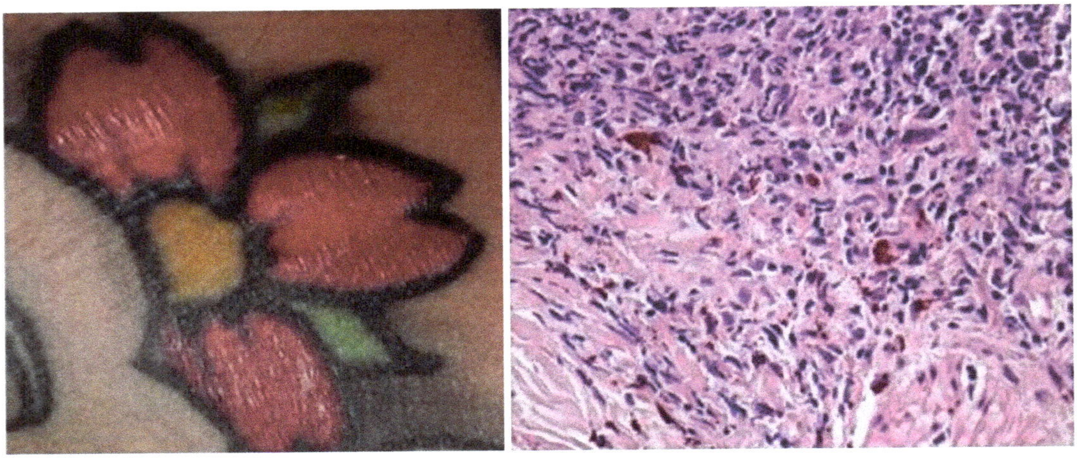

Fig. 29.9 Pseudolymphomatous reaction on a red tattoo and relative histology with the presence of red color exogenous pigment in the background of reactive lymphoid hyperplasia in the superficial and medium dermis [47]

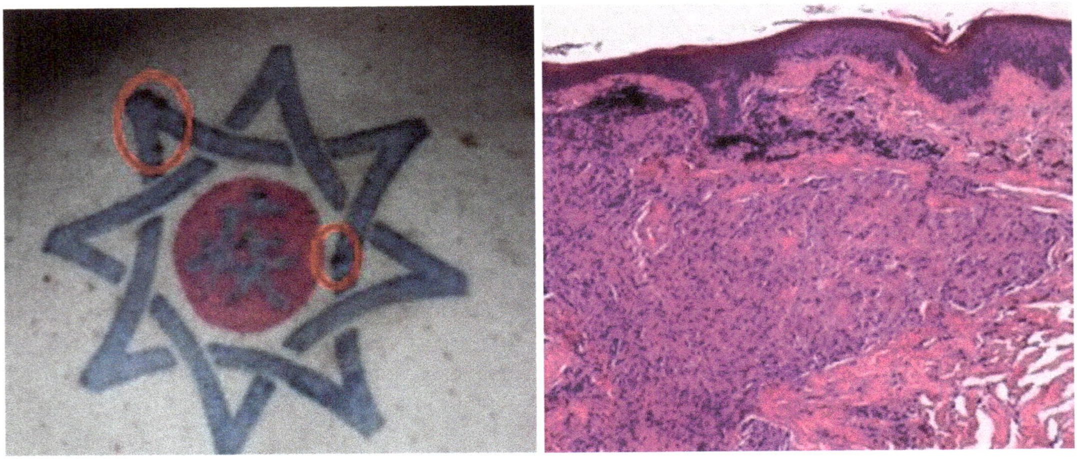

Fig. 29.10 Foreign body granulomatous reaction on a black tattoo and relative histology with granulomatous depositions of exogenous pigment in the background of granulomatous-productive inflammation of the dermal stroma [47]

29.5.3 Diagnosis

Clinical diagnosis is usually straightforward as the tattoo reactions are obviously evident.

Histopathology helps to confirm the diagnosis and reveals the type of reaction. Granulomatous reaction shows chronic inflammatory cell infiltrate with scattered exogenous tattoo pigments. Swiss-cheese pattern is particularly seen because of oil solvent mixing with tattoo substances. Relatively high rate of granulomatous reaction is attributed to an allergic reaction to oil solvent. To detect the tattoo components, a biopsy specimen should be analyzed by electron microscopy and energy-dispersive X-ray spectroscopy (SEM-EDS) (Fig. 29.13) [43–46, 54].

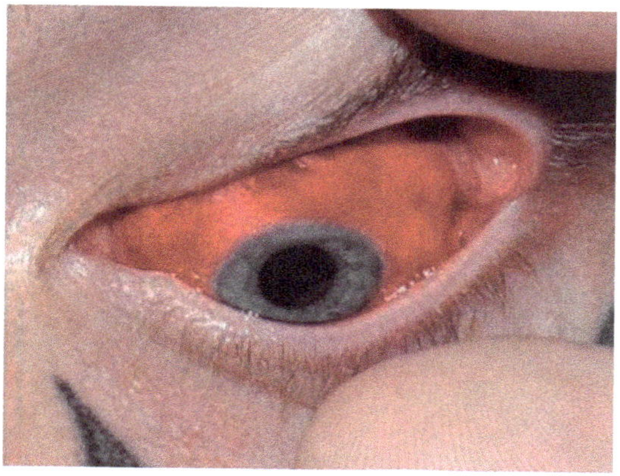

Fig. 29.11 Left eye showing three distinct areas of conjunctival swelling indicating red tattoo granulomas. The patient having undergone episcleral tattooing 7 weeks previously [53]

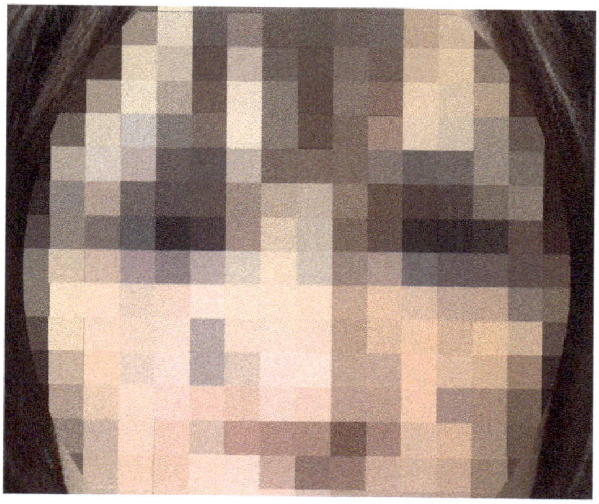

Fig. 29.12 Patient with periorbital granulomas 30 years after acupuncture done. Acupuncture trigger points and sites of granuloma formation. Granulo mas are seen at sites labeled (**a**)–(**f**), which correspond to common acupuncture trigger points: (**a**) jingming, (**b**) tongziliao, (**c**, **d**) taiyang, (**e**) bitong, and (**f**) quanliao [54]

29.5.4 Treatment

- Mild skin reactions may help with anti-inflammatory drugs (NSAIDs), that can reduce pain and inflammation.
- Anti-histamine drugs such as cetirizine, fexofenadine can reduce symptoms of minor allergic reactions such as small red bumps or rash.
- Small granulomatous lesions are treated with topical and/or intralesional steroids; however, for bigger granulomas, it is important to remove the lesion. For refractory skin eruptions unresponsive to medical therapy, surgical or laser treatment may be considered. The laser of choice is the Q-Switched Nd:YAG laser capable of emitting two different wavelengths at 1064 nm (useful for dark blue and black pigment) and 532 nm (useful for removal of red, orange, and purple tattoo pigments). The Q-Switched Nd:YAG system releases high energy in extremely short times (max 6 ns), producing a "photoacoustic" effect that breaks down the derma cells containing the tattoo pigment [56, 57].

29.6 Essential Features

- The common forms of chemical granuloma include Cocaine abuse, Berryliosis seen in industrial workers, Talcosis (Silicosis) due to talcum powder use, and Tattooing.
- Cocaine snorting is associated with a peculiar type of drug-induced chronic rhinitis, loss of nasal hair, crusting, epistaxis slowly progressing to a destruction of nasal, palatal, and pharyngeal tissues. These characteristic lesions due to cocaine abuse are commonly called cocaine-induced midline destructive lesions (CIMDL).
- The mainstay of treatment is anti-inflammatory medicines and reconstruction such as closure of the oroantral fistula.
- A berylliosis is a form of metal poisoning caused by the inhalation of beryllium dust or vapors in industrial workers. It manifests in two forms—Acute Berylliosis (Acute Beryllium Disease) and Chronic Berylliosis (Chronic Beryllium Disease—CBD).
- Acute berylliosis is characterized by severe pneumonitis usually associated with upper respiratory infection causing sore throat, rhinitis, and tracheobronchitis.
- Chronic beryllium disease (CBD) is a granulomatous lung disorder characterized by pulmonary granulomas, interstitial fibrosis and

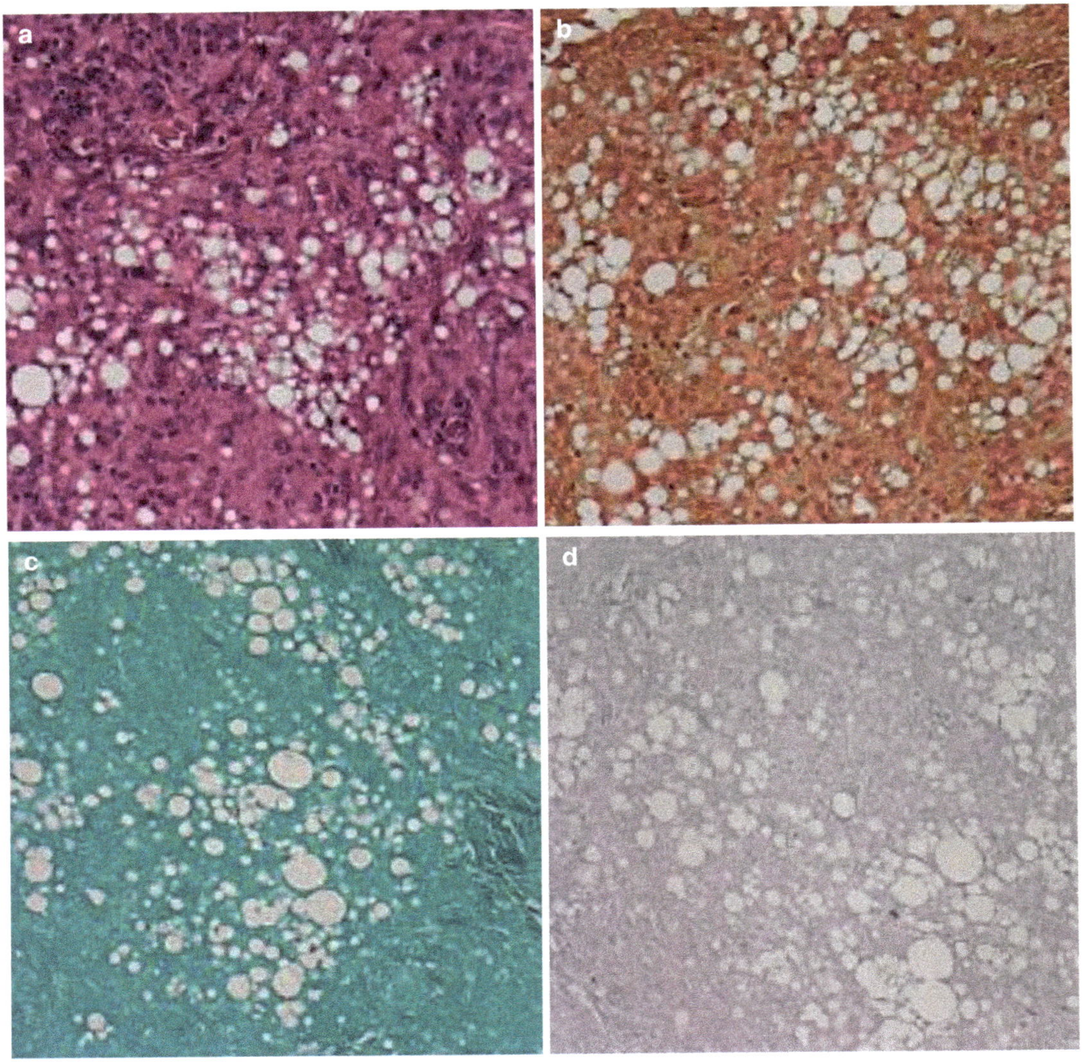

Fig. 29.13 Hematoxylin and eosin stain (**a**) revealing fibrovascular tissue containing granulomatous inflammation with foci of clear spaces consistent with silicone oil or other foreign material. No organisms are seen on gram stain (**b**), Grocott's methenamine silver stain (**c**), or acid-fast staining (**d**) [54]

may be associated with upper airway granulomas.

- There is currently no cure for CBD. Symptomatic treatment with corticosteroids, mucolytics, antihistaminic medicines, and breathing support is recommended. Upper respiratory tract granulomas can be excised surgically.
- Pulmonary talcosis is most commonly seen secondary to occupational exposure or intravenous (IV) drug abuse and, occasionally, in excessive use of cosmetic talc.
- Pulmonary talcosis is associated with histological patterns of diffuse interstitial fibrosis, nodular fibrosis, and foreign body granulomatosis. It may also cause sinonasal granulomas, laryngeal granulomas, silicosis and silicotuberculosis, malignant neoplasms of the respiratory tract, including nasopharynx, lung, bronchial and tracheal cancers.

- Cerebellar talcosis is a rare but severe condition caused by intravenous use of talc contaminated drugs.
- Histopathology typically reveals the foreign material deposits of intravascular talcosis have varying morphologies such as plate-like polarizable material, needle-like morphology, or commonly found asteroid bodies.
- Steroids and immunosuppressants are frequently used with varying results. Lung transplantation is an option reserved for patients with end-stage disease.
- Tattooing is a common practice worldwide. In addition to serving a broad range of decorative functions, tattooing also includes permanent makeup and reconstructive dermatological/surgical applications.
- Various tattoo reactions are dermatitis, lichenoid reaction, pseudolymphomatous reaction, and granulomatous reaction.
- Mild reactions respond well to oral and intralesional steroids. For severe cases, surgical excision of the tattoo with laser is preferred.

References

1. Gawin FH. Cocaine abuse and addiction. J Fam Pract. 1989;29:193–7.
2. Adlaf EM, et al. Alcohol, tobacco, and illicit drug use amongst Ontario adults. 1977-1996. Survey by the Addiction Research Foundation.
3. Laskin DM. Looking out for the cocaine abuser. J Oral Maxillofac Surg. 1993;51:111.
4. Lee CY, et al. Medical and dental implications of cocaine abuse. J Oral Maxillofac Surg. 1991;49:290–3.
5. Goldstein FJ. Toxicity of cocaine. Compendium. 1990;11:710, 712, 714-6.
6. United Nations Office on Drugs and Crime (UNODC). World Drug Report 2018. United Nations publication, Sales No. E.18.XI.9. Vienna: UNODC; 2018.
7. Sastry RC, et al. Palatal perforation from cocaine abuse. Otolaryngol Head Neck Surg. 1997;116:565–6.
8. Sousa O, Rowley S. Otorhinolarygologic symptoms caused by the intranasal abuse of cocaine. Report of a case. Rev Med Panama. 1994;19:55–60.
9. Schweitzer V. Osteolytic sinusitis and pneumomediastinum: deceptive otolarygologic complications of cocaine abuse. Laryngoscope. 1986;96:206–10.
10. Smith JC, et al. Midline nasal and hard palate destruction in cocaine abusers and cocaine's role in midline nasal and rhinologic practice. Ear Nose Throat J. 2002;81:172–7.
11. Woolverton WL, Johnson KM. Neurobiology of cocaine abuse. Trends Pharmacol Sci. 1992;13:193–200.
12. Blanco GF, et al. Acute cardiac events temporally related to cocaine abuse. N Engl J Med. 1986;315:1438–43.
13. Barrientos J, et al. Surgical treatment of cocaine-induced palatal perforations: report of three cases and literature review. J Clin Exp Dent. 2021;13(2):e201–6. https://doi.org/10.4317/jced.57730. Published online 2021 Feb 1.
14. Kapila YL, Kashani H. Cocaine-associated rapid gingival recession and dental erosion. A case report. J Periodontol. 1997;68:485–8.
15. Parry J, et al. Mucosal lesions due to oral cocaine use. Br Dent J. 1996;180:462–4.
16. Newman NM, et al. Bilateral optic neuropathy and osteolytic sinusitis. Complications of cocaine abuse. JAMA. 1988;259:72–4.
17. Sawicka EH, Trosser A. Cerebrospinal fluid rhinorrhoea after cocaine sniffing. Br Med J (Clin Res Ed). 1983;286:1476–7.
18. Rampi A, et al. Cocaine-induced midline destructive lesions: a real challenge in oral rehabilitation. Int J Environ Res Public Health. 2021;18(6):3219. https://doi.org/10.3390/ijerph18063219. Published online 2021 Mar 20.
19. Kampaman KM. New medications for the treatment of Cocaine Dependence. Psychiatry. 2005;2(12):44–8.
20. Nagaoka K, et al. Significant improvement from chronic beryllium disease following corticosteroid pulse therapy. Ind Health. 2006;44:296–301.
21. Fontenot AP, Maier LA. Genetic susceptibility and immune-mediated destruction in beryllium-induced disease. Trends Immunol. 2005;26:543–9.
22. Rossman MD. Chronic beryllium disease: diagnosis and management. Environ Health Perspect. 1996;5:945–7.
23. Middleton DC. Chronic beryllium disease: uncommon disease, less common diagnosis. Environ Health Perspect. 1998;12:765–7.
24. Culver DA, Dweik RA. Chronic beryllium disease. Clin Pul Med. 2003;10:72–9.
25. Newman LS, et al. The natural history of beryllium sensitization and chronic beryllium disease. Environ Health Perspect. 1996;5:937–43.
26. Newman LS, et al. Significance of the blood beryllium lymphocyte proliferation test. Environ Health Perspect. 1996;5:953–6.
27. Henderson WJ, et al. Ingestion of talc particles by cultured lung fibroblasts. Environ Res. 1975;9(2):173–8. https://doi.org/10.1016/0013-9351(75)90061-4.
28. Marchiori E, et al. Pulmonary talcosis: imaging findings. Lung. 2010;188(2):165–71. https://doi.org/10.1007/s00408-010-9230-y.
29. Griffith CC, et al. Intravascular talcosis due to intravenous drug use is an underrecognized cause of pulmonary hypertension. Pulm Med. 2012;2012:617531. https://doi.org/10.1155/2012/617531. Published online 2012 May 7.

30. Jones RN, et al. Disease related to non-asbestos silicates 'Talc' pneumoconiosis. In: Parkes WN, editor. Occupational lung disorders. 3rd ed. Oxford: Butterworth-Heinemann; 1994. p. 536–50.
31. Ward S, et al. Talcosis associated with IV abuse of oral medications: CT findings. Am J Roentgenol. 2000;174(3):789–93. https://doi.org/10.2214/ajr.174.3.1740789.
32. Mukhopadhyay S, Gal AA. Granulomatous lung disease: an approach to the differential diagnosis. Arch Pathol Lab Med. 2010;134(5):667–90.
33. Ganesan S, et al. Embolized crospovidone (poly[N-vinyl-2-pyrrolidone]) in the lungs of intravenous drug users. Modern Pathol. 2003;16(4):286–92.
34. Walley VM, et al. Foreign materials found in the cardiovascular system after instrumentation or surgery (including a guide to their light microscopic identification). Cardiovasc Pathol. 1993;2(3):157–85.
35. Arnett EN, et al. Intravenous injection of talc containing drugs intended for oral use. A cause of pulmonary granulomatosis and pulmonary hypertension. Am J Med. 1976;60(5):711–8.
36. Roberts WC. Pulmonary talc granulomas, pulmonary fibrosis, and pulmonary hypertension resulting from intravenous injection of talc-containing drugs intended for oral use. Baylor Univ Med Center Proc. 2002;15:260–1.
37. Oreški I, Grgić MV. Unilateral talc-induced intranasal tissue necrosis – a case report. Ann Otolaryngol Rhinol. 2018;5(5):1224.
38. Omar NB, et al. Cerebellar talcosis following posterior reversible encephalopathy syndrome in an intravenous methamphetamine abuser. Surg Neurol Int. 2021;12:2. https://doi.org/10.25259/SNI_616_2020. Published online 2021 Jan 5.
39. Kahn J. A cloud of smoke: the complicated death of a 9/11 hero. The New Yorker. 2008.
40. Nguyen T-P, et al. Pulmonary talcosis in an immunocompromised patient. Case Rep Med. 2016;2016:4678637. https://doi.org/10.1155/2016/4678637. Published online 2016 Jun 30.
41. Mortimer NJ, et al. Red tattoo reactions. Clin Exp Dermatol. 2003;28:508–10.
42. Lee JS, et al. Basal cell carcinoma arising in a tattooed eyebrow. Ann Dermatol. 2009;21:281–4.
43. Hogsberg T, et al. Tattoo inks in general usage contain microparticles. Br J Dermatol. 2011;165:1210–8.
44. Laumann AE. History and epidemiology of tattoos and piercings. Legislation in the United States. In: Dermatologic complications with body art. 2009. p. 1–11.
45. Goldstein N. Tattoos defined. Clin Dermatol. 2007;25(4):417–20. https://doi.org/10.1016/j.clindermatol.2007.05.015.
46. Hutton Carlsen K, Serup J. Patients with tattoo reactions have reduced quality of life and suffer from itch. Skin Res Technol. 2015;21(1):101–7. https://doi.org/10.1111/srt.12164.
47. Bassi A, et al. Tattoo-associated skin reaction: the importance of an early diagnosis and proper treatment. BioMed Res Int. 2014;2014:Article ID 354608, 7 pages. https://doi.org/10.1155/2014/354608
48. Mataix J, Silvestre JF. Cutaneous adverse reactions to tattoos and piercings. Actas Dermo Sifiliográficas Engl Ed. 2009;100(8):643–56.
49. Jacob CI. Tattoo-associated dermatoses: a case report and review of the literature. Dermatol Surg. 2002;28(10):962–5.
50. Lubeck G, Epstein E. Complications of tattooing. Calif Med. 1952;76(2):83–5.
51. Cruz FAM, et al. Reactions to the different pigments in tattoos: a report of two cases. An Bras Dermatol. 2010;85(5):708–11. https://doi.org/10.1590/S0365-05962010000500019.
52. Sowden JM, et al. Red tattoo reactions: X-ray microanalysis and patch-test studies. Br J Dermatol. 1991;124(6):576–80. https://doi.org/10.1111/j.1365-2133.1991.tb04954.x.
53. Brodie J, et al. A case of episcleral tattooing – an emerging body modification trend. BMC Ophthalmol. 2015;15:95. https://doi.org/10.1186/s12886-015-0095-y. Published online 2015 Aug 8.
54. Pirakitikulr N, et al. Periorbital silicone granulomatosis 30 years after acupuncture. Case Rep Ophthalmol Med. 2020;2020:6323646. https://doi.org/10.1155/2020/6323646. Published online 2020 Jun 24.
55. Barrett J. Acupuncture and facial rejuvenation. Aesthetic Surg J. 2005;25(4):419–24. https://doi.org/10.1016/j.asj.2005.05.001.
56. Kent KM, Graber EM. Laser tattoo removal: a review. Dermatol Surg. 2012;38(1):1–13. https://doi.org/10.1111/j.1524-4725.2011.02187.x.
57. Taylor CR, et al. Treatment of tattoos by q-switched ruby laser: a dose-response study. Arch Dermatol. 1990;126(7):893–9. https://doi.org/10.1001/archderm.1990.01670310055007.

30 Foreign Body Granuloma

Abstract

Foreign body granuloma is granulomatous inflammatory changes due to the presence of foreign/exogenous material. It can be traumatic or iatrogenic. Among the commonly encountered foreign bodies encountered due to trauma are glass, metal, and wood in nature. Iatrogenic exogenous materials may include dental materials, retained sutures, and cosmetic filler substances, such as hyaluronic acid and silicon. Variable clinical features include localized erythema, induration, pigment alteration, nodules/papules at the site of cutaneous injury. Over time, lesions may become ulcerated and colonized secondarily by bacteria. Deep fungal or bacterial infection and abscess may develop if foreign material gets contaminated with microorganisms. Lesion may ulcerate with extrusion of foreign material (e.g., transepidermal elimination of suture material long after surgery). Foreign material may migrate via lymphatics to regional lymph nodes, leading to nodal granulomas and palpable lymphadenopathy. The utility of imaging modalities is based upon features of foreign body (e.g., composition, size, orientation, duration of its presence and anatomic site). Complete excision with removal of the foreign body is often curative. Superinfected lesions may require antimicrobial therapy with drainage of abscess.

30.1 Background

The foreign body granuloma is a response of biological tissue to any foreign material in the tissue [1]. The foreign body is the most common source of localized granulomatous inflammation. Foreign bodies can penetrate soft tissues through open wounds, lacerations, or through accidents iatrogenically. Among the commonly encountered foreign bodies encountered due to trauma are glass, metal, and wood in nature. Iatrogenic exogenous materials may include dental materials, retained sutures, and cosmetic filler substances—such as hyaluronic acid and silicon. Foreign body reaction consists of protein adsorption, macrophages, multinucleated foreign body giant cells (macrophage fusion), fibroblasts, and angiogenesis [1, 2].

30.2 Etiopathogenesis

There are numerous endogenous and exogenous substances which may trigger foreign body reactions. Foreign body is an exogenous substance not inherently native to the body (e.g., suture material) or foreign to a specific body part (e.g., urate crystals in the skin). Relatively common endogenous sources include hair fibers, keratin aggregates and lipids derived from cholesterol deposits and fat emboli [3]. Exogenous materials

S. V. Nemade, K. J. Shinde, *Granulomatous diseases in Otorhinolaryngology, Head and Neck*,
https://doi.org/10.1007/978-981-16-4047-6_30

may include an array of commonly used dental materials, retained sutures and cosmetic filler substances. Nowadays, in an attempt to prevent esthetic changes as a result of aging, the use of injectable soft tissue fillers (STFs) is increasingly observed. Cosmetic filler materials commonly used are hyaluronic acid and silicon used for labial, peri-labial augmentation, nose reshaping, cheek, and chin augmentation [4]. Hyaluronic acid and silicon are also used in vocal fold augmentation phonosurgery [4, 5]. Even though STFs are biologically inert, their injection can result in the formation of granulomas. These granulomas can result from an inflammatory or autoimmune tissue response [5, 6].

30.2.1 Etiological Factors [5–9]

Accidental:

- Wood splinters
- Blast injury
- Motor vehicle accident

Surgical Procedures:

- Surgical sutures
- Gelfoam

Iatrogenic:

- Hyaluronic acid fillers
- Bovine collagen fillers
- Silicone
- Paraffin for tissue augmentation

Foreign body granuloma can occur at any age and initially begins with acute inflammation at the site of entry of the foreign material. This is often followed by apparent resolution of the lesion. However, after a period of weeks, months, or even years, a chronic inflammatory reaction can ensue, presenting as a red or red-brown, inflamed, indurated papule, plaque, or nodule. Additional clinical findings may include cellulitis, abscess, edema, ulceration, and erythema [7, 8].

The formation of a foreign body granuloma begins with neutrophils attracted to the site of entry. When the neutrophils are unable to engulf the foreign material, macrophages are attracted to the site. Macrophages become active and secrete cytokines once they have phagocytosed the foreign material. The secreted cytokines attract more macrophages and peripheral monocytes to the site of entry, and this process forms a chronic granuloma. Macrophages may fuse together to form multinucleated giant cells [8, 9].

Two basic categories of etiologic factors are recognized as inducers of granulomatous inflammatory responses. The first comprises inert substance that is unable to incite any specific inflammatory or immune response. These are artificially termed foreign body typed agents, and although non-immunogenic, their chemical properties render them able to generate granulomas which differ in evolution, dynamics, duration, severity, and involution rates from infectious type [10].

30.3 Clinical Features

- Foreign body granuloma may have varied presentation. It may present as a nodular mass, erythema, localized or generalized edema, induration, pigment alteration or papules at the site of injury [2]. Over time, lesions may become ulcerated and colonized secondarily by bacteria.
- Deep fungal or bacterial infection and abscess may develop if foreign material gets contaminated with fungal organisms (e.g., wood splinters).
- The lesion may later become painful and ulcerate with extrusion of foreign material (e.g., transepidermal elimination of suture material long after surgery).
- Foreign material may migrate via lymphatics to regional lymph nodes, leading to nodal granulomas and palpable lymphadenopathy [4, 5].
- "Migratory" granulomas are due to visible dermatologic lesions remote from the initial site of injury [24].

In oral cavity, the gingiva is the most common site followed by the tongue. Clinically localized change in gingival color, especially at the interdental papilla, ulceration, or diffuse erythema, is noticeable [10]. In the nose, the nasal septum and inferior turbinate are the most common sites. It presents with nasal obstruction, pain, and sometimes epistaxis. Rarely foreign bodies may get impacted in the maxillary sinus during road traffic accidents, leading to foreign body granuloma formation (Fig. 30.1). It may present with sinusitis not responding to antimicrobial treatment. Other common sites of involvement during road traffic injury are lips, palate, and soft tissues of the face (muscles and parotid gland) (Fig. 30.2). Tracheobronchial foreign body granulomas have also been reported, although they are rare [5, 6].

FBG due to Soft tissue fillers (STFs): STFs such as Hyaluronic acid and silicon may cause granulomas (Figs. 30.3 and 30.4), nodularity, migration, and chronic cellulitis [16, 17, 20].

In ear, the most common site for FB granuloma is the external canal skin. It presents with otalgia, decreased hearing, and ear discharge in case of secondary infection. Foreign body may travel to the middle ear through the perforated tympanic membrane leading to middle ear granuloma formation [8, 11, 14].

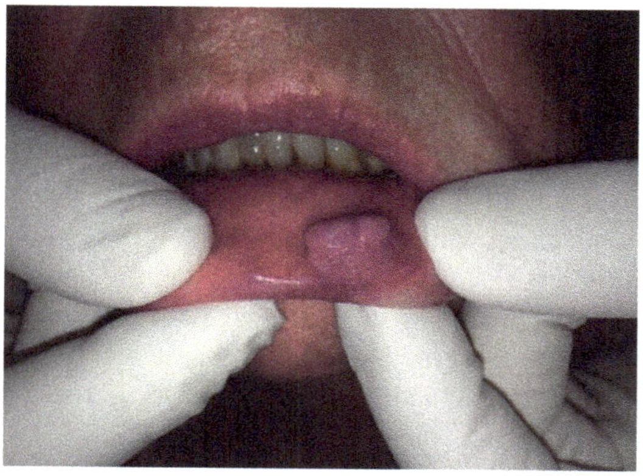

Fig. 30.1 (**a**) Presence of a free, well-defined, rounded nodule on the left lateral border of the tongue due to foreign body granuloma. (**b**) Ultrasonography showing a circumscribed nodular lesion. The echographic aspect was suggestive of a foreign body inside, suggesting an image compatible with a thorn, with granuloma formation [17]

FB granuloma due to surgical sutures may be seen after head-neck surgeries. Small indurated granulomas are seen at the incision site, which may liquefy with serous discharge. Secondary infection may lead to purulent discharge [7, 8].

In patients with penetrating injury, the nature of foreign body determines the clinical behavior. Inert objects such as steel and glass may not cause significant inflammation. Removal of organic foreign bodies such as wood pieces and fish bones is mandatory because they provide a good medium for microbial agents, and this usually leads to secondary infection with abscess and fistula formation [15, 18].

30.4 Diagnosis

30.4.1 Histopathology

Histopathologically, the presence of well formed, often non-caseating granuloma exhibiting proliferation of fibroblasts and endothelial cells with a mixed inflammatory infiltrate consisting of lymphocytes, plasma cells, histiocytes, few polymorphonuclear leucocytes & few giant cells confirms the diagnosis (Fig. 30.5). In many cases, the foreign material is readily evident on microscopic examination (Fig. 30.4b, c) [6]. Vacuoles corresponding to the filler material are frequently found, particularly with silicone [16].

Foreign body is often refractile but may or may not be polarizable; examination with polarized light is useful component of granulomatous dermatitis workup. Periodic acid Schiff (PAS) and Gomori silver methenamine (GMS) stains are useful to rule out secondary deep fungal infection [16, 17].

30.4.2 Imaging

Radiographs—The visibility of different materials on plain radiographs depends on their ability to attenuate X-rays. Hence, it may not always be useful. Metallic objects, except aluminum are opaque on radiographs, as are most animal bones and all glass foreign bodies [7].

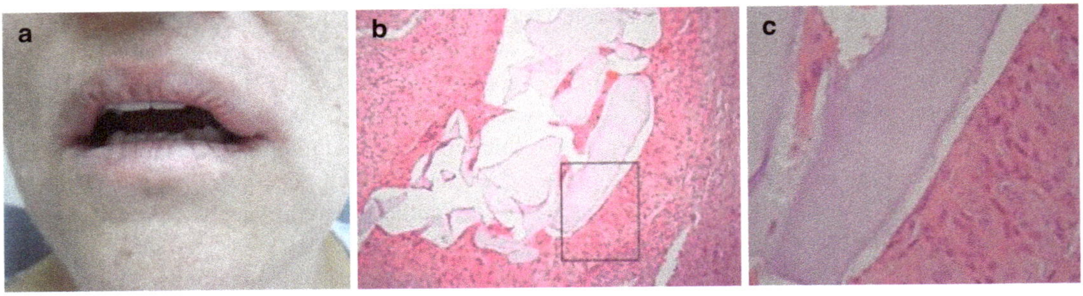

Fig. 30.2 Foreign body granulomas in the right parotid gland. (**a**) Intraoperative image showing needle location of glass pieces and the granulomas around the pieces. (**b**) Glass pieces removed. (**c**) Preoperative photo showing right facial paralysis. (**d**) Postoperative photo showing improvement in facial nerve function. (**e**) Complete eye closure achieved after excision of foreign body granulomas

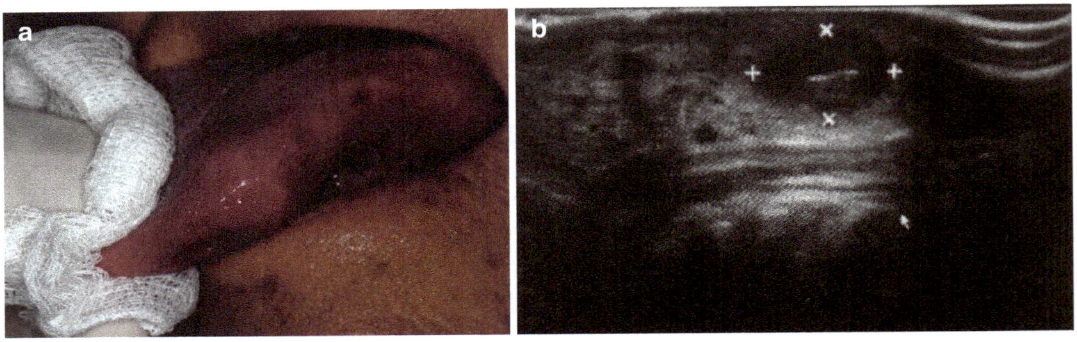

Fig. 30.3 Exophytic nodule on the lower lip. Patient had received hyaluronic acid injections in the lower lip 1.5 years before [16]

Ultrasonography—It is particularly helpful in the detection of foreign body in subcutaneous soft tissues or tongue. The echographic aspects of foreign body image help in suspecting the foreign body material (Fig. 30.1b) [17].

CT scan—It can delineate most of the foreign bodies well (Figs. 30.6 and 30.7), however, it may not distinguish plastic material from soft tissues. Depending on their relative densities although it may show signs of infection or other chronic reactions [4, 7, 8].

MRI is the preferred imaging technique to locate plastic foreign bodies embedded in soft tissues [5, 8, 12].

Confocal laser scanning is a newer method of identifying the microscopic changes within the tissues where the foreign body is embedded. It helps in providing improved tissue images, bi-dimensional pictures with better resolution at the cellular level, and in particular, a three-dimensional imaging and reconstruction is possible (Fig. 30.7) [13].

30.5 Treatment

The definitive treatment is excision of the granuloma along with the removal of the foreign body (Fig. 30.8). Infected lesions may require antimicrobial therapy with drainage of the abscess. Supportive therapy with anti-inflammatory analgesics, topical and/or intralesional corticosteroid treatment may be warranted [6–9].

For foreign body granuloma secondary to soft tissue fillers, intralesional steroids represent the first line of treatment, sparing systemic steroids for recurrent lesions in doses higher than those used before locally. Excision of

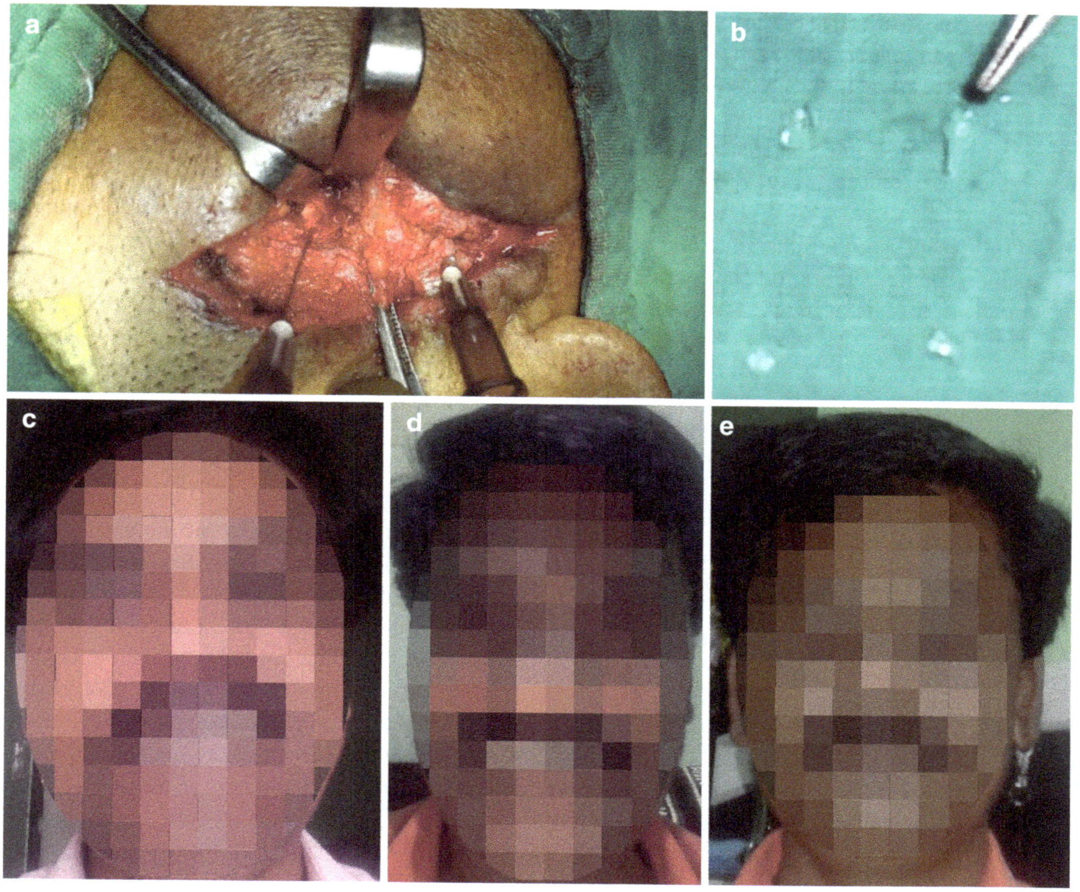

Fig. 30.4 Extraoral view of the submucosal nodule on the upper left labial mucosa. Hyaluronic acid filler injections were done 6 months before the nodule. A pool of amorphous basophilic material corresponding to hyaluronic acid lined by epithelioid macrophages is observed [(**b**) hematoxylin-eosin stain, original magnification ×100, (**c**) hematoxylin-eosin stain, original magnification ×200] [16]

FBGs secondary to STFs is difficult, especially when they appear as multiple nodules or as a diffuse swelling. Granulomas can migrate throughout multiple layers of soft tissue, often necessitating the removal of thick sections of tissue. However, when it presents as a single nodule, excisional biopsy is both diagnostic and therapeutic [16, 22].

Adjuvant therapy: Tetracycline antibiotics, especially minocycline (200 mg/day), have been used successfully for their anti-inflammatory, immunomodulating, antigranulomatous properties, as well as their mycobacterial coverage. 5-Fluorouracil and isotretinoin have been proven effective in patients refractory to steroid treatment [23, 24].

30.6 Essential Features

- Granulomatous inflammatory changes due to the presence of foreign/exogenous material.
- Offending agents may be grouped as follows:
  - Iatrogenic: suture, surgical adhesive.
  - Cosmetic: silicon, lipid, zirconium, cutaneous bleaching agents, bovine collagen,

injectable fillers including hyaluronic acid and many others.
 – Traumatic: metallic or non-metallic splinters, shrapnel, arthropod bite/mouthparts, sea urchin spine, cactus glochids/spines, hair, or keratin from ruptured cysts or follicles.
- May present as a nodular mass/papules, erythema, edema, induration and/or ulceration, abscess at the site of injury. May be associated

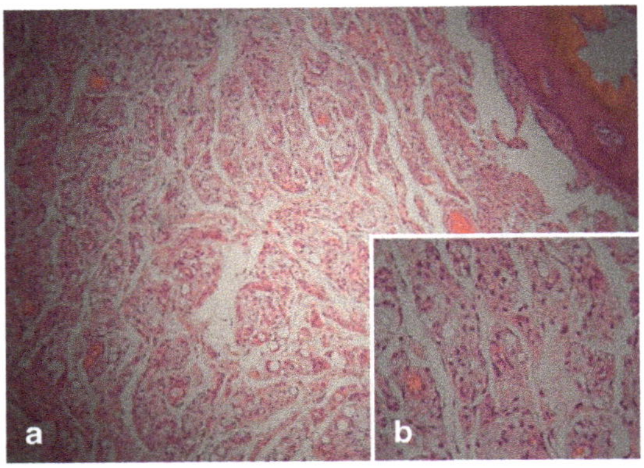

Fig. 30.5 FB granulomatous reaction seen on Histopathology: Multiple clear cystic spaces of varying size intermixed with epithelioid macrophages with vacuolated cytoplasm in a fibrous connective tissue stroma are observed [(**a**) hematoxylin-eosin stain, original magnification ×100, (**b**) hematoxylin-eosin stain, original magnification ×200] [16]

with regional lymphadenopathy with nodal granulomas.
- Lesion may heal only to later become painful and ulcerate with extrusion of foreign material (e.g., transepidermal elimination of suture material long after surgery).
- Foreign material may migrate via lymphatics to regional lymph nodes, leading to nodal granulomas and palpable lymphadenopathy.
- Radiography is useful to locate only radio-opaque foreign body. Computed Tomography is helpful to delineate all foreign bodies, however, it may not differentiate plastic material from soft tissue. MRI is particularly reliable to locate the plastic foreign body.
- Confocal laser scanning is a newer method of identifying the microscopic changes within the tissues where the foreign body is embedded.
- Histopathologically the presence of well formed, often non-caseating granuloma exhibiting proliferation of fibroblasts and endothelial cells with mixed inflammatory infiltrate.
- Complete excision with removal of the foreign body is often curative.
- Infected lesions may require antimicrobial therapy with drainage of the abscess.

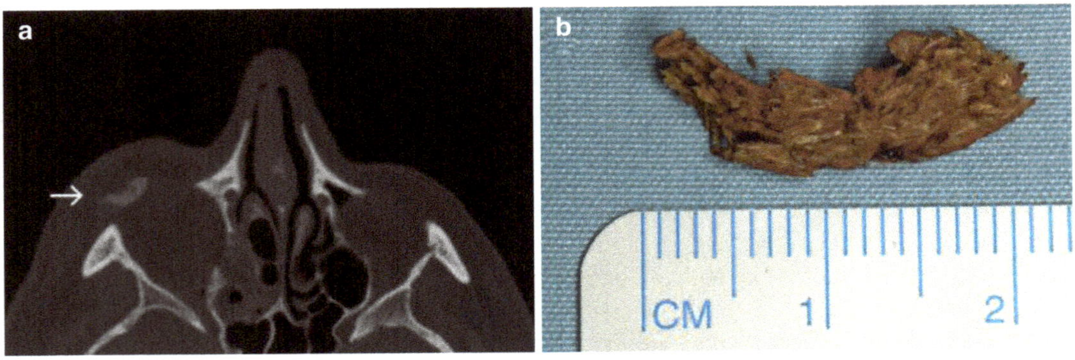

Fig. 30.6 Chipboard wood. (**a**) An axial CT image displaying a hyperdense structure dislocated in periorbital soft tissues inferior and anterior to the right globe (arrow). Hyperdensity of the foreign object, in this case, is likely due to its industrial processing. (**b**) A photograph of a chipboard fragment after its removal from the soft tissues [21]

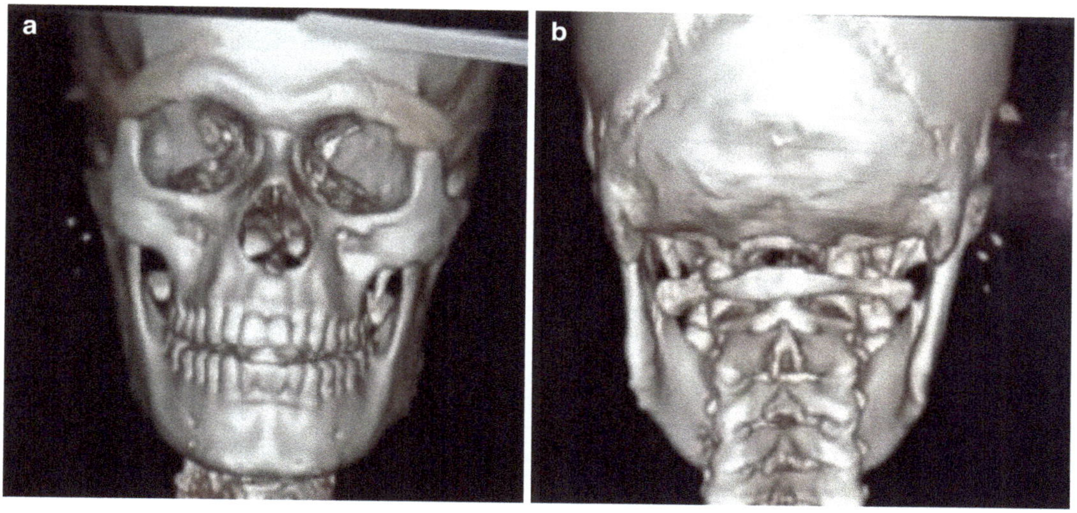

Fig. 30.7 (a, b) 3D reconstruction CT showing glass pieces in the right parotid region

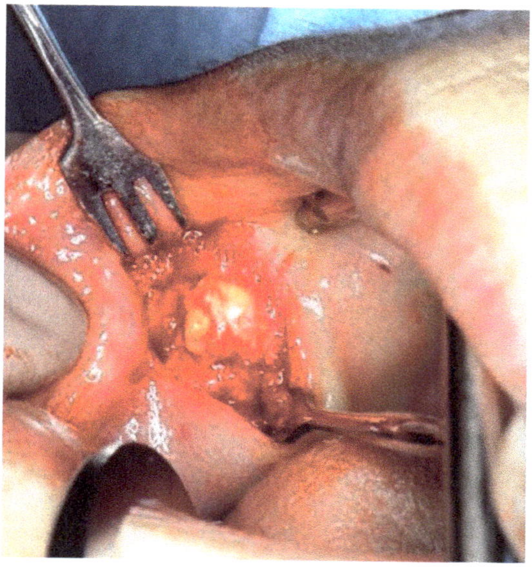

Fig. 30.8 Intraoperative photograph while removal of silicon granuloma [19]

References

1. Rapini RP, Bolognia JL, Jorizzo JL. Dermatology: 2-Volume Set. St. Louis: Mosby; 2007. p. 1443. ISBN 978-1-4160-2999-1.
2. Ratner BD, et al. Biomaterials science. 2nd ed. p. 296–304.
3. Sumanth KN, Karen B. Glass embedded in labial mucosa for 20 years. Indian J Dent Res. 2008;19(2):160–1. https://doi.org/10.4103/0970-9290.40473.
4. El-Khalawany M, et al. Dermal filler complications: a clinicopathologic study with a spectrum of histologic reaction patterns. Ann Diagn Pathol. 2015;19:10–5.
5. Owosho AA, et al. Orofacial dermal fillers: foreign body reactions, histopathologic features, and spectrometric studies. Oral Surg Oral Med Oral Pathol Oral Radiol. 2014;117:617–25.
6. Murakami K, et al. Buccal silicone granuloma caused by the dental infection. Case Rep Dent. 2020;2020:Article ID 8834475, 7 pages. https://doi.org/10.1155/2020/8834475.
7. Robinson PD, Rajayogeswaran V. Unlikely foreign bodies in unusual facial sites. Br J Oral Maxillofac Surg. 1997;35:36–9. https://doi.org/10.1016/S0266-4356(97)90006-1.
8. McCaughey AD. An unusual infraorbital foreign body. Br J Oral Maxillofac Surg. 1988;26:426–9.
9. Westermark AH. Spontaneous removal of foreign bodies from the maxillary sinus. Br J Oral Maxillofac Surg. 1989;47:75–7.
10. Mariano M. The experimental granuloma. A hypothesis to explain the persistence of the lesion. Rev Inst Med Trop Sao Paulo. 1995;37(2):161–76. https://doi.org/10.1590/S0036-46651995000200012.
11. Henry RC. Infra orbital penetrating foreign body. Br J Oral Surg. 1971;8:192.
12. Krishnan A. Trismus caused by a retained foreign body in an adult. Oral Surg Oral Med Oral Pathol. 1992;73:546–7.
13. Michele S, Alberta L. Oral pulse granuloma: histological findings by confocal laser scanning microscopy. Ultrastruct Pathol. 2009;33(4):155–9.
14. Law S, Watters GW. Penetrating oral foreign body presenting as an aural polyp. J Laryngol Otol. 1997;3111:749–51.

15. Krimmel M, et al. Wooden foreign bodies in facial injury: a radiological pitfall. Int J Oral Maxillofac Surg. 2001;30:445–7.
16. Tamiolakis P, et al. Report of two cases and review of the literature. J Clin Exp Dent. 2018;10(2):e177–84. https://doi.org/10.4317/jced.54191. Published online 2018 Feb 1.
17. Pereira RMA, et al. Foreign body granuloma in the tongue by a pequi spine. Case Rep Dent. 2020;2020:8838250. https://doi.org/10.1155/2020/8838250. Published online 2020 Nov 10.
18. Henry RC. Infra orbital penetrating foreign body. Br J Oral Surg. 1971;8:192.
19. Murakami K, et al. Buccal silicone granuloma caused by the dental infection. Case Rep Dent. 2020;2020:Article ID 8834475, 7 pages. https://doi.org/10.1155/2020/8834475.
20. Chasan PE. The history of injectable silicone fluids for soft-tissue augmentation. Plast Reconstruct Surg. 2007;120(7):2034–40.
21. Voss JO, et al. Imaging foreign bodies in head and neck trauma: a pictorial review. Insights Imaging. 2021;12:20. https://doi.org/10.1186/s13244-021-00969-9. Published online 2021 Feb 15.
22. Lee JM, Kim YJ. Foreign body granulomas after the use of dermal fillers: pathophysiology, clinical appearance, histology features, and treatment. Arch Plast Surg. 2015;42:232–9.
23. Arin MJ, et al. Silicone granuloma of the face treated with minocycline. J Am Acad Dermatol. 2005;52(2 Suppl 1):53–6.
24. Teuber SS, et al. Severe migratory granulomatous reactions to silicone gel in 3 patients. J Rheumatol. 1999;26(3):699–704.

31 Pyogenic Granuloma

Abstract

Pyogenic granuloma is commonly occurring non-neoplastic reactive lesion of the oral cavity. Clinically it is characterized by localized solitary nodule reddish or pink in color with a sessile or pedunculated base. Low-grade chronic irritation, trauma, and hormonal imbalances are said to be the main etiology for pyogenic granuloma, which results in the overzealous proliferation of vascular type of connective tissue. It shows predilection for gingiva and is usually slow growing, but sometimes shows a rapid growth. The disease progresses in three phases—cellular phase, capillary phase/vascular phase, and involutionary phase. Histopathologically, the pyogenic granuloma is classified into lobular capillary hemangioma (LCH) and non-lobular capillary hemangioma (non-LCH). LCH type shows numerous blood vessels organized into lobular aggregates, whereas the non-LCH type does not show any such organization and resembles granulation tissue. The involutionary phase shows healing of the lesion and is characterized by extensive fibrosis in the connective tissue. Surgical excision is the treatment of choice. After surgical excision of gingival lesions, deep curettage of the underlying tissue is recommended to prevent recurrence. Excision can be done by using the laser with the advantage of painless procedure and minimum blood loss.

Synonyms

Telangiectatic Granuloma, Pregnancy tumor, granuloma pyogenicum, botryomycosis hominis, granuloma pediculatum benignum, benign vascular tumor, vascular epulis, Crocker and Hartzell's disease [1, 2].

31.1 Background

Pyogenic granuloma is a non-neoplastic soft tissue lesion of the oral cavity occurring as a result of inflammatory reaction. Pyogenic granuloma was first identified by Poncet and Dor in 1897, who described it as a vascularised mass and named it "Human Botryomycosis" [3]. It was given its present name by Crocker in 1903. However, some researchers believe that Hartzell in 1904 introduced the term "pyogenic granuloma" that is widely used in the literature, although it does not accurately express the clinical or histopathologic features [4, 5]. The term pyogenic granuloma is being used now to describe this lesion, but it is considered to be a misnomer as it is neither infective nor a true granuloma. Due to its vascularity, the term

S. V. Nemade, K. J. Shinde, *Granulomatous diseases in Otorhinolaryngology, Head and Neck*,
https://doi.org/10.1007/978-981-16-4047-6_31

"Telangiectatic Granuloma" has also been proposed [2]. Angelopoulos proposed the term "hemangiomatous granuloma" that accurately expresses the histopathologic picture (hemangioma-like) and the inflammatory nature (granuloma) of oral pyogenic granuloma [5]. Gingiva is the commonest site of presentation. Extragingivally, it can occur on the lips, tongue, buccal mucosa and palate [5].

31.2 Epidemiology

According to Cawson et al., oral pyogenic granuloma is relatively common. It represents 0.5% of all skin nodules in children. The pregnancy tumor variant of pyogenic granuloma occurs in up to 5% of pregnancies [6]. Esmeili et al. in their review, stated that hyperplastic reactive lesions represent as a group the most common oral lesions, excluding caries, periodontal, and periapical inflammatory disease. In this group, the second most common group is represented by hyperplastic reactive gingival/alveolar lesions, including inflammatory gingival hyperplasia, oral pyogenic granuloma, peripheral giant-cell lesion and peripheral cemento-ossifying fibroma [7].

Oral pyogenic granuloma occurs over a wide age range of 4.5–93 years, with highest incidence in the second and fifth decades, and females are slightly more affected than males [1].

31.3 Etiopathogenesis

Low-grade chronic irritation, trauma, and hormonal imbalances are said to be the main etiology for pyogenic granuloma, which results in the overzealous proliferation of a vascular type of connective tissue. Poor oral hygiene leading to accumulation of plaque and calculus and overhanging restorations are said to be the most common precipitating factors. Other etiological agents include the use of certain immunosuppressive drugs and oral contraceptives. Nonspecific bacterial infection is thought to be a secondary involvement rather than being the main etiology of this lesion [8, 9].

Some investigators consider pyogenic granuloma as a "reactive" or "reparative" tumor process. Regezi et al. suggest that pyogenic granuloma represents an exuberant connective tissue proliferation to a known stimulus or injuries like calculus or foreign material within the gingival crevice [10].

The key to wound healing is the formation of granulation tissue, and this includes the migration of inflammatory cells, migration and proliferation of vascular endothelial cells and fibroblasts and synthesis of extracellular matrix. Such processes of wound healing seem to be controlled by various kinds of cytokines. Out of these cytokines—role of growth factors, particularly bFGF—a heparin-binding angiogenic protein, has been found to be highly mitogenic for capillary endothelial cells and to induce angiogenesis [11].

Yung et al. suggested hormonal influence on the basis of the observation that pregnancy tumor that occurs in pregnant women also arises from the gingiva and has the same microscopic appearance [12]. On the basis of these observations, gingiva can be regarded as another "target organ" for direct action of estrogen and progesterone. The levels of estrogen and progesterone are markedly elevated in pregnancy and could therefore exert a greater effect on the endothelium of oral pyogenic granuloma. However, pyogenic granuloma occurs almost as often in males as females; for this reason, a hormonal basis is doubtful [1, 12].

Pyogenic granuloma is classified as:

1. Non-lobular capillary haemangioma (pedunculated form)—77%
2. Lobular Capillary Haemangioma (sessile form)—66% [13]

31.4 Clinical Features

Pyogenic granuloma occurred more commonly in females and located at gingival and extragingival sites. Extragingivally, it can occur on the lips, tongue, buccal mucosa and palate. It can present with a wide array of clinical appearances, ranging from a sessile lesion or pedunculated mass ranging from few millimeters to centimeters in size and are usually slow growing and asymptomatic. Pyogenic granulomas generally are soft, painless, and pink, purplish, to red in color depending on the vascularity of the lesion (Fig. 31.1) [14–16].

Pyogenic granuloma frequently occurs during pregnancy, especially during the second and third trimesters, wherein it is referred to as "pregnancy tumor." Increased levels of estrogen and progesterone modify the vascular response to local irritants that lead to the occurrence of the lesion. Histopathologically, pregnancy tumor has features similar to pyogenic granuloma [16].

The course of the lesion can be described as "early," "established," and "healing" type. The color of the lesion also varies and is dependent on the vascularity of the lesion in relation to its clinical course. The early lesions are usually pinkish in color and resemble the normal mucosal color. Established lesions are reddish to purplish due to the increased vascularity, whereas the late healing type presents as pinkish to whitish mass due to fibrosis. These different phases of pyogenic granuloma can be appreciated on the microscopic level as well. The natural course of this lesion can be categorized into three distinct phases, namely, (1) cellular phase, (2) capillary phase/vascular phase, and (3) involutionary phase [17].

31.5 Diagnosis

31.5.1 Histopathology

This is the gold standard investigation. The microscopic picture of pyogenic granuloma, in general, shows exuberant granulation tissue, which is covered by atrophic/hyperplastic epithelium that may be ulcerated at times and reveals fibrinous exudates. The presence of numerous endothelium-lined vascular spaces and proliferation of fibroblasts and budding endothelial cells are the characteristic features of pyogenic granuloma. The presence of mixed inflammatory cell infiltration is also observed (Fig. 31.2) [17, 18].

Cawson et al. have described two variants of pyogenic granuloma depending on the rate of proliferation and vascularity, namely, (1) lobular capillary hemangioma and (2) non-lobular capillary hemangioma [6]. The LCH type of pyogenic granuloma is characterized by proliferating blood vessels organized in lobular aggregates, whereas the non-LCH type shows high vascular proliferation resembling granulation tissue [6, 17].

Sternberg et al. suggested three distinct phases to describe the course of pyogenic granuloma. The "early phase" reveals a compact cellular stroma with little lumen formation. The next phase described as the capillary phase, reveals lobules that are highly vascular with abundant intralumi-

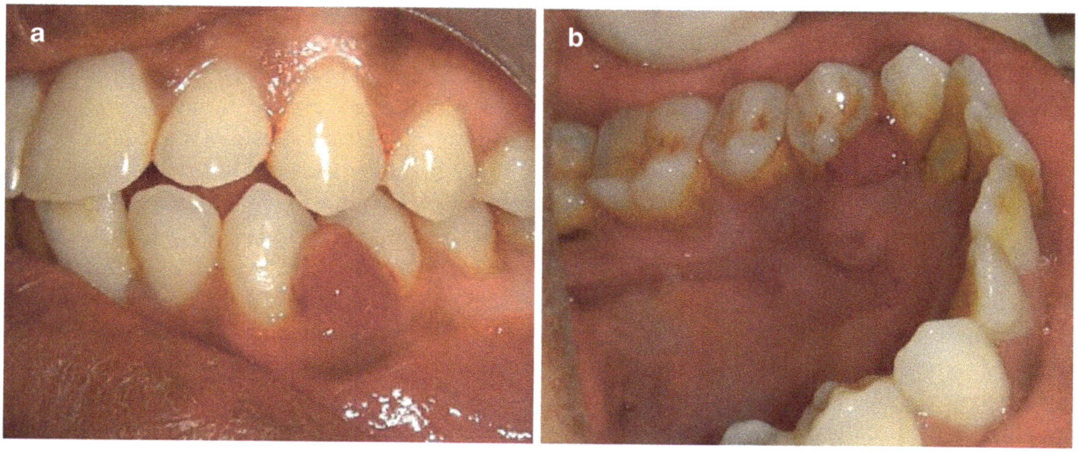

Fig. 31.1 Exophytic and hemorrhagic lesion in the lower canine-premolar region. (**a**) Buccal view and (**b**) lingual view [14]

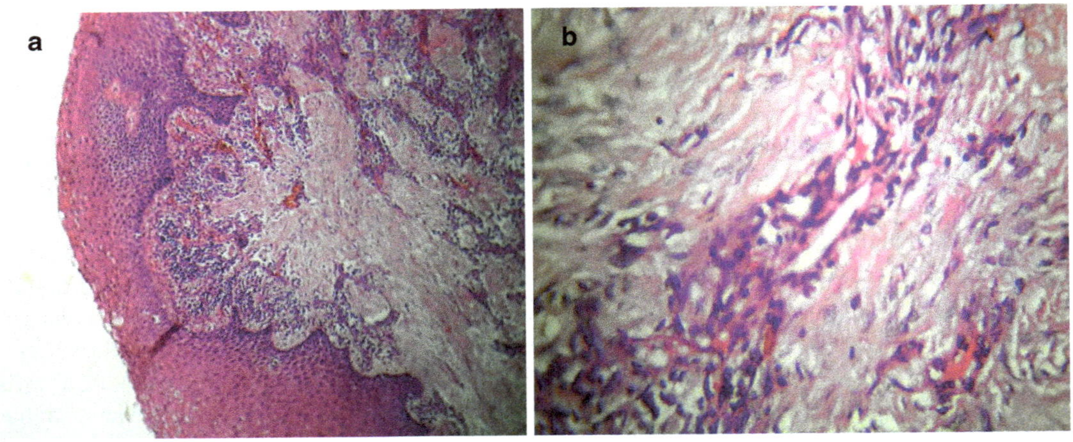

Fig. 31.2 (**a**) Scanning view showing hyperplastic parakeratinized stratified squamous epithelium and (**b**) connective tissue with numerous endothelial cell lined capillaries and dense fibrous stroma (H&E, 50×) [17]

nal red blood cells. The final phase, referred to as "involutionary phase," shows intra-and perilobular fibrosis. This phase is suggestive of the healing phase of pyogenic granuloma [6, 17].

31.5.2 Immunohistochemistry

Pyogenic granuloma lesions express factor VIII-related antigen positivity in the endothelial cells lining large vessels but are negative in the cellular areas. Enhanced expression of the bFGF, Tie-2, anti-CD34 and anti-alpha SMA antibodies, and vascular morphogenesis factors such as angiopoietin-1, angiopoietin-2, ephrinB2, and ephrinB4 is often evident. There is also the expression of inducible nitric oxide synthase, increased expression of vascular endothelial growth factor, low apoptotic rate expression of Bax/Bcl-2 proteins and strong expression of phosphorylated mitogen-activated protein kinase [19].

31.5.3 Imaging

Imaging carries a minimal role in the diagnosis of pyogenic granuloma. Orthopantomogram (OPG) may show localized alveolar bone resorption in rare instances of large and long-standing gingival tumors [5].

31.6 Treatment

There are different methods that have been used to treat pyogenic granuloma like excisional biopsy, liquid nitrogen spray, flash lamp pumped pulsed dye laser, corticosteroids, injection of absolute alcohol, use of sclerosing agent like monoethanolamine oleate, carbon dioxide laser, Nd:YAG laser, Er:YAG laser, etc. [13].

Surgical excision is the most effective treatment of choice. After surgical excision of gingival lesions, deep curettage of the underlying tissue is recommended. Excision with 2 mm margins at its clinical periphery and to a depth to the periosteum or to the causative agent. Any foreign body, calculus, or defective restoration should be removed as part of the excision [1, 20].

Excision can be done by using the laser. It achieves a painless postoperative period with almost no blood loss. The lasers that can be used for the excision treatment are neodymium-doped yttrium aluminum garnet (Nd:YAG) laser, diode lasers, erbium-doped YAG (Er:YAG) laser, flash lamp pulsed dye laser [13, 21].

Recurrence rate varies between 5% and 15% depending on the conservative or wide local excision. Gingival cases show a much higher recurrence rate than lesions from other oral mucosal sites; however pyogenic granuloma lacks infiltrative or malignant potential. Sapp et al. stated that oral pyogenic granulomas have a relatively high rate of recurrence after simple excision [1, 22].

31.7 Essential Features

- Pyogenic granuloma is a non-neoplastic soft tissue lesion of the oral cavity.
- It is mostly affecting the gingiva and very rarely other sites of the oral cavity such as lip, tongue, and buccal mucosa.
- The etiological factors are low-grade chronic irritation, trauma, and hormonal imbalances.
- The disease progresses in three phases—cellular phase, capillary phase/vascular phase, and involutionary phase.
- Presents as an exophytic mass with smooth or ulcerative surface. Though, sometimes the lesion appears as a small erythematous papule on a pedunculated or sessile base.
- Pyogenic granuloma frequently occurs during wherein it is referred to as "pregnancy tumor."
- Histopathologically, two variants of pyogenic granuloma are described depending on the rate of proliferation and vascularity, namely, (1) lobular capillary hemangioma type (2) non-lobular capillary hemangioma type. The LCH type of pyogenic granuloma is characterized by proliferating blood vessels organized in lobular aggregates, whereas the non-LCH type shows high vascular proliferation resembling granulation tissue.
- Surgical excision is the treatment of choice. After surgical excision of gingival lesions, deep curettage of the underlying tissue is recommended to prevent recurrence. Excision can be done by using the laser with the advantage of painless procedure and minimum blood loss.

References

1. Kamal R, et al. Oral pyogenic granuloma: various concepts of etiopathogenesis. J Oral Maxillofac Pathol. 2012;16(1):79–82. https://doi.org/10.4103/0973-029X.92978.
2. Kamal R, Dahiya P, Puri A. Oral pyogenic granuloma: various concepts of etiopathogenesis. J Oral Maxillofac Pathol. 2012;16(1):79–82.
3. Poncet A, Dor L. Botryomycose humaine. Revue de Chirurgie. 1897;18:996–1003.
4. Bhaskar SN, Jacoway JR. Pyogenic granuloma – clinical features, incidence, histology, and result of treatment: report of 242 cases. J Oral Surg. 1966;24:391–8.
5. Angelopoulos AP. Pyogenic granuloma of the oral cavity: statistical analysis of its clinical features. J Oral Surg. 1971;29:840–7.
6. Cawson RA, et al. Lucas pathology of tumors of oral tissues. 5th ed. Missouri: Mosby; 1998. p. 252–4.
7. Esmeili T, et al. Common benign oral soft tissue masses. Dent Clin North Am. 2005;49:223–40.
8. Martins-Filho PRS, et al. Aggressive pregnancy tumor (pyogenic granuloma) with extensive alveolar bone loss mimicking a malignant tumor: case report and review of literature. Int J Morphol. 2011;29(1):164–7.
9. Vilmann A, et al. Pyogenic granuloma: evaluation of oral conditions. Br J Oral Maxillofac Surg. 1986;24(5):376–82.
10. Regezi JA, et al. Oral pathology: clinical pathologic considerations. 4th ed. Philadelphia, PA: WB Saunders; 2003. p. 115–6.
11. Murata M, et al. Dynamic distribution of basic fibroblast growth factor during epulis formation: an immunohistochemical study in an enhanced healing process of the gingiva. J Oral Pathol Med. 1997;26:224–32.
12. Yih WY, et al. Expression of estrogen receptors in desquamative gingivitis. J Periodontol. 2000;71:482–7.
13. Yadav RK, et al. Non-invasive treatment of pyogenic granuloma by using Nd:YAG laser. BMJ Case Rep. 2018;2018:bcr2017223536. https://doi.org/10.1136/bcr-2017-223536. Published online 2018 Aug 9.
14. Chandrashekar B. Minimally invasive approach to eliminate pyogenic granuloma: a case report. Case Rep Dent. 2012;2012:Article ID 909780, 3 pages.
15. Sachdeva SK. Extragingival pyogenic granuloma: an unusual clinical presentation. J Dent. 2015;16(3 Suppl):282–5.
16. Steelman R, Holmes D. Pregnancy tumor in a 16-year-old: case report and treatment considerations. J Clin Pediat Dent. 1992;16(3):217–8.
17. Marla V, et al. The histopathological spectrum of pyogenic granuloma: a case series. Case Rep Dent. 2016;2016:Article ID 1323798, 6 pages.
18. Shafer WG, et al. Shafer's textbook of oral pathology. 4th ed. Philadelphia, PA: WB Saunders; 1983.
19. Sato H, et al. Expression of the endothelial receptor tyrosine kinase Tie2 in lobular capillary hemangioma of the oral mucosa: an immunohistochemical study. J Oral Pathol Med. 2002;31:432–8.
20. Marx RE, Stern D. Oral and maxillofacial pathology: a rationale for diagnosis and treatment. Chicago, IL: Quintessence Publishing; 2003. p. 21–3.
21. Rai S, et al. Laser: a powerful tool for treatment of pyogenic granuloma. J Cutan Aesthet Surg. 2011;4:144–7. https://doi.org/10.4103/0974-2077.85044.
22. Sapp JP, et al. Contemporary oral and maxillofacial pathology. 2nd ed. Missouri: Mosby; 1997. p. 318–22.

Part VII

Diseases with Secondary Granulomatous Manifestations

32 Relapsing Polychondritis

Abstract

Relapsing polychondritis is a severe systemic immune-mediated disease characterized by an episodic and progressive inflammatory condition with progressive destruction of cartilaginous structures. The multiple clinical presentations and episodic nature of relapsing polychondritis cause a significant diagnosis delay. The most common initial clinical picture is chondritis of the ears associated with pain, erythema, and edema, followed by chondritis of the nose. Chondritis of chondro-costal joints and upper airways, scleritis and episcleritis, arthralgia, and various mucocutaneous lesions can subsequently occur. Repeated inflammation can lead to the destruction of the cartilage and deformity of the nose, ears and respiratory tract. Tracheobronchomalacia and ascending aorta involvement are the most feared complications. The current diagnosis of relapsing polychondritis is clinical, based on Michet et al. criteria. Anti-inflammatory drugs, colchicine or dapsone, along with low-dose glucocorticoid therapy, is preferred for mild disease. Corticosteroids combined with an immunosuppressive or immunomodulatory agent may reduce the frequency and severity of relapses in severe cases.

Synonyms

Atrophic polychondritis, systemic chondromalacia, chronic atrophic polychondritis, Meyenburg-Altherr-Uehlinger syndrome, generalized chondromalacia [1, 2].

32.1 Background

Relapsing polychondritis (RP) is a multi-systemic condition with secondary granulomatous manifestations. In 1923, Jaksch Wartenhorst published the first description and gave the name of polychondropathy to this disease. In 1960, Pearson et al. proposed its currently accepted name, "relapsing polychondritis" [1]. It is characterized by repeated episodes of inflammation and destruction of cartilage. This can lead to joint deformity and can be life-threatening if the respiratory tract, heart valves, or blood vessels are affected. The exact mechanism is unknown, but it is thought to be related to immune-mediated degeneration of proteins that are abundant in cartilage. About one third of people with RP might be associated with other autoimmune diseases, vasculitis and hematologic disorders. Systemic vasculitis is the most common association with RP, followed by rheumatoid arthritis and systemic lupus erythematosus [2, 3].

S. V. Nemade, K. J. Shinde, *Granulomatous diseases in Otorhinolaryngology, Head and Neck*,
https://doi.org/10.1007/978-981-16-4047-6_32

32.2 Epidemiology

Relapsing polychondritis occurs as often in men as in women. The global annual incidence is about 3.5 cases per million. The highest incidence is between the ages of 40 and 50 years, but it may occur at any age [4]. Relapsing polychondritis has a ubiquitous distribution with documented cases in all ethnic groups, but most patients appear to be of Caucasian origin [1].

32.3 Etiopathogenesis

Relapsing polychondritis is an autoimmune disease in which the body's immune system begins to destroy the cartilage tissues in the body. It has been postulated that both cell-mediated immunity and humoral immunity are responsible [4, 5].

Cartilage inflammation (chondritis) that is relapsing is very characteristic of the disease and is required for the diagnosis of RP. These recurrent episodes of inflammation over the course of the disease may result in breakdown and loss of cartilage, leading to deformity [6].

32.4 Clinical Features

Constitutional Symptoms:
These symptoms consist of asthenia, fever, anorexia, and weight loss. They mostly occur during a severe disease flare [6, 7].

Ear Nose Throat Involvement:
Perichondritis involving auricular cartilage is seen in 20% of patients during initial presentation and 90% of patients at some point [3]. Inflammation may alternate between either ear during a relapse. The entire pinna except the ear lobe is swollen, red, or less often purplish, warm, and tender (Fig. 32.1a, b). Sparing the ear lobe

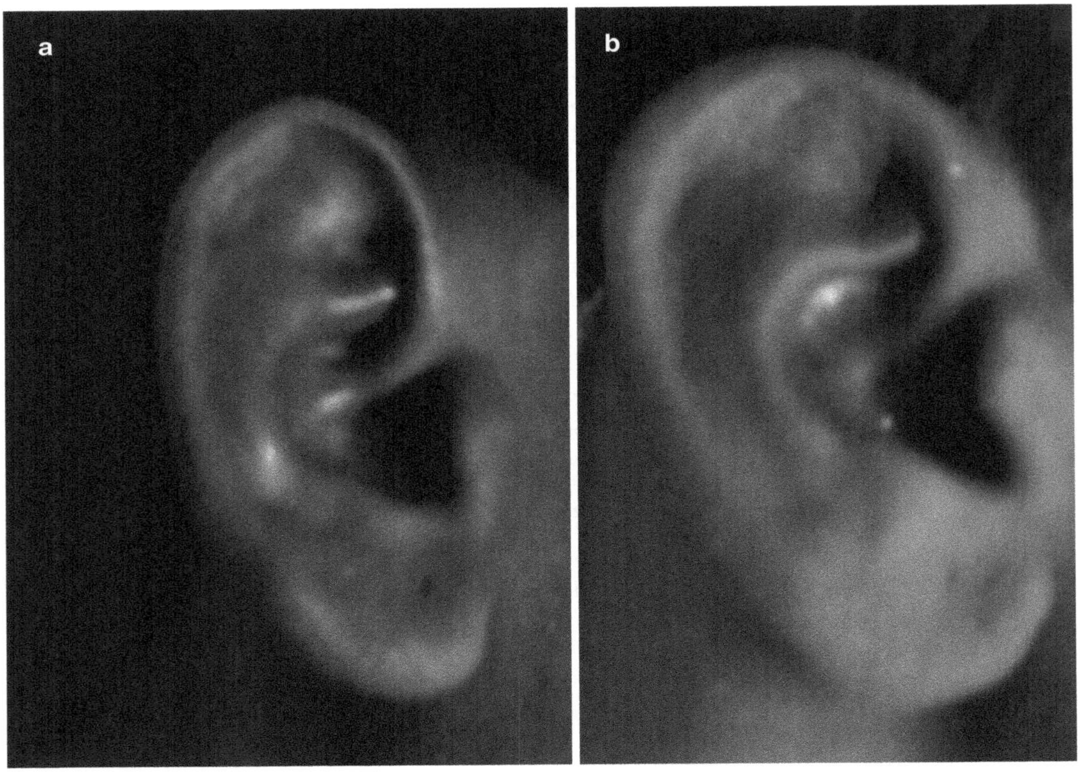

Fig. 32.1 (a) and (b) Perichondritis typically sparing the ear lobe

(due to the absence of cartilage) is a peculiar feature (Figs. 32.1 and 32.2). Because of the destruction of cartilage, after several episodes, cauliflower ear deformity may result. These cauliflower ear deformities occur in about 10% of patients with RP (Fig. 32.2) [6].

The pinna may be either floppy or hardened by calcifications of the scar tissue that replaces the cartilage.

Involvement of lateral cartilages of nasal framework and collapse of the nasal septum may lead to external deformity (saddle nose deformity), which is painless but irreversible. Atrophic rhinitis is often associated with cartilage destruction [6].

The inflammation of the laryngotracheobronchial cartilages may be severe and life-threatening. It causes one-third of all deaths among persons with RP. Laryngeal chondritis manifests as pain above the thyroid gland and dysphonia with a hoarse voice or transient aphonia. Because this disease is relapsing, recurrent laryngeal inflammation may result in laryngomalacia or laryngeal stenosis presenting with inspiratory dyspnea, dry cough, wheezing and choking. It may require tracheostomy to restore airway patency [2, 6, 9].

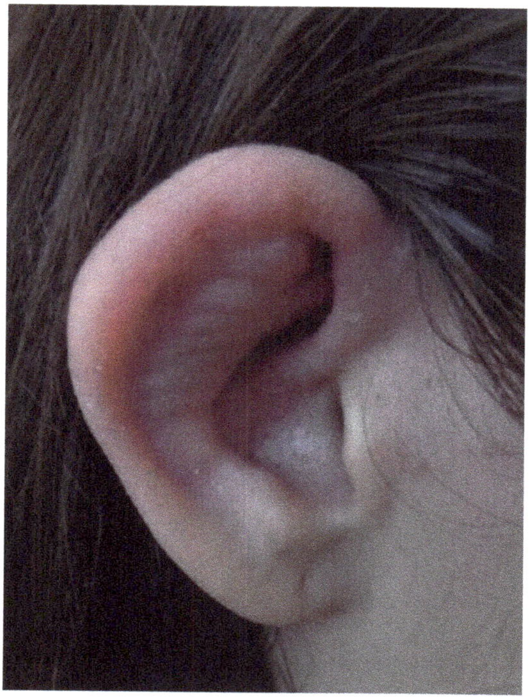

Fig. 32.2 Cauliflower ear. Swelling and erythema of the cartilaginous part of the ear, sparing the lobule which lacks cartilage [8]

Tracheobronchial involvement may or may not be accompanied by laryngeal chondritis and is potentially the most severe manifestation of RP. The symptoms are dyspnea, wheezing, a non-productive cough, and recurrent, sometimes severe, lower respiratory tract infections. Obstructive respiratory failure may develop as the result of either permanent tracheal or bronchial narrowing or chondromalacia with the expiratory collapse of the tracheobronchial tree. The initial symptoms of dry cough, wheezing are usually mistaken for asthma [2, 6, 9].

Audiovestibular involvement: Sensorineural hearing loss is the most common audiovestibular symptom associated with relapsing polychondritis (when vasculitis of the auricular artery or its cochlear branch occurs), although conductive hearing loss may also be present (attributed to the expansion of the inflammatory procedure to the middle ear and eustachian tube). Hearing loss may present in sudden, slowly, rapidly progressive or fluctuating form and is mostly bilateral and asymmetric. Vestibular symptoms, tinnitus, and aural fullness can be found in few patients, thus mimicking other primary inner ear disorders such as Meniere's disease [10].

Other System Involvement:

- Involvement of ribs may cause costoperichondritis, joint pain due to arthritis and chondritis, eye involvement manifests as episcleritis, scleritis, conjunctivitis, uveitis, and cataract [7].
- Neurological—The involvement of the peripheral or central nervous system is relatively rare and only occurs in 3% of persons affected with RP and is sometimes seen in a relation to concomitant vasculitis. The most common neurological manifestation is V and VII cranial nerve palsy. VIII nerve involvement leads to Sensorineural hearing loss. Hemiplegia, ataxia, myelitis, and polyneuropathy may also occur [6, 7].
- Renal involvement manifests as glomerulonephritis or glomerulosclerosis.

- Skin and mucous membranes—20–30% of people with relapsing polychondritis have skin involvement, including aphthous ulcers, genital ulcers, and a number of non-specific skin rashes, including erythema nodosum, livedo reticularis, and erythema multiforme [6].
- Cardiovascular system—Relapsing polychondritis may cause inflammation of the aorta. It can also cause aortic valve regurgitation in 4–10% and mitral valve regurgitation in 2% of patients [4, 6].

32.5 Diagnosis

There are several clinical criteria used to diagnose this disease. McAdam et al. introduced the clinical criteria for RP in 1976. These clinical criteria had later been expanded by Damiani et al. in 1979 and finally Michet et al. modified them in 1986 [2, 11, 12].

Authors	Criteria	Conditions required
McAdam et al.	• Bilateral auricular chondritis • Nasal chondritis • Respiratory tract chondritis • Non-erosive seronegative polyarthritis • Ocular inflammation • Audiovestibular damage	3 out of 6 criteria
Damiani et al.	• Bilateral auricular chondritis (A) • Nasal cartilage inflammation (A) • Respiratory tract chondritis (A) • Non-erosive sero-negative polyarthritis (A) • Ocular inflammation (A) • Audiovestibular involvement (A) • Histologic confirmation (B) • Positive response to corticosteroids or dapsone (C)	3 (A) criteria OR 1 (A) and (B) OR 2 (A) criteria and (C)
Michet et al.	• Auricular cartilage inflammation (A) • Nasal cartilage inflammation (A) • Laryngotracheal cartilage inflammation (A) • Ocular inflammation (B) • Hearing loss (B) • Vestibulary dysfunction (B) • Sero-negative arthritis (B)	2 out of 3 (A) criteria OR 1 out of 3 (A) criteria and 2 (B) criteria

Laboratory Tests and Serology:
Patients presenting with acute episodes often have high levels of inflammatory markers such as erythrocyte sedimentation rate or C-reactive protein. Patients often have cartilage-specific antibodies present during acute relapsing polychondritis episodes. Antinuclear antibody reflexive panel, rheumatoid factor, and antiphospholipid antibodies are tests that may assist in the evaluation and diagnosis of autoimmune connective-tissue diseases [12, 13].

Imaging:
FDG positron emission tomography (PET) may be useful to detect the condition early. Other imaging studies, including MRI, CT scans, and X-rays, may reveal inflammation and/or damaged cartilage facilitating diagnosis [13, 14].

Histopathology:
Biopsy of the cartilage tissue (of the ear or nose) may show chondrolysis, chondritis, and perichondritis [15]. Mixed inflammatory infiltrates (lymphocytes, plasma cells, neutrophils, occasional eosinophils) extending into cartilage with the blurring of the interface between cartilage and adjacent soft tissue are the typical features. Cartilage shows loss of normal basophilia, loss of chondrocytes and destruction of lacunar architecture at advancing edge of inflammation with cartilage replaced by fibrous tissue (Fig. 32.3) [8, 15].

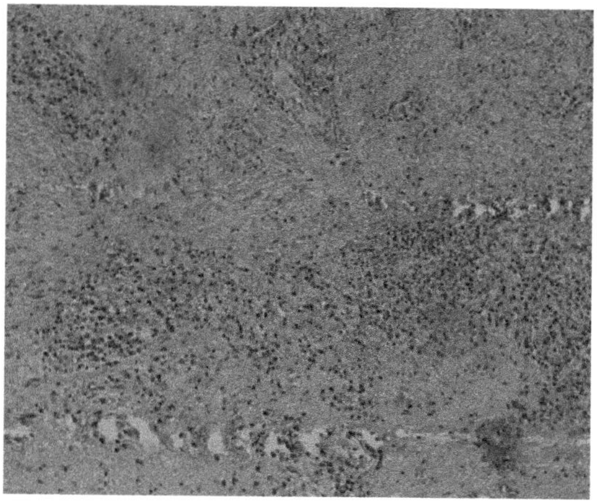

Fig. 32.3 The inflammatory cells infiltrate, including lymphocytes, plasma cells, and histiocytes, infiltrate the degenerative cartilage. H&E, ×100 [8]

Other Tests:

- Pulmonary function tests—It is useful to do a complete set of pulmonary function tests, including inspiratory and expiratory flow-volume loops. Patterns consistent with either extrathoracic or intrathoracic obstruction (or both) may occur in this disease. Pulmonary function tests (flow-volume loops) provide a useful noninvasive means of quantifying and following the degree of extrathoracic airway obstruction in relapsing polychondritis [13, 15].
- Bronchoscopy may confirm mucosal inflammation, airway stenosis, or tracheobronchomalacia, but it has to be performed with caution because of the fragility of the airway wall and risk of perforation. Sometimes, respiratory tract involvement demands reconstruction surgery, which is also associated with serious risk because inflamed tissues may collapse during the operating procedure, and it may be complicated by infection [16].
- In audiovestibular involvement, audiometry and electrocochleography (ECochG) can diagnose the extent of inner ear dysfunction.

32.6 Treatment

Pharmacotherapy:

- Medical treatment of RP depends on disease severity and extension of the disease.
- For patients with nasal, auricular, and articular chondritis but no visceral involvement, non-steroidal anti-inflammatory drugs, colchicine, or dapsone along with Low-dose glucocorticoid (5-25 mg/day) therapy is often required. Dapsone is effective in doses from 25 mg/day to 200 mg/day [4, 17].
- For patients with large airway, ocular, cardiovascular, neurologic, or renal disease, the initial treatment is determined by the assessment of disease severity. For those with relatively mild involvement, oral glucocorticoids can be initially used. In patients with potentially severe manifestations (severe laryngeal or tracheobronchial chondritis, very recent and abrupt onset of sensorineural hearing loss, or systemic vasculitis with poor prognosis factors), methylprednisolone bolus therapy (15 mg/kg/day) combined with an immunosuppressive or immunomodulatory agent can be beneficial as an initial therapy [4, 11, 17].
- Intratympanic corticosteroids injection is found to be effective in sensorineural hearing loss. Doses may be tapered off after the relapse, but most patients require permanent low-dose corticosteroids. Long-term corticosteroids may reduce the frequency and severity of relapses [1].
- Corticosteroid-dependent or resistant diseases and/or life-threatening diseases are an indication for immunosuppressive or immunomodulatory drugs. Their addition is necessary to control the disease activity or to spare corticosteroid dose and adverse events. Among these, colchicine, dapsone, methotrexate, cyclophosphamide, cyclosporine, chlorambucil, azathioprine, mycophenolate mofetil, intravenous immunoglobulin, minocycline, and leflunomide have been shown to be effective [1, 18].

- Emerging treatment options include the use of immunomodulatory agents such as infliximab, etanercept, adalimumab, and abatacept. Tocilizumab has shown utility in patients with disease unresponsive to TNF antagonists. Allogeneic and autologous hematopoietic stem cell transplantation remains a controversial subject but may be of potential utility in refractory cases [19].
- The disease severity at presentation was assessed by using the Relapsing Polychondritis Disease Activity Index (RPDAI). This scoring system takes into account the disease manifestations in a 28 day period [20].

Surgical Management:

- Respiratory tract involvement is associated with poor prognosis in RP patients. Strictures, mucosal edema, and cartilage collapse can lead to fatal airway obstruction, which requires tracheostomy and is a poor prognostic sign. Tracheobronchomalacia may need airway stenting. Thereafter, tracheal dilatation, stenting, or reconstruction surgeries in the case of extensive lesions are sometimes necessary to save the patient. However, the risk of surgical procedures on inflamed and fragile tissue is high. Pneumothorax and pneumomediastinum are adverse events described after stenting [1].
- In the case of sensorineural hearing loss, cochlear implants can restore hearing [1, 18].
- Saddle nose deformity can be corrected by reconstructive surgeries with a bone graft from the iliac crest; autoimmune nature of chondritis contraindicates cartilage grafting due to expected cartilage destruction [1].
- Heart valve replacement surgeries and aortic aneurysm surgery have been proposed to many patients [1].

The life expectancy of patients with RP may be reduced due to its progressive nature, however due to the advent of better therapeutic modalities and early diagnosis, the survival at 8 years may be as high as 94% [21].

32.7 Essential Features

- Relapsing polychondritis, an autoimmune disease, is a relapsing disease with progressive degeneration of cartilage throughout the body with secondary granulomatous manifestations.
- No gender preference, common in 1940s to 1960s, although it affects all ages.
- Ninety percent have perichondritis involving auricular cartilage, usually bilateral, with swelling, erythema, and tenderness. Ear lobes are typically spared due to the absence of cartilage.
- Cause floppy pinna or cauliflower ear deformity.
- Atrophic rhinitis, nasal septal destruction and saddle-node deformity may be seen. Recurrent laryngeal chondritis may lead to stenosis and airway obstruction.
- Michet's clinical criteria for diagnosis requires 2 of 3 of the following—(a) recurrent chondritis of both auricles; (b) chondritis of upper respiratory tract including larynx or tracheal cartilage; And 1 of 4 of the following (a) ocular inflammation (b) Sensorineural hearing loss (c) vestibular dysfunction (d) seronegative arthritis.
- High levels of inflammatory markers such as erythrocyte sedimentation rate or C-reactive protein.
- CT, MRI, and PET scan may reveal inflammation and/or damaged cartilage facilitating diagnosis.
- Histopathology reveals Mixed inflammatory infiltrate (lymphocytes, plasma cells, neutrophils, occasional eosinophils) extending into cartilage with the blurring of the interface between cartilage and adjacent soft tissue.
- Bronchoscopy may confirm mucosal inflammation, airway stenosis, or tracheobronchomalacia.
- Anti-inflammatory drugs, colchicine or dapsone, along with Low-dose glucocorticoid therapy, is preferred for mild disease. Corticosteroids combined with an immunosuppressive or immunomodulatory agent may

reduce the frequency and severity of relapses in severe cases.

- Tracheostomy, tracheal dilatation, airway stenting or reconstruction for airway obstruction Reconstructive surgery rhinoplasty and auroplasty may be required.

References

1. Lekpa FK, Chevalier X. Refractory relapsing polychondritis: challenges and solutions. Open Access Rheumatol. 2018;10:1–11. https://doi.org/10.2147/OARRR.S142892. Published online 2018 Jan 9.
2. Cantarini L, et al. Diagnosis and classification of relapsing polychondritis. Journal of Autoimmunity. 2014;48-49:53–9.
3. Langford CA. Harrison's principles of internal medicine. 19th ed. New York, NY: McGraw-Hill; 2015. p. 389: Relapsing Polychondritis. ISBN 978-0-07-1802161.
4. Chopra R, Chaudhary N, Kay J. Relapsing polychondritis. Rheumat Dis Clinics North Am. 2013;39(2):263–76.
5. Relapsing polychondritis: autoimmune disorders of connective tissue. Merck Manual Home Health Handbook.
6. Puéchal X, et al. Relapsing polychondritis. Joint Bone Spine : Revue du Rhumatisme. 2014;81(2):118–24.
7. Davies HR, Kelsall AR. Atrophic polychondritis with the report of a case. Ann Rheumat Dis. 1961;20(2):189–93.
8. Sosada B, et al. Relapsing polychondritis. Case Rep Dermatological Med. 2014;2014:Article ID 791951, 4 pages. https://doi.org/10.1155/2014/791951.
9. Mohammad A, et al. Relapsing polychondritis: reversible airway obstruction or asthma. Clin Exp Rheumatol. 2008;26:938–40.
10. Ralli M, et al. Audiovestibular symptoms in systemic autoimmune diseases. J Immunol Res. 2018; ID 5798103.
11. Damiani JM, Levine HL. Relapsing polychondritis–report of ten cases. Laryngoscope. 1979;89(6 Pt 1):929–46.
12. Michet CJ Jr, et al. Relapsing polychondritis. Survival and predictive role of early disease manifestations. Ann Intern Med. 1986;104(1):74–8.
13. McAdam LP, et al. Relapsing polychondritis: prospective study of 23 patients and a review of the literature. Medicine. 1976;55(3):193–215.
14. Dubey S, et al. Respiratory subtype of relapsing polychondritis frequently presents as difficult asthma: a descriptive study of respiratory involvement in relapsing polychondritis with 13 patients from a single UK centre. ERJ Open Res. 2021;7(1):00170-2020. https://doi.org/10.1183/23120541.00170-2020. Published online 2021 Feb 15.
15. Stone JH. CURRENT rheumatology diagnosis & treatment. 3rd ed. New York, NY: McGraw-Hill; 2013. Chapter 28, Relapsing Polychondritis.
16. Tillie-Leblond I, et al. Respiratory involvement in relapsing polychondritis. Clinical, functional, endoscopic, and radiographic evaluations. Medicine (Baltimore). 1998;77:168–76.
17. Emmungil H, Zehra ydın S. Relapsing polychondritis. Eur J Rheumatol. 2015;2(4):155–9. https://doi.org/10.5152/eurjrheum.2015.0036. Published online 2015 Dec 1.
18. Chang-Miller A, et al. Renal involvement in relapsing polychondritis. Medicine (Baltimore). 1987;66(3):202–17.
19. Sharma A, et al. Relapsing polychondritis: clinical presentations, disease activity and outcomes. Orphanet J Rare Dis. 2014;9:198. https://doi.org/10.1186/s13023-014-0198-1. Published online 2014 Dec 20.
20. Arnaud L, et al. The Relapsing Polychondritis Disease Activity Index: development of a disease activity score for relapsing polychondritis. Autoimmun Rev. 2012;12:204–9. https://doi.org/10.1016/j.autrev.2012.06.005.
21. Trentham DE, Le CH. Relapsing polychondritis. Ann Intern Med. 1998;129:114–22. https://doi.org/10.7326/0003-4819-129-2-199807150-00011.

Langerhans Cell Histiocytosis (LCH) 33

Abstract

"Langerhans cell histiocytosis" (LCH) describes a spectrum of clinical presentations ranging from a single bone lesion or trivial skin rash to an explosive disseminated disease. The pathogenesis of histiocytosis has been unclear and controversial, with arguments supporting both inflammatory and neoplastic causes. It can be unifocal, multifocal involving a single organ system or disseminated. In multisystem disease, the organs involved in decreasing order of frequency are bone, skin, bone marrow, lymph nodes, liver, spleen, oral mucosa, lung, central nervous system/pituitary, and gastrointestinal tract. Brain involvement can result in a neurodegenerative syndrome and pituitary involvement can present with diabetes insipidus. Sinonasal and nasopharyngeal granulomas are secondary to osseous lesions in the skull base. Oral cavity ulcers and granulomas are secondary to maxillary or mandibular involvement. Imaging continues to play an important role in the diagnosis and treatment monitoring of histiocytosis. Regardless of clinical severity, LCH lesions share the common histology of CD1a dendritic cells with characteristic morphology among an inflammatory infiltrate. The clinical outcome has improved markedly over the past decades through empiric therapeutic strategies. Intralesional steroids or curettage may be sufficient for single-system disease and isolated bone lesions. Multifocal/multisystem disease is treated with systemic chemotherapy (vinblastine, prednisone, mercaptopurine).

Synonyms Histiocytosis X, eosinophilic granuloma, Hand–Schuller–Christian disease, Letterer–Siwe disease [1, 2].

33.1 Background

Langerhans cell histiocytosis (LCH) is a rare disease of the family of histiocytosis characterized by the accumulation of histiocytic cells in various tissues. The first report of the disease was made in 1865, when "Thomas Smith" described the case of a child with impetigo and osseous lesions in the cranium [1]. Since then, several reports of children with a picture of exophthalmia, osseous lesions, and diabetes insipidus have appeared, amongst which those described by "Hand," "Schuller," and "Christian," who named one of the forms of the disease [2]. In 1924, "Letterer" and "Siwe" described a more severe and lethal form of the visceral disease which consisted of cutaneous lesions, hepatosplenomegaly, lymphadenopathy, and pneumonia [1, 2]. In 1953, "Lichtenstein" gathered the several clinical forms under the name histiocytosis X, and later, in

S. V. Nemade, K. J. Shinde, *Granulomatous diseases in Otorhinolaryngology, Head and Neck*,
https://doi.org/10.1007/978-981-16-4047-6_33

1973, "Nezelof" modified it to Langerhans cell histiocytosis [1].

> The manifestations in the head and neck are the most common and their diagnosis becomes difficult once it simulates other more common diseases such as malignant otitis externa, acute mastoiditis, and gingivitis, bone tumors, other sinonasal granulomas [1–3].

33.2 Epidemiology

The incidence of the LCH is estimated as 3–5 cases per million children. There is a slight predominance of the male sex at an overall proportion of 1.5:1. The age range of the disease is mainly pediatric, although in the literature there are reports of the disease in adults [3, 4]. The incidence peak is from 1 to 3 years of age and the patients with focal lesions are generally older (0.1–15.1 years) than those with multisystemic disease (0.09–14.8 years) [5].

33.3 Etiopathogenesis

It is not yet known whether it results from a genetic defect or an abnormal response to the infection, trauma, or autoimmune phenomenon. There has been considerable debate whether LCH represents an inflammatory or a neoplastic disease. The discovery of recurrent mutations in the mitogen-activated protein kinase (MAPK) pathway (i.e., BRAF and MAP2K1 mutations) indicates that it is a neoplastic disease [6, 7]. It is characterized by osteonecrosis and osteolysis. In the soft tissue and organ involvement, it typically shows eosinophilic granuloma formation. Recently, the Histiocyte Society has published a revised classification of histiocytoses in which LCH is sub-classified according to the site of manifestation and organ involvement: single system LCH, lung LCH, and multisystem LCH with or without risk organ involvement (risk organs: liver, spleen, bone marrow) [7, 8].

33.4 Clinical Features

The most frequent is the osseous affection (78% of the patients), more common in the cranial vault, temporal bone followed by the femur, orbit, and spine. Diabetes insipidus is the most frequent endocrinopathy in the LCH, with reports of up to 50% of the cases. There may be maxillomandibular affection leading to gingival ulceration, mucous bleeding, or early dental loss in very young children [2].

Ear–Nose–Throat involvement:
Ear and temporal bone involvement occurs in 14–61% of children with LCH, but only a few cases have been reported in adults [9, 10]. Ear involvement can be in the form of chronic otitis externa or otitis media, external ear canal mass or polyp, postauricular swelling, conductive hearing loss and rarely facial paralysis, and vertigo [11]. External canal polyps with the destruction of posterior canal wall are common presentation. Because the disease is predominant in children, hearing loss is not a much-reported symptom, but when tested it is invariably associated with conductive hearing loss. The inner ear lesions are very rare, as the otic capsule is highly resistant to invasion by granulomatous tissue [12, 13].

Laryngeal involvement is usually associated with multisystem disease. It presents as supraglottic granulomatous mass (Fig. 33.1) [14].

Oral cavity and oropharyngeal involvement are secondary to osseous lesions in the maxilla or mandible with associated mucosal ulceration and granuloma formation.

Sinonasal and nasopharyngeal granulomas have been reported with extensive skull base involvement and intracranial, intraorbital spread [13, 15].

Other system involvement:
The following sites can also be involved, particularly in multisystem disease (in order of decreasing frequency): bone, skin, bone marrow, lymph

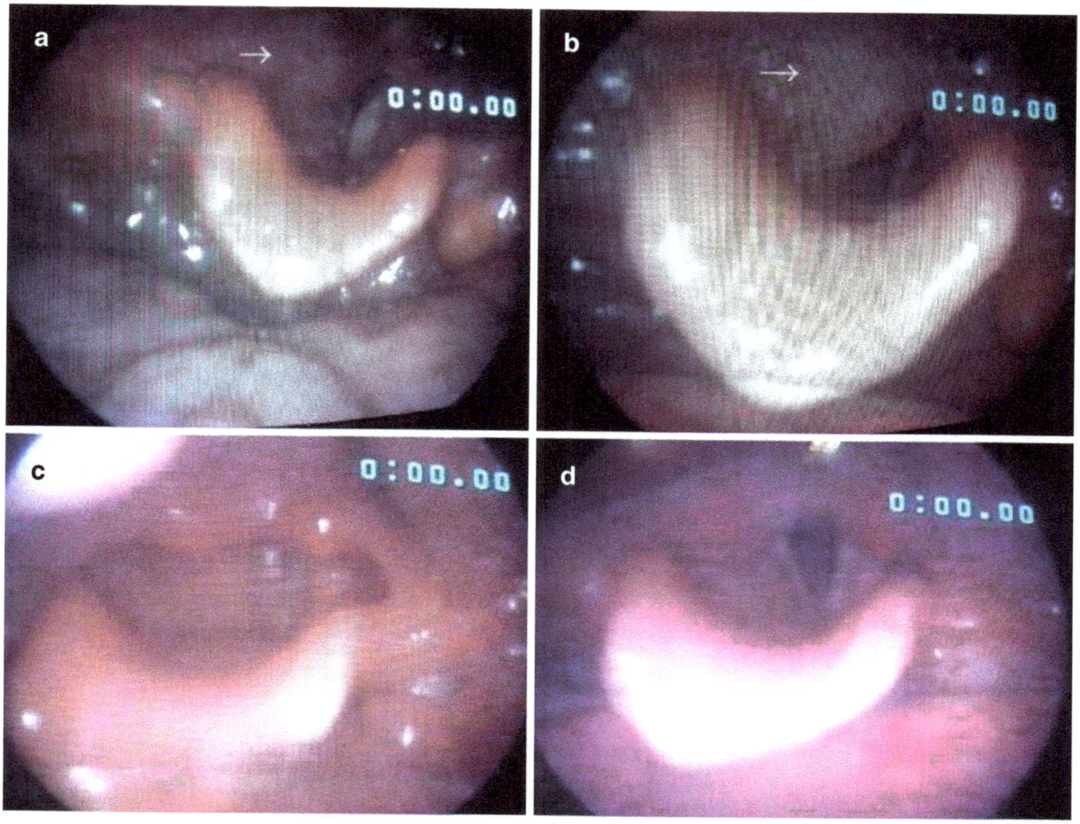

Fig. 33.1 The stroboscopic view of the laryngeal lesion before [upper row: (**a**), (**b**)] and after [lower row: (**c**), (**d**)] radiotherapy [14]

nodes, liver, spleen, lung, central nervous system/pituitary, and gastrointestinal tract [14, 16].

Cutaneous involvement—Cutaneous lesions are verified in up to 50% of the patients and maybe the only sign of the disease or evidence of multisystemic involvement. One of the most common forms is the rash, in addition to the cutaneous infiltrates. Petechias, nodes, or papules is also common. The preferential location is the middle line of the trunk and the flexor areas of the limbs. The scalp has erythematous lesions that may evolve into petechias that ulcerate and form crusts; these are not pruriginous lesions and there may be alopecia.

Pulmonary involvement—It is observed in 20–40% of the patients and manifests clinically with cough, tachypnea, dyspnea, or even pneumothorax. It is strongly associated with smoking [17]. In addition to this, the radiological images show a micronodular or cystic infiltrate. The lung function tests reveal a restrictive pulmonary disease and a reduced pulmonary volume [14].

Gastrointestinal lesions may cause GI bleeding. In the hepatic involvement, the aminotransferases and less commonly, the bilirubins increase. The hematological alterations suggest a lesion in the bone marrow or in the spleen [14, 15].

CNS manifestations of LCH include granulomatous lesions in the extra-axial regions (e.g., pituitary gland and meninges) or in the intra-axial parenchymal regions and neurodegenerative LCH. Pituitary-hypothalamic involvement of LCH is the most common form, reported in 84% of patients with LCH with CNS involvement, and is more frequent in multisystem LCH. Diabetes insipidus can be the first clinical sign of LCH, especially in adult patients [9, 16, 18].

33.5 Diagnosis

Imaging:

Plain radiograph—It is helpful in the early detection of pulmonary lesions. It may show a combination of cysts and nodules with centrilobular distribution and upper and middle lung predominance, classically sparing the costophrenic angle. Initial manifestation with pneumothorax is reported in 15% of patients with LCH, and pneumothorax can be recurrent [15, 19].

CT scan—The typical radiological appearance of LCH is a shining lesion, with sclerotic margins and a beveled edge, with homogeneous soft-tissue masses enhancing uniformly with the administration of intravenous contrast (Fig. 33.2) [15]. High-resolution CT findings are helpful in the diagnosis of LCH. In the early stage of pulmonary LCH, nodules of varying sizes with indistinct margins (1–10 mm), mainly in a peribronchovascular distribution, are visualized. Some nodules may demonstrate cavitation [19].

MRI scan—It is most effective for brain lesions. WB(whole-body)-MRI has excellent lesion detectability, with a sensitivity of 99.0% for overall LCH lesions, and a sensitivity of 98.8% for skeletal LCH lesions. LCH lesions are T1 hypointense to isointense, T2 hyperintense, and T1 contrast enhancing (Fig. 33.3) [20].

Bone scintigraphy can also reveal other lesions, particularly in complex bones.

PET-CT scan—PET-CT is another option for determining the extent of LCH in the initial evaluation and follow-up because it can assess the physiological activity of the LCH lesion [19].

Histopathology:

Tissue diagnosis is the gold standard to confirm the diagnosis. It shows Langerhans' cells associated with granulation tissue and inflammatory

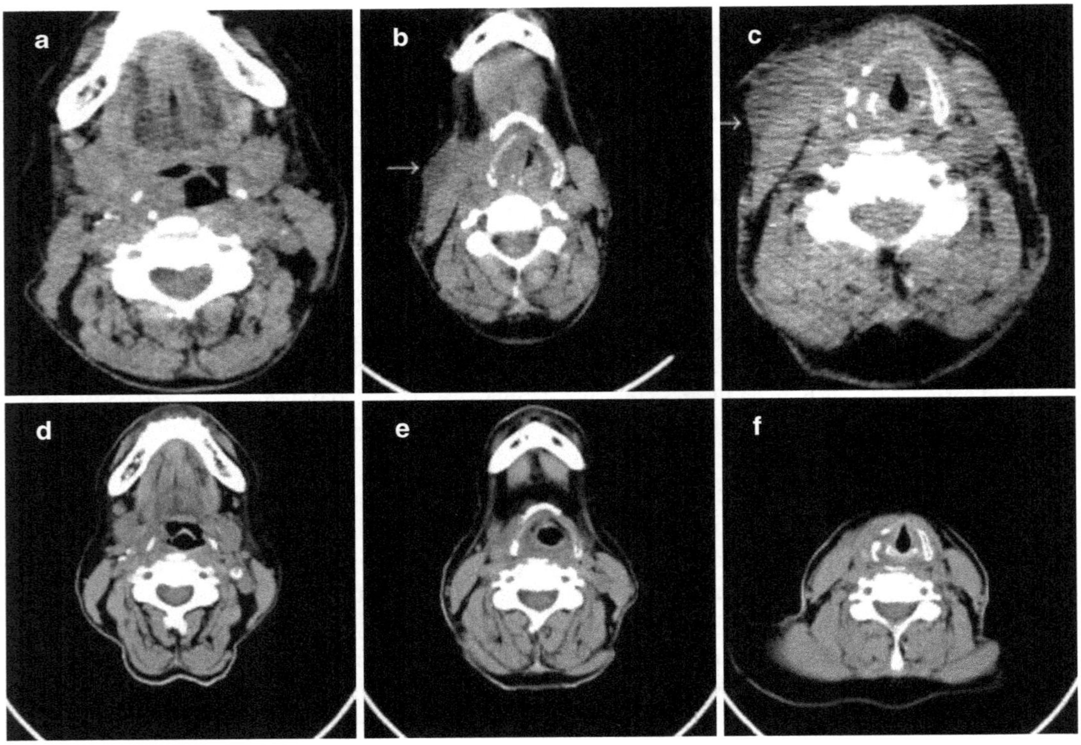

Fig. 33.2 Cervical CT scan of the laryngeal mass before [upper row: (**a**), (**b**), and (**c**)] and after [lower row: (**d**), (**e**), and (**f**)] radiotherapy [14]

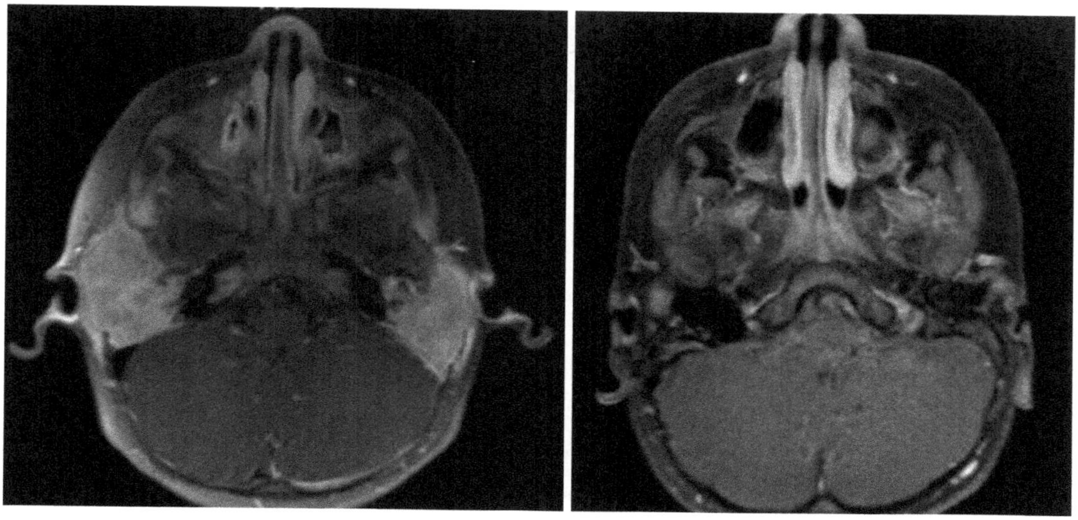

Fig. 33.3 Axial view of post-contrasted T1 MRI images. Left—the image shows the heterogeneous enhancing lesion in the temporal bone area bilaterally. Right—the image shows the decreased enhancement of the temporal bone lesions post-salvage protocol [15]

infiltrate consisting of lymphocytes, plasma cells, giant cells, and abundant eosinophils (Fig. 33.4) [22]. Langerhans cells are the macrophages with characteristic X bodies (Birbeck granules) within. Langerhans' or X bodies are an ultrastructural feature in 90% of patients. They are identical to the granules in Langerhans' epidermal cells and consist of intracytoplasmic rod, plate, or cup-like pentalaminar structures. The presence of these tennis racket-shaped ultrastructural Birbeck granules is diagnostic of the disorder. They have surface adenosine triphosphate activity identifiable by gold fluorescence.

Langerhan's cells are readily found in the nasal secretions, oral secretions, ear discharge, and bronchoalveolar lavage, and this technique may make biopsy unnecessary. However, biopsy still remains the gold standard investigation for this disease [21–23].

Immunohistochemistry:

Langerhans cells show strong positivity by IHC studies for S100 protein, CD1a and CD68 (Fig. 33.5) [23].

Other investigations:

- Complete blood count: cytopenias suggest bone marrow involvement.
- Bone marrow biopsy/aspiration is recommended in patients with cytopenia. Hepatic involvement is associated with raised aminotransferases and less commonly, the bilirubins increase.
- The pulmonary function tests reveal a restrictive pulmonary disease and a reduced pulmonary volume [24, 25].
- Endoscopy to rule out gastrointestinal involvement in patients with evidence of malabsorption.

33.6 Treatment

Treatment of LCH depends on the pattern of the disease. Localized disease may be treated with surgical excision and intralesional steroids [16, 21]

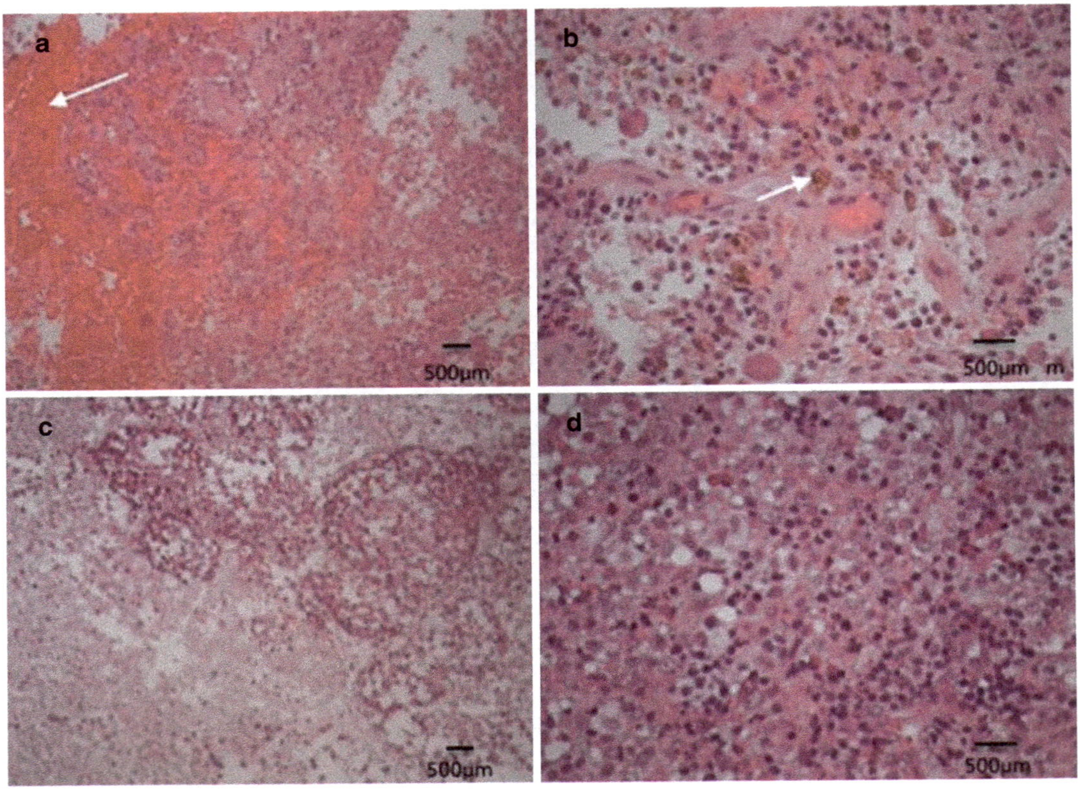

Fig. 33.4 Histopathology image with image (**a**): Dense infiltrate of Langerhans-type histiocytes and eosinophilic cells with many red blood cells (×200) (**b**): A large amount of hemosiderin and macrophages which contained hemosiderin (×400) (**c**): A large amount of necrotic tissue within the tumor cells (×200); (**d**): A large proliferation of Langerhans cells, eosinophils, and neutrophils as well as lymphocytes with scattered plasma cells and blood cells (×400) [21]

- Skin limited LCH: Therapies include topical steroids, nitrogen mustard, or imiquimod; surgical resection of isolated lesions; phototherapy; systemic methotrexate, 6-mercaptopurine, vinblastine/vincristine, thalidomide, cladribine, and/or cytarabine. Commonly used therapy is topical steroids with oral methotrexate (20 mg/m^2 weekly) and 6-mercaptopurine (50 mg/m^2/day), then the dose of immunosuppressant should be adjusted as per the need for myelosuppression. Patients with deep ulcerative LCH lesions who do not respond to oral therapy may require systemic chemotherapy [21, 26, 27].
- Single bone lesions: Isolated bone lesions can be effectively treated with curettage, intralesional corticosteroids, and/or oral chemotherapy [26, 27].
- High risk/disseminated LCH: The current standard of care for patients with high-risk LCH is 1 year of therapy with vinblastine/prednisone/mercaptopurine [27].
- If patients have a refractory or recurrent disease with vinblastine/prednisone, subsequent treatment with cytarabine or clofarabine may be effective [27].
- Radiotherapy for LCH has been reported to have high rates of local control and symptomatic improvement. However, there is evidence of short-term and long-term morbidity when children are treated with low-dose irradiation. Doses used for the treatment of LCH range

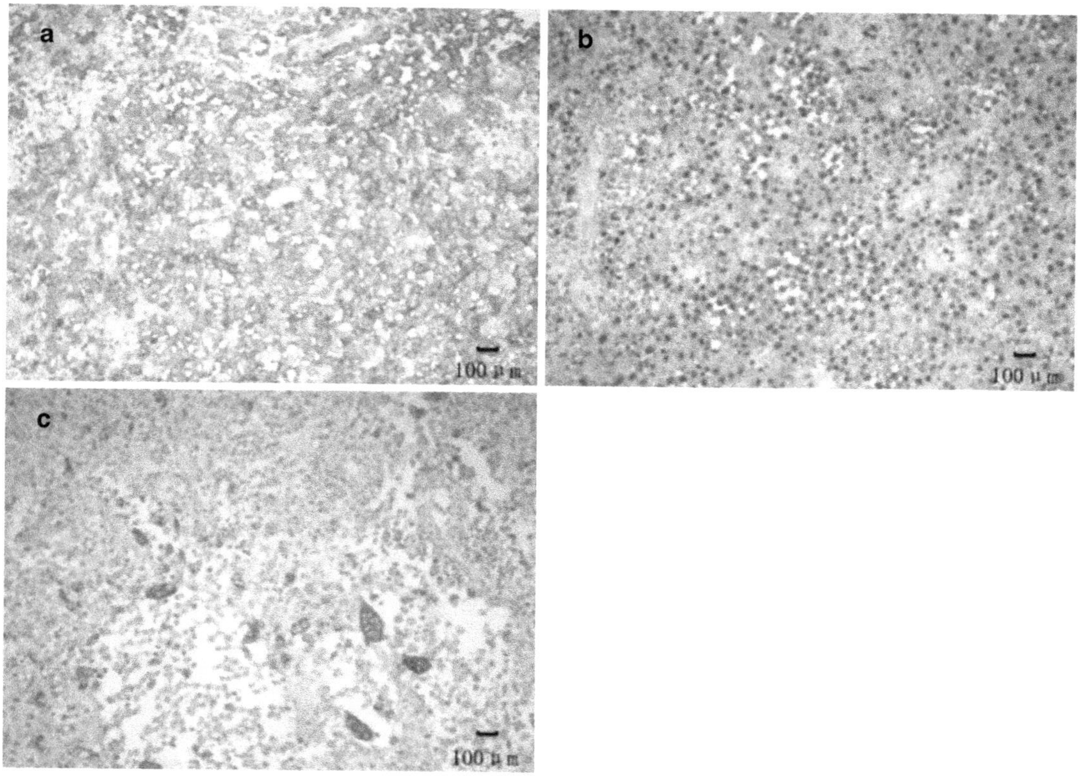

Fig. 33.5 Immunohistochemistry stain: (**a**): CD 1a positive (×200), (**b**): S100 positive (×200), (**c**): CD68 positive (×200)' [21]

from 2.5 to a very high 45 Gy (median, 10 Gy) [28].

- Smoking cessation is advised for pulmonary Langerhans cell histiocytosis. Follow-up is monitored with a PET/CT to be taken 2 and 6 months after the start of the chemotherapy. After six cycles of chemotherapy, the patient clinically shows complete soft tissue healing [21].

33.7 Essential Features

- Langerhans cell histiocytosis is a clonal proliferation of cells that morphologically and immunophenotypically resemble Langerhans cells.
- More common in childhood (1–3 years old) and involves nodal and extranodal sites (most common site is bone)
- Can be unifocal, multifocal but involving a single organ system or involve multiple organs (disseminated).
- The most common sites involved are bone (78% of patients) and adjacent soft tissue; more common in the cranial vault, temporal bone followed by the femur, orbit, and spine.
- External canal polyps with the destruction of the posterior canal wall are common presentations. Manifests with ear discharge, conductive hearing loss, and rarely facial paralysis. The inner ear lesions are very rare and seen secondary to granuloma formation.

- Sinonasal and nasopharyngeal granulomas are secondary to osseous lesions in the skull base. Oral cavity ulcers and granulomas are secondary to maxillary or mandibular involvement.
- The following sites can also be involved, particularly in multisystem disease (in order of decreasing frequency): bone, skin, bone marrow, lymph nodes, liver, spleen, oral mucosa, lung, central nervous system/pituitary, and gastrointestinal tract
- Brain involvement can result in a neurodegenerative syndrome; pituitary involvement can present with diabetes insipidus
- Imaging studies aid the diagnosis
  - Plain Radiograph/CT: solitary or multiple punched-out lytic lesions without sclerotic rim is diagnostic.
  - PET-CT scan
  - MRI: T1 hypointense to isointense, T2 hyperintense lesions. Also helpful in brain lesions.
- Histopathology reveals Langerhans' cells with Birbeck granules within and associated with granulation tissue and inflammatory infiltrate consisting of lymphocytes, plasma cells, giant cells, and abundant eosinophils
- Langerhans cells show strong positivity by Immunohistochemistry with S100 protein, CD1a and CD68.
- Surgical resection with intralesional steroids may be sufficient for single-system disease. Curettage may be sufficient for isolated bone lesions.
- Multifocal/multisystem disease is treated with systemic chemotherapy (vinblastine, prednisone, mercaptopurine)
- Radiotherapy has been reported to have high rates of local control.

References

1. Egeler RM. Historical review – the Langerhans cell histiocytosis X files revealed. Br J Haematol. 2002;116:3–9.
2. DiNardo LJ, Wetmore RF. Head and neck manifestations of histiocytosis-X in children. Laryngoscope. 1989;99:721–4.
3. Minkov M, et al. Langerhans cell histiocytosis in neonates. Pediatr Blood Cancer. 2005;45(6):802–7.
4. Fuertes Cabero S, et al. Usefullnes of bone scintigraphy for staging in a case of histiocytosis of the temporal bone. Rev Esp Med Nucl. 2005;24(1):45–7.
5. Cajade Frías JM, et al. Unifocal eosinophilic granuloma of the temporal bone (Langerhans cell histiocytosis). Acta Otorrinolaringol Esp. 2000;51(6):525–9.
6. Brown NA, et al. High prevalence of somatic MAP2K1 mutations in BRAF V600Enegative Langerhans cell histiocytosis. Blood. 2014;124(10):1655–8.
7. Badalian-Very G, et al. Recurrent BRAF mutations in Langerhans cell histiocytosis. Blood. 2010;116(11):1919–23.
8. Emile JF, et al. Revised classification of histiocytoses and neoplasms of the macrophage-dendritic cell lineages. Blood. 2016;127(22):2672–81.
9. McCaffrey TV, McDonald TJ. Histiocytosis X of the ear and temporal bone: review of 22 cases. Laryngoscope. 1979;89(11):1735–42.
10. Arico M, et al. Langerhans cell histiocytosis in adults: report from the International Registry of the Histiocyte Society. Eur J Cancer. 2003;39(16):2341–8.
11. Whitaker EG, et al. Multifocal Langerhans' cell histiocytosis involving bilateral temporal bones, lungs, and hypothalamus in an adult. Skull Base Surg. 1999;9(1):51–6.
12. Hudson WR, Kenan PD. Otologic manifestations of histiocytosis X. Laryngoscope. 1969;25:678–93.
13. Hashimoto K, et al. Pagetoid self-healing Langerhans cell histiocytosis in an infant. Pediatr Dermatol. 1999;16(2) 121–7.
14. Jahandideh H, et al. Laryngeal Langerhans cell histiocytosis presenting with neck mass in an adult woman. Case Rep Otolaryngol. 2016;2016:2175856. https://doi.org/10.1155/2016/2175856. Published online 2016 Apr 5.
15. Alhaidri NE, et al. Temporal bone Langerhans cell histiocytosis: an uncommon bilateral presentation. Cureus. 2021;13(1):e12732. https://doi.org/10.7759/cureus.12732. Published online 2021 Jan 16.
16. Nelson BL. Langerhans cell histiocytosis of the temporal bone. Head Neck Pathol. 2008;2(2):97–8.
17. Aricò M, et al. Langerhans cell histiocytosis in adults. Report from the International Registry of the Histiocyte Society. Eur J Cancer. 2003;39(16):2341–8. https://doi.org/10.1016/s0959-8049(03)00672-5.
18. Prayer D, et al. MR imaging presentation of intracranial disease associated with Langerhans cell histiocytosis. AJNR Am J Neuroradiol. 2004;25(5):880–91.
19. Obert J, et al. 18F-fluorodeoxyglucose positron emission tomography-computed tomography in the management of adult multisystem Langerhans cell histiocytosis. Eur J Nucl Med Mol Imaging. 2017;44:598–610. https://doi.org/10.1007/s00259-016-3521-3.
20. Kim JR, et al. Comparison of whole-body MRI, bone scan, and radiographic skeletal survey for

lesion detection and risk stratification of Langerhans Cell Histiocytosis. Sci Rep. 2019;9:317. https://doi.org/10.1038/s41598-018-36501-1. Published online 2019 Jan 22.
21. Wu C, et al. MR imaging features of orbital Langerhans cell histiocytosis. BMC Ophthalmol. 2019;19:263. https://doi.org/10.1186/s12886-019-1269-9. Published online 2019 Dec 19.
22. Ha SY, et al. Lung involvement in Langerhans cell histiocytosis: prevalence, clinical features, and outcome. Pediatrics. 1992;89(3):466–9.
23. Marioni G, et al. Langerhans' cell histiocytosis: temporal bone involvement. J Laryngol Otol. 2001;115(10):839–41.
24. Donadieu J, et al. Medical management of Langerhans cell histiocytosis from diagnosis to treatment. Expert Opin Pharmacother. 2012;13(9):1309–22.
25. Saliba I, et al. Langerhans' cell histiocytosis of the temporal bone in children. Int J Pediatric Otorhinolaryngol. 2008;72(6):775–86.
26. Allen CE, et al. Neurodegenerative central nervous system Langerhans cell histiocytosis and coincident hydrocephalus treated with vincristine/cytosine arabinoside. Pediatr Blood Cancer. 2010;54(3):416–23.
27. Simko SJ, et al. Clofarabine salvage therapy in refractory multifocal histiocytic disorders, including Langerhans cell histiocytosis, juvenile xanthogranuloma and Rosai-Dorfman disease. Pediatr Blood Cancer. 2014;61(3):479–87.
28. Kotecha R, et al. Clinical outcomes of radiation therapy in the management of Langerhans cell histiocytosis. Am J Clin Oncol. 2014;37(6):592–6.

Systemic Lupus Erythematosus (SLE) 34

Abstract

Systemic lupus erythematosus (SLE) is a chronic autoimmune disease characterized by the production of autoantibodies and the deposition of immune complexes, affecting a wide range of organs. Genetic factors, environmental factors and hormonal factors are believed to contribute to the occurrence of SLE. However, the pathogenesis of SLE is complex and remains unknown. Though not a granulomatous disease, it may have secondary granulomatous manifestations. Clinically, lupus is a disease with an unpredictable course involving flares and remissions, where cumulative damage over time significantly interferes with the quality of life and adversely affects organ function. It can affect almost any organ system, although it mainly involves the skin, joints, kidneys, blood cells, and nervous system. Its presentation and course are highly variable, ranging from indolent to fulminant. The diagnosis of SLE is based on a combination of clinical findings and laboratory evidence. The American College of Rheumatology (ACR) and the European League Against Rheumatism (EULAR) published new criteria for the classification of SLE in 2019. Management of SLE often depends on the individual patient's disease severity and disease manifestations, although hydroxychloroquine has a central role for long-term treatment in all SLE patients.

Synonyms

Disseminated lupus erythematosus, LE syndrome, Libman-Sacks disease, lupus, SLE [1, 2].

34.1 Background

Systemic lupus erythematosus (SLE) is an autoimmune disorder characterized by antibodies to nuclear and cytoplasmic antigens, multisystem inflammation, protean clinical manifestations, and relapsing and remitting course. Though not a granulomatous disease, it may have secondary granulomatous manifestations. In 1872 Kaposi subdivided lupus into discoid and systemic forms and introduced the concept of systemic disease with a potentially fatal outcome. In 1902, Sequira and Balean published a large series of patients with discoid and systemic LE and provided clinical and pathologic details of a young woman who died of glomerulonephritis [3]. Common symptoms include arthritis, fever, chest pain, hair loss, oral ulcers, lymphadenopathy, fatigue, and a red butterfly rash commonly seen on the face. Often there are periods of illness, called flares, and periods of remission during which there are few symptoms. More than 90% of cases of SLE occur in women, frequently starting at childbearing age [1, 2].

S. V. Nemade, K. J. Shinde, *Granulomatous diseases in Otorhinolaryngology, Head and Neck*,
https://doi.org/10.1007/978-981-16-4047-6_34

34.2 Epidemiology

The female-to-male ratio peaks at 11:1 during the childbearing years. Worldwide, the prevalence of SLE varies. The highest rates of prevalence have been reported in Italy, Spain, Martinique, and the United Kingdom Afro-Caribbean population; overall prevalence rates ranged from 4.3 to 45.3 per 100,000, and the overall incidence ranges from 0.9 to 3.1 per 100,000 per year [2, 4].

34.3 Etiopathogenesis

SLE is an autoimmune disorder characterized by multisystem inflammation with the generation of autoantibodies. Although the specific cause of SLE is unknown, multiple factors are associated with the development of the disease, including genetic, epigenetic, ethnic, immunoregulatory, hormonal, and environmental factors [2, 5–7]. HLA class I, class II, and class III genes are associated with SLE, but only classes I and II contribute independently to increased risk of SLE [8]. SLE tends to run in families, but the inheritance pattern is usually unknown. In rare cases, SLE can be inherited in an autosomal recessive pattern. SLE is regarded as a prototype disease due to the significant overlap in its symptoms with other autoimmune diseases [3].

Pathogenesis of granuloma formation in SLE is still unclear. It was regarded as a response to tissue injury and considered as a manifestation of allergic tissue reaction. Formation of granuloma occurs in response to a persistent stimulus and has also been linked with TNF and induction of host matrix metalloproteinase (MMPs) production in tuberculosis. Animal studies showed proliferative glomerulonephritis was associated with infiltrating kidney macrophages, renal expression of IFN-inducible genes and MMPs, which were mediated IFN. Granuloma formation in SLE may be due to the persistence of apoptotic bodies and/or various cytokines and MMPs. It may also support the role of type IV mediated injury in the pathogenesis of SLE [4, 9, 10].

34.4 Clinical Features

SLE is a chronic inflammatory disease that can affect almost any organ system, although it mainly involves the skin, joints, kidneys, blood cells, and nervous system. Its presentation and course are highly variable, ranging from indolent to fulminant.

Cutaneous manifestations: Cutaneous lesions are reported during the course of SLE in 76% of patients [11]. Malar rash, photosensitivity, discoid lupus are the common presentations.

- Malar rash is characterized by erythema over the cheeks and nasal bridge (but sparing the nasolabial folds (Fig. 34.1), which is in contrast to the rash of dermatomyositis). It lasts from days to weeks and is occasionally painful or pruritic [13, 14].
- Photosensitive rash is often macular or diffusely erythematous in sun-exposed areas of the face, arms, or hands and generally persists for more than 1 day. Discoid rash occurs in 20% of patients with SLE and can result in disfiguring scars [13].
- The discoid rash can present as erythematous patches with keratotic scaling over sun-exposed areas of the skin [13].
- Lupus profundus (LP) is a form of cutaneous lupus erythematosus, which may be a unique manifestation or appear before or after the

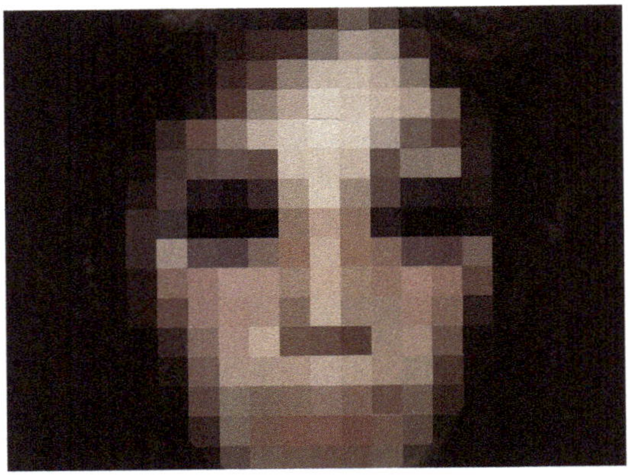

Fig. 34.1 Photograph showing malar rash sparing nasolabial fold [12]

clinical onset of SLE. Lupus profundus consists of deep brawny indurations, or subcutaneous nodules occur under normal or, less often, involved skin; the overlying skin may be erythematous, atrophic, ulcerated, and, on healing, may leave a depressed scar (Fig. 34.2). The most common sites of involvement are proximal extremities, particularly the lateral aspects of the arms and shoulders, face, thighs, buttocks, trunk, breast, and scalp [12].

Ulcers/mucocutaneous involvement: It is associated with mucosal or mucocutaneous ulcers (Fig. 34.3).

Lymphadenopathy: It has been reported in 23–34% of patients with SLE. Despite being frequent manifestation, lymphadenopathy is not included in the ACR criteria for the diagnosis of SLE. Lymphadenopathy has even been reported as the first clinical manifestation of SLE in children. Lymphadenopathy is very common in children due to variety of etiologies and hence may pose a delay in the diagnosis of SLE. Lymph nodes in SLE are usually soft, non tender, mobile, generalized and of varying size [14, 15].

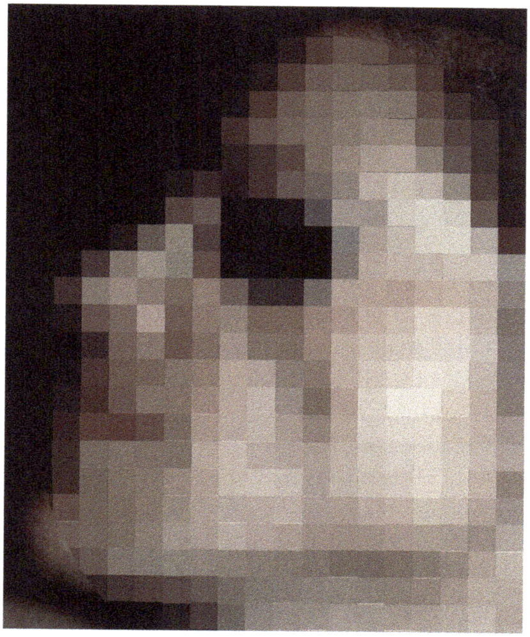

Fig. 34.2 Lupus profundus [12]

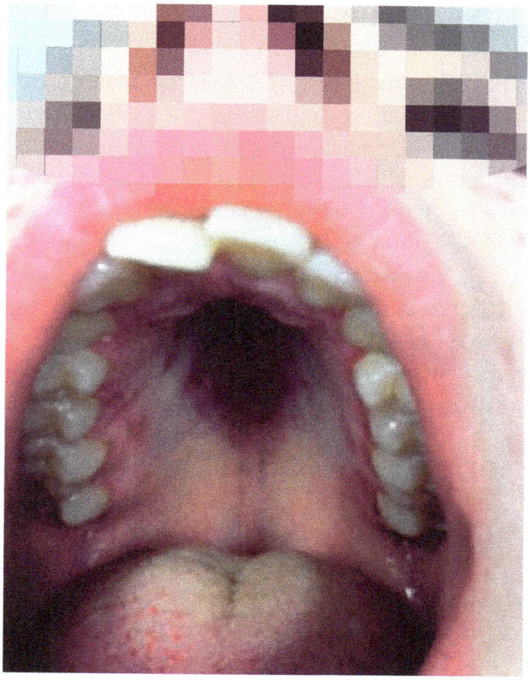

Fig. 34.3 Palatal ulcers in SLE [12]

Other manifestations [16]:

- Constitutional (fatigue, fever, arthralgia, weight changes)
- Musculoskeletal (arthralgia, arthropathy, myalgia, arthritis, avascular necrosis)
- Renal (acute or chronic renal failure, acute nephritic disease)
- Neuropsychiatric (seizure, psychosis)
- Pulmonary (pleurisy, pleural effusion, pneumonitis, pulmonary hypertension, interstitial lung disease)
- Gastrointestinal (nausea, dyspepsia, abdominal pain)
- Cardiac (pericarditis, myocarditis)
- Hematologic (cytopenias such as leukopenia, lymphopenia, anemia, or thrombocytopenia)

In adults, Raynaud pleuritis and sicca are twice as common as in children and adolescents [1].

The classic presentation of a triad of fever, joint pain, and rash in a woman of childbearing age should prompt investigation into the diagnosis of SLE [17, 18].

34.5 Diagnosis

The diagnosis of SLE is based on a combination of clinical findings and investigations. Familiarity with the diagnostic criteria helps clinicians to recognize SLE and to subclassify this complex disease based on the pattern of target-organ manifestations.

The American College of Rheumatology (ACR) established 11 criteria in 1982, which were revised in 1997 [18, 19] a person has SLE if any 4 out of 11 symptoms are present simultaneously or serially on two separate occasions.

1. Malar rash (rash on cheeks); sensitivity = 57%; specificity = 96%.
2. Discoid rash (red, scaly patches on the skin that cause scarring); sensitivity = 18%; specificity = 99%.
3. Serositis: Pleuritis or pericarditis; sensitivity = 56%; specificity = 86% (pleuritis is more sensitive; pericarditis is more specific).
4. Oral ulcers (includes oral or nasopharyngeal ulcers); sensitivity = 27%; specificity = 96%.
5. Arthritis: nonerosive arthritis of two or more peripheral joints, with tenderness, swelling, or effusion; sensitivity = 86%; specificity = 37%.
6. Photosensitivity (exposure to ultraviolet light causes rash or other symptoms of SLE flare-ups); sensitivity = 43%; specificity = 96%.
7. Blood—hematologic disorder—hemolytic anemia (low red blood cell count), leukopenia (white blood cell count <4000/μl), lymphopenia (<1500/μl), or thrombocytopenia (<100,000/μl) in the absence of offending drug; sensitivity = 59%; specificity = 89%. Hypocomplementemia is also seen due to either consumption of C3and C4 by immune complex-induced inflammation or to congenitally complement deficiency, which may predispose to SLE.
8. Renal disorder: More than 0.5 g/day protein in the urine or cellular casts seen in urine under a microscope (proteinuria); sensitivity = 51%; specificity = 94%.
9. Antinuclear antibody test positive; sensitivity = 99%; specificity = 49%.
10. Immunologic disorder: Positive anti-Smith, anti-ds DNA, antiphospholipid antibody, or false-positive serological test for syphilis; sensitivity = 85%; specificity = 93%. Presence of anti-ss DNA in 70% of cases (though also positive with rheumatic disease and healthy persons).
11. Neurologic disorder: Seizures or psychosis; sensitivity = 20%; specificity = 94%.

The American College of Rheumatology (ACR) and the European League Against Rheumatism (EULAR) published new criteria for the classification of SLE in 2019 [7, 12, 13]. These criteria represent current concepts of SLE and have excellent specificity and sensitivity. They replace the 1997 ACR criteria for SLE diagnosis [14].

The ACR/EULAR classification requires an antinuclear antibody (ANA) titer of at least 1:80 on HEp-2 cells or an equivalent positive test at least once. If that is present, 22 "additive weighted" classification criteria are considered, comprising seven clinical domains (constitutional, hematological, neuropsychiatric, mucocutaneous, serosal, musculoskeletal, renal) and three immunologic domains (antiphospholipid antibodies, complement proteins, SLE-specific antibodies) [15, 16]. Each criterion is assigned points ranging from 2 to 10. Patients with at least one clinical criterion and 10 or more points are classified as having SLE [7].

Laboratory studies used in the diagnosis of SLE are as follows [15, 16]:

- CBC with differential count
- Serum creatinine
- Urine analysis with microscopy
- ESR or CRP
- Liver function tests
- Creatine kinase assay
- Spot protein/spot creatinine ratio
- Autoantibody tests: Antinuclear antibody (ANA) testing and anti-extractable nuclear antigen (anti-ENA) form the mainstay of serologic testing for SLE. Clinically the most widely used method is indirect immunofluorescence (IF). The pattern of fluores-

cence suggests the type of antibody present in the serum. Direct immunofluorescence can detect deposits of immunoglobulins and complement proteins in the patient's skin. When skin not exposed to the sun is tested, a positive direct IF (the so-called lupus band test) is evidence of systemic lupus erythematosus [15].

34.5.1 Cytology and Histopathology

FNAC of the cervical lymph node is often suggestive of granulomatous lymphadenopathy showing clusters of epithelioid cells in a lymphoid background. It is better demonstrated with the Wright stain (Fig. 34.4).

More commonly, lymph node biopsies in SLE show reactive follicular hyperplasia, which is considered a nonspecific feature. Atypical lymphoproliferation found in the lymph node biopsies of SLE were classified as reactive follicular hyperplasia with giant follicles, aspects similar to Castleman's disease, atypical paracortical hyperplasia with lymphoid follicles, and atypical immunoblastic and lymphoplasmacytic proliferation. Histopathology with H & E staining usually shows epithelioid granuloma admixed with several eosinophils, lymphocytes, and plasma cells (Fig. 34.5). Lymphoid follicles with prominent germinal center are seen [14, 20].

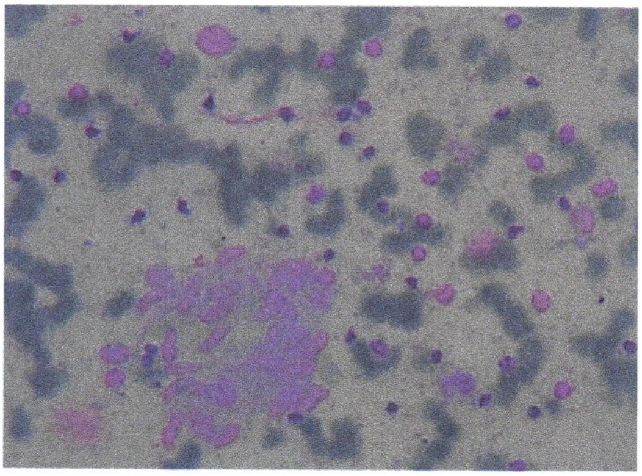

Fig. 34.4 Photomicrograph of FNAC of a cervical lymph node. FNAC smear showing clusters of epithelioid cells in a lymphoid background (Wright stain, ×100) [14]

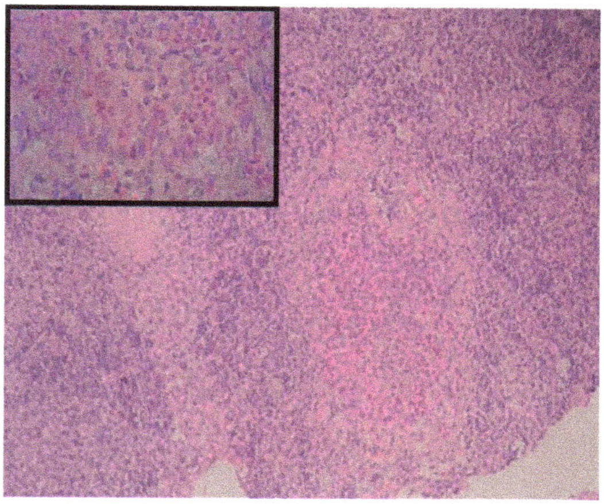

Fig. 34.5 Photomicrograph of a cervical lymph node biopsy. Lymph node biopsy showing epithelioid granuloma admixed with eosinophils, lymphocytes, and plasma cells (H&E stain, ×40). Inset showing epithelioid granuloma in higher magnification (H&E stain, ×400) [14]

34.5.2 Lupus Band Test

The deposition of immunoglobulin and/or complements at the dermoepidermal junction is a histological feature of SLE. Examination of tissue may be done on lesional skin or on nonlesional skin. Nonlesional skin biopsies may be performed on sun-exposed or nonexposed areas. Testing of nonlesional, nonexposed skin is termed the lupus band test. By immunohistology, approximately 70% of patients with various subtypes of SLE show a positive lupus band test when skin biopsies are performed in normal-appearing skin (Fig. 34.6) [12].

34.5.3 Imaging

The following imaging studies may be used to evaluate patients with suspected SLE [15, 21]:

- Ultrasonography of the abdomen to rule out hepatic, splenic granulomas
- Joint radiography
- Chest radiography and chest CT scan
- Echocardiography
- Brain MRI/MRA
- Cardiac MRI

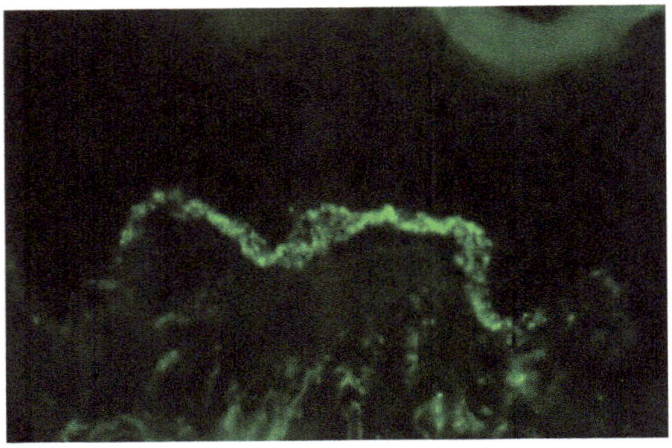

Fig. 34.6 Lupus band test [12]

Procedures that may aid diagnosis in patients with suspected SLE include the following [16, 17]:

- Arthrocentesis
- Lumbar puncture
- Renal biopsy

34.6 Treatment

Medications used to treat SLE manifestations include the following [16, 17, 22]:

- Antimalarials (hydroxychloroquine—HCQ).
- Corticosteroids (methylprednisolone, prednisone)—short-term use is recommended.
- Nonbiologic DMARDS: Cyclophosphamide, Methotrexate, Azathioprine, Mycophenolate, Cyclosporine.
- Nonsteroidal anti-inflammatory drugs (NSAIDS—ibuprofen, naproxen, diclofenac).
- Biologic DMARDs (disease-modifying antirheumatic drugs): Belimumab, Rituximab, and/or IV immune globulin.

34.6.1 First-Line Standard Treatment

(A) Antimalarial Agents

In every patient with SLE, treatment with antimalarials is recommended unless there are contraindications. The action of antimalarials is based on, among other factors, the inhibition of activation of intracellular toll-like receptors. Apart from their good efficacy against arthritis and LE-specific skin lesions, antimalarials maintain SLE in remission. Furthermore, the positive impact of antimalarials on lipid and glucose metabolism has been described, as well as a reduction of thromboembolisms with a favorable influence on cardiovascular risk in SLE, and antineoplastic effects have been reported.

HCQ $\leq$ 6.0–6.5 mg/kg ideal body weight/day OR Chloroquine $\leq$3.5–4.0 mg/kg ideal body weight/day

(Calculation of ideal body weight: Men—[Height minus 100] minus 10% and Women—[Height minus 100] minus 15%)

The optimal efficacy of antimalarials is often not observed before 3–6 months of therapy. LE-specific skin lesions, however, may respond after 4–6 weeks.

Based on the experience of experts, the continuation of hydroxychloroquine treatment during pregnancy is recommended, as SLE patients on hydroxychloroquine show lower disease activity and fewer exacerbations and need lower doses of glucocorticoids at the time of birth. Hydroxychloroquine can also be continued during breastfeeding [22–26].

(B) Topical Treatment

Glucocorticoids are the topical treatment of choice for skin lesions in SLE. Class IV glucocorticoids (clobetasol) can be applied to the scalp, palms, and soles, whereas in other areas, only class II (methylprednisolone aceponate) and class III (mometasone furoate) glucocorticoids are recommended. Due to the adverse effects (atrophy, teleangiectasia, perioral dermatitis), glucocorticoids should be administered only intermittently and not long term, particularly not for butterfly rash [23, 24].

(C) Immunosuppressive Treatment

In patients without organ-threatening manifestations (LE-specific skin lesions, arthritis, pleurisy), long-term treatment with antimalarials is sufficient. Due to the delayed onset of action of antimalarials, most patients temporarily need additional, short-term effective medication, usually non-steroidal anti-inflammatory drugs or glucocorticoids.

Methylprednisolone 500–750 mg i.v. on 3 consecutive days; then glucocorticoids per orally 0.5 mg/kg body weight/day for 4 weeks with subsequent tapering. Maintenance with 5.0–7.5 mg/day prednisone is preferred [25, 26].

Steroid sparing medications are:

- Azathioprine (2–3 mg/kg body weight/day), Methotrexate (15–20 mg/week preferably s.c.), mycophenolate mofetil (2 g/day), Cyclophosphamide—Total dose of 3 g (6 × 500 mg every 2 weeks). Immunosuppresion is usually required for 3 months.
- Methotrexate may have a favorable effect on joint and skin lesions and on general disease activity.
- For patients who respond to initial treatment, the recommended maintenance therapy is lower immunosuppression, with either mycophenolate mofetil/mycophenolic acid or azathioprine for at least 3 years in combination with low-dose prednisone. Thereafter, a gradual reduction of the medication can be attempted, beginning with tapering glucocorticoids [25, 26].

34.6.2 Adjunct Treatment

It is required in patients having autoantibody-positive SLE with high disease activity, intolerance of other treatments for SLE, or an unacceptably high need for glucocorticoids, despite standard treatment [25, 26].

34.6.3 Biologic DMARDs (Disease-Modifying Antirheumatic Drugs)

Belimumeab (10 mg/kg body weight i.v. infusion [over 1 h] initially, then after 14 days and subsequently every 4 weeks) is the preferred drug. The most frequently occurring adverse effects include nausea, diarrhea, and bacterial and viral infections (e.g., bronchitis, cystitis, and pharyngitis), as well as hypersensitivity/infusion reactions. Data on the efficacy of belimumab in routine clinical practice are limited [25].

Prophylactic measures such as ultraviolet (UV) light protection and abstinence from smoking should be explained to the patient [25].

34.7 Essential Features

- Systemic lupus erythematosus (SLE or lupus) is a potentially fatal systemic autoimmune disease that predominantly affects women of childbearing age.
- It is not a granulomatous disease but with secondary granulomatous manifestations.
- SLE is a chronic inflammatory disease that can affect almost any organ system, although it mainly involves the skin, joints, kidneys, blood cells, and nervous system.
- Cutaneous lesions are reported during the course of SLE in 76% of patients. Malar rash, photosensitivity, discoid lupus are the common presentations.
- Lupus profundus consists of deep brawny indurations or subcutaneous granulomatous nodules commonly affecting extremities and the face.
- Lymphadenopathy occurs in 23–34% of patients with SLE.
- Constitutional symptoms include fatigue, fever, arthralgia, and weight changes.
- The classic presentation of a triad of fever, joint pain, and rash in a woman of childbearing age should prompt investigation into the diagnosis of SLE.
- Diagnosis of SLE can be challenging. It is aided by the established diagnostic criteria by the American College of Rheumatology (ACR) and the European League Against Rheumatism (EULAR) in 2019.
- Antinuclear antibody (ANA) testing and anti-extractable nuclear antigen (anti-ENA) form the mainstay of serologic testing for SLE.

- FNAC of the cervical lymph node is often suggestive of granulomatous lymphadenopathy showing clusters of epithelioid cells in a lymphoid background. It is better demonstrated with Wright stain.
- Lupus Band Test demonstrates the deposition of immunoglobulin and/or complements at the dermoepidermal junction.
- The goal of treatment in SLE is to prevent organ damage and achieve remission. The choice of treatment is dictated by the organ system/systems involved and the severity of involvement and ranges from minimal treatment (NSAIDs, antimalarials) to intensive treatment (cytotoxic drugs, corticosteroids).
- Patient education, physical and lifestyle measures and emotional support play a central role in the management of SLE.

References

1. Costa-Reis P, Sullivan KE. Genetics and epigenetics of systemic lupus erythematosus. Curr Rheumatol Rep. 2013;15(9):369.
2. D'Cruz DP, et al. Systemic lupus erythematosus. Lancet. 2007;369(9561):587–96.
3. Smith CD, Cyr M. The history of lupus erythematosus. From Hippocrates to Osler. Rheum Dis Clin North Am. 1988;14(1):1–14.
4. Ramakrishnan L. Revisiting the role of the granuloma in tuberculosis. Nat Rev Immunol. 2012;12(5):352–66.
5. Livingston B, et al. Differences in clinical manifestations between childhood-onset lupus and adult-onset lupus: a meta-analysis. Lupus. 2011;20(13):1345–55.
6. Rahman A, David A. Isenberg "Review Article: Systemic Lupus Erythematosus". N Engl J Med. 2008;358(9):929–39.
7. Aringer M, et al. European League Against Rheumatism/American College of Rheumatology classification criteria for systemic lupus erythematosus. Ann Rheum Dis. 2019;78(9):1151–9.
8. Martens HA, et al. An extensive screen of the HLA region reveals an independent association of HLA class I and class II with susceptibility for systemic lupus erythematosus. Scand J Rheumatol. 2009;38(4):256–62.
9. Teilum G. Miliary epithelloid-cell granulomas in lupus erythematosus disseminatus. Acta Pathol Microbiol Scand. 1945;22(1):73–9.
10. Triantafyllopoulou A, et al. Proliferative lesions and metalloproteinase activity in murine lupus nephritis mediated by type I interferons and macrophages. Proc Natl Acad Sci U S A. 2010;107(7):3012–7. https://doi.org/10.1073/pnas.0914902107.
11. Duan L, et al. Treatment of bullous systemic lupus erythematosus. J Immunol Res. 2015;2015:Article ID 167064, 6 pages. https://doi.org/10.1155/2015/167064.
12. Uva L, et al. Cutaneous manifestations of systemic lupus erythematosus. Autoimmune Dis. 2012;2012:Article ID 834291, 15 pages. https://doi.org/10.1155/2012/834291.
13. Firestein GS, et al. Kelley's textbook of rheumatology. 8th ed. Philadelphia, PA: Saunders Elsevier; 2008.
14. Shrestha D, et al. Systemic lupus erythematosus and granulomatous lymphadenopathy. BMC Pediatr. 2013;13:179. https://doi.org/10.1186/1471-2431-13-179. Published online 2013 Nov 5.
15. Neto NS, et al. Lymphadenopathy and systemic lupus erythematosus. Bras J Rheumatol. 2010;50(1):96–101.
16. Lisnevskaia L, et al. Systemic lupus erythematosus. Lancet. 2014;384(9957):1878–88.
17. Davis LS, Reimold AM. Research and therapeutics—traditional and emerging therapies in systemic lupus erythematosus. Rheumatology. 2017;56(Suppl 1):i100–13.
18. Murphy G, Isenberg D. Effect of gender on clinical presentation in systemic lupus erythematosus. Rheumatology (Oxford, England). 2013;52(12):2108–15.
19. Tiffin N, et al. A diverse array of genetic factors contribute to the pathogenesis of systemic lupus erythematosus. Orphanet J Rare Dis. 2013;8:2.
20. Weinstein A, et al. Antibodies to native DNA and serum complement (C3) levels. Application to diagnosis and classification of systemic lupus erythematosus. Am J Med. 1983;74(2):206–16.
21. Rahman A, Isenberg DA. Systemic lupus erythematosus. N Engl J Med. 2008;358(9):929–39.
22. Ruiz-Irastorza G, et al. Systemic lupus erythematosus. Lancet. 2001;357(9261):1027–32.
23. Revision of Rheumatology.org's diagnostic criteria. Rheumatology.org. 2011-06-08.
24. Edworthy SM, et al. Analysis of the 1982 ARA lupus criteria data set by recursive partitioning methodology: new insights into the relative merit of individual criteria. J Rheumatol. 1988;15(10):1493–8.
25. Kuhn A, et al. The diagnosis and treatment of systemic lupus erythematosus. Dtsch Arztebl Int. 2015;112(25):423–32. https://doi.org/10.3238/arztebl.2015.0423. Published online 2015 Jun 19.
26. Bertsias G, et al. EULAR recommendations for the management of systemic lupus erythematosus. Report of a Task Force of the EULAR Standing Committee for International Clinical Studies Including Therapeutics. Ann Rheum Dis. 2008;67:195–205.

Rheumatoid Arthritis

35

Abstract

Rheumatoid arthritis (RA), which is a common autoimmune disorder that is characterized by systemic inflammatory polyarthritis, affects approximately 1% of the global population. It is characterized by the formation of both articular and extra-articular lesions with a predilection for small joints. It causes varied head and neck manifestations with emphasis on the larynx. Laryngeal findings range from cricoarytenoid joint fixation and neuropathy of the recurrent laryngeal nerve, to myositis and the presence of laryngeal nodules. Temporomandibular joint involvement is clinically observed in 50–60% of patients with RA. Rheumatoid nodules are common extra-articular findings occurring in 20% of rheumatoid arthritis patients. They develop most commonly subcutaneously in pressure areas (elbows and finger joints) and may occasionally affect internal organs including pleura, lungs, meninges, larynx, and in other connective tissues elsewhere in the body. Common symptoms are malaise, fatigue, musculoskeletal pain, then joint involvement; joints are warm, swollen, painful, stiff in the morning. Diagnosis is based on criteria proposed by the American College of Rheumatology, imaging and histopathology of rheumatoid nodules. Pharmacotherapy, physiotherapy, occupational therapy, counselling, and surgery form the mainstay of treatment. The medical treatment consists of administering steroids, non-steroid anti-inflammatory drugs (NSAID), Disease-modifying antirheumatic drugs (DMARDs), and Tumor necrosis factor-alpha inhibitors (TNF-alpha inhibitors).

35.1 Background

Rheumatoid arthritis (RA) is a destructive autoimmune disease involving small joints usually of the hands and feet first and then all over the body. It is a chronic disease with remissions and exacerbations and often leads to disability. It is characterized by the formation of both articular and extra-articular lesions with a predilection for small joints. The otolaryngologic features of RA are protean and ill-defined, with joint involvement being the most significant. These include the temporomandibular joint, the cricoarytenoid joint, cricothyroid joint, middle ear ossicular joints, and cervical spine. Small bones of the hand are affected first (MCP, PIP joints of hands and feet), then wrist, elbow, knee.

The first recognized description of R was made in 1800 by "Dr. Augustin Jacob Landre-Beauvais" (1772–1840) of Paris. The name "rheumatoid arthritis" itself was coined in 1859 by British rheumatologist "Dr. lfred Baring

S. V. Nemade, K. J. Shinde, *Granulomatous diseases in Otorhinolaryngology, Head and Neck*,
https://doi.org/10.1007/978-981-16-4047-6_35

Garrod." The term rheumatoid arthritis is based on the Greek word meant for watery and inflamed joints [1, 2].

35.2 Epidemiology

Rheumatoid arthritis is a common autoimmune disease that affects 3% of the adult population and up to 35 per 100,000 of the pediatric population. Onset is most frequent during middle age, peaks at ages 10–29 years, and in the menopausal age. Women are affected 2.5 times as frequently as men [1, 3].

35.3 Etiopathogenesis

RA primarily starts as a state of persistent cellular activation leading to autoimmunity and immune complexes in joints and other organs where it manifests. The initial site of disease is the synovial membrane, where swelling and congestion lead to infiltration by immune cells. Three phases of progression of RA are an initiation phase (due to non-specific inflammation), an amplification phase (due to T cell activation), and chronic inflammatory phase, with tissue injury resulting from the cytokines, IL-1, TNF-alpha, and IL-6 [4].

First stage: Inflammation initiates. In this stage autoantibodies to IgGFc, known as rheumatoid factors and ACPA (Anti-citrullinated protein antibody) help in the diagnosis of RA, with ACPA having an 80% specificity [5].

Second stage: Once the generalized abnormal immune response has become established—which may take several years before any symptoms occur—plasma cells derived from B lymphocytes produce rheumatoid factors and ACPA of the IgG and IgM classes in large quantities. These activate macrophages through Fc receptor and complement binding, which is part of the intense inflammation in RA [6]. This contributes to local inflammation in a joint, specifically the synovium with edema, vasodilation, and entry of activated T cells, mainly CD4 in microscopically nodular aggregates and CD8 in microscopically diffuse infiltrates. Synovial macrophages and dendritic cells function as antigen-presenting cells by expressing MHC class II molecules, which establishes the immune reaction in the tissue [7].

Third stage: The disease progresses by forming granulation tissue at the edges of the synovial lining, pannus with extensive angiogenesis and enzymes causing tissue damage. The synovium thickens, cartilage and underlying bone disintegrate, and the joint deteriorates, with raised calprotectin levels serving as a biomarker of these events [8]. Cytokines and chemokines attract and accumulate immune cells, i.e., activated T and B cells, monocytes and macrophages from activated fibroblasts, in the joint space. By signaling through RANKL and RANK, they eventually trigger osteoclast production, which degrades bone tissue [8]. Viral infections such as rubella, human parvovirus B19 (B19), cytomegalovirus (CMV), human T cell leukemia virus 1, and HIV often cause an acute onset of polyarthritis and are considered to be important in the pathogenesis of RA. The presence of B19 DNA has been demonstrated in RA. Although the expression of B19 protein or its isolation from the affected organ is critical to know the role of the virus in vivo, these have remained unelucidated [9].

35.4 Clinical Features

Symptoms of RA include:

- pain, swelling, and stiffness in more than one joint
- symmetrical joint involvement
- joint deformity
- unsteadiness while walking
- malaise
- fever
- loss of function and mobility
- weight loss

Laryngeal involvement:

This is the most common ENT manifestation of RA. Laryngeal findings range from cricoarytenoid joint fixation and neuropathy of the recurrent laryngeal nerve, to myositis and the presence of laryngeal nodules [8, 10].

In the acute phase, patients may complain of burning, foreign body sensation in the throat, and difficulty in swallowing. In chronic cases, the cricoarytenoid joint (CAJ) is usually affected with resultant fixation, and severe distress may warrant emergency tracheotomy. In cases of minimal involvement of the joint, the mobility of the vocal cord may not be impaired and hence both phonation and breathing are unaffected. When the inflammation is moderate and one joint is involved, patients may have persistent respiratory discomfort, shortness of breath, and a decrease in exercise tolerance. In cases of bilateral involvement of the joints, the clinical presentation will depend on the position of the vocal cords. If both vocal cords are immobile and cannot assume the phonatory position, that is, near-total adduction, patients will present with stridor, vocal fatigue, inability to sustain phonation, and at times aphonia [4, 10]. The laryngoscopic findings include mucosal edema, myositis of the intrinsic laryngeal muscles, hyperemia, inflammation and swelling of the arytenoids (Fig. 35.1), interarytenoid mucosa, aryepiglottic folds and epiglottis, and impaired mobility or fixation of the cricoarytenoid joint. Other laryngoscopic findings include the presence of inflammatory masses or rheumatoid nodules (Bamboo nodes) in the larynx and pharynx. In 1987, the American Rheumatism Association has included submucosal nodules in the laryngeal tissue in the revised criteria for the classification of rheumatoid arthritis. The nodules can present as submucosal and/or subcutaneous masses in patients with autoimmune diseases [8, 10, 11].

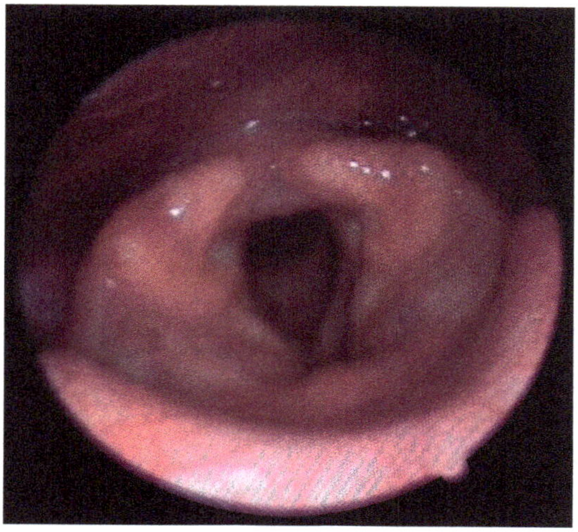

Fig. 35.1 Nasopharyngeal fiberoptic endoscopic view of the larynx showing edema and deformity of both arytenoid cartilages during deep inspiration in a 37-year-old man with advanced rheumatoid arthritis [11]

Bamboo nodes were initially described by Hosako et al. in a female patient with lupus erythematosus. Endoscopic visualization shows transversally arranged cystic yellowish bamboo nodes in the submucosal space of the middle portion of the vocal folds. Similar to other laryngeal lesions in patients with RA, these nodes are more often seen in patients with an active disease rather than inactive and correlates with antibody deposits. These lesions are seen more commonly in females with a history of phonotraumatic behavior and gastroesophageal reflux disease. In selected patients with autoimmune diseases, these laryngeal lesions have been reported in almost 80–100% of the cases [8, 10].

Four causes of vocal cord immobility in RA:

1. Fixation of cricoarytenoid joint.
2. Presence of rheumatoid nodule in either the vocalis muscle and/or near the CAJ hindering its mobility.
3. Abductor muscle paralysis: Severe demyelination and degeneration of the recurrent laryngeal and vagus nerves together with atrophy of the laryngeal muscles with or without obliterative arteritis of the vasa vasorum.
4. Cervicomedullary compression due to rheumatoid involvement of the cervical spine [8, 10].

   Another laryngeal manifestation of RA is cricothyroid joint arthritis. In cases of involvement of the cricothyroid joint, patients will complain of limited vocal range.

Ear involvement:

Sensory-neural hearing loss (SNHL) is a common finding in patients with RA involving the cochlea. Rarely RA may involve incudomalleolar joint leading to impaired ossicular mobility and conductive hearing loss [12, 13].

Temporomandibular joint involvement:
Temporomandibular joint (TMJ) involvement in rheumatoid arthritis (RA) is not uncommon. Temporomandibular joint involvement is clinically observed in 50–60% of patients with RA (Fig. 35.2). The most frequent physical examination finding, a "click" in the joint upon opening of the mouth, is found in almost 50% of the patients. The most frequently observed radiological finding is synovial proliferation [15].

RA commonly involves interphalangeal joints leading to deformities such as ulnar deviation of fingers, hyperextension, or hyperflexion of joints (Figs. 35.3 and 35.4).

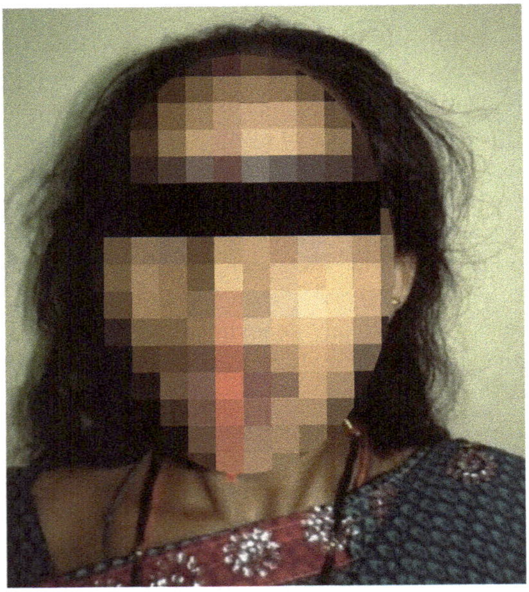

Fig. 35.2 Photograph showing deviation of mandible toward right side [14]

Rheumatoid nodules:
Rheumatoid nodules are common extra-articular findings occurring in 20% of rheumatoid arthritis patients. They develop most commonly subcutaneously in pressure areas (elbows and finger joints) and may lead to deformity. It occasionally affects internal organs including the pleura, lungs, meninges, larynx, and in other connective tissues elsewhere in the body [16, 17].

35.5 Diagnosis

Diagnostic criteria:
In 2010, the American College of Rheumatology recommended the following criteria for diagnosing RA:

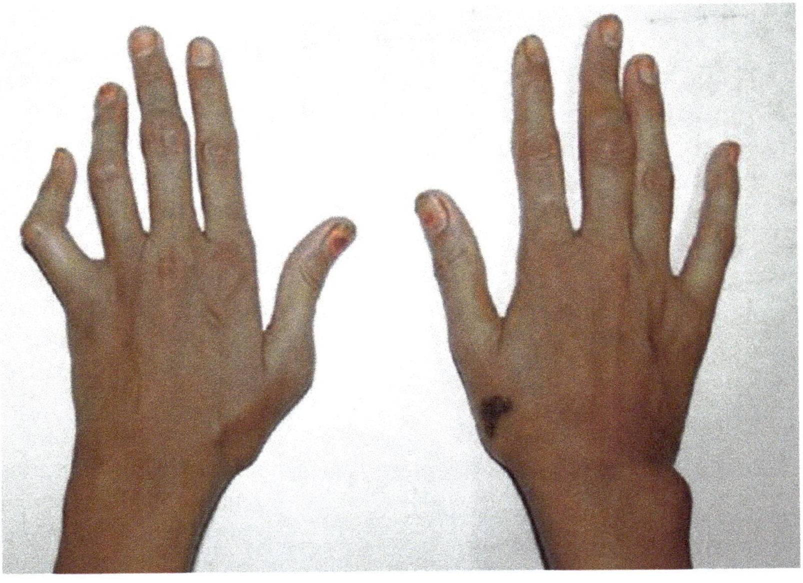

Fig. 35.3 Showing minor joint deformity with a stiffness of the interphalangeal joints of the hand [14]

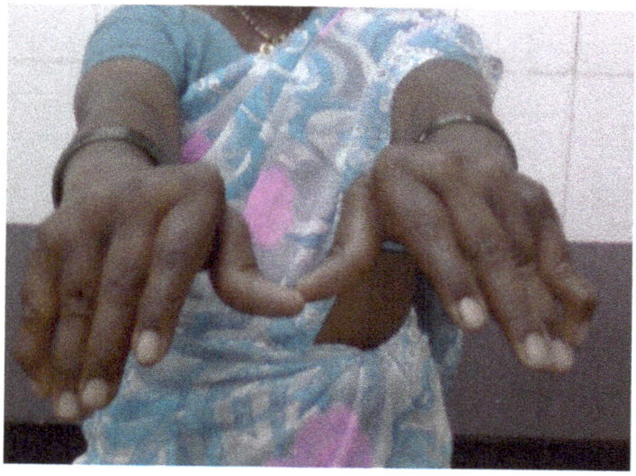

Fig. 35.4 Rheumatoid arthritis involving interphalangeal joints of the hand causing deformity

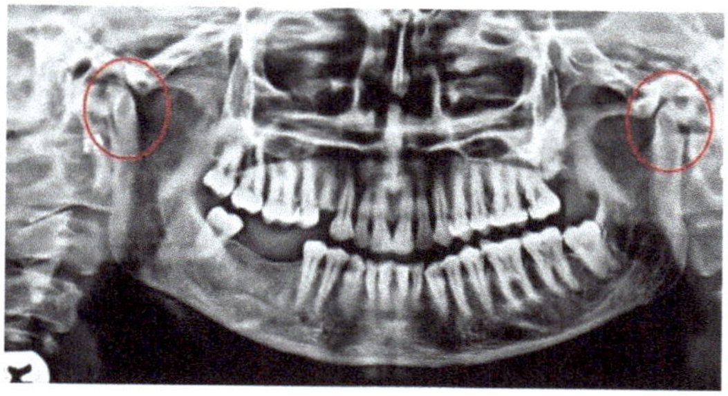

Fig. 35.5 Panoramic view showing irregular erosion on right and left side of condyle with flattening of articular eminence [14]

- Swelling is present in at least one joint, and it does not have another cause.
- At least one blood test indicates the presence of RA.
- Symptoms have been present for at least 6 weeks [13, 18, 19].

Electromyography is a useful test to differentiate between CAJ fixation and paralysis secondary to recurrent laryngeal nerve injury [11, 20].

Imaging:
Radiography, CT, or MRI of a joint can help to identify what type of arthritis is present and monitor the progress of RA over time. CT and MRI are particularly helpful in delineating rheumatoid nodules.

- Radiography: joint effusions, juxta-articular osteopenia, erosions, and narrowing of joint space (Figs. 35.5 and 35.6); destruction of tendons, ligaments, and joint capsules are the common findings. X-rays of the hands and feet are generally performed when many joints are affected. In RA, there may be no changes in the early stages of the disease or the x-ray may show juxta-articular osteopenia near the joint, soft tissue swelling, reduced joint space. As the disease advances, there may be bony erosions and subluxation. X-ray of the hand may reveal radial deviation of the wrist, ulnar deviation of digits, or swan-neck finger abnormalities.
- High-resolution computerized tomography of neck is also helpful for the early detection of CAJ arthritis. The most common findings are increased density of the joint, narrowing of the joint space, ankylosis, and vocal fold thickening. It also better delineates the rheumatoid nodules in the oropharynx, hypopharynx, and larynx (Fig. 35.7) [13, 18, 19].

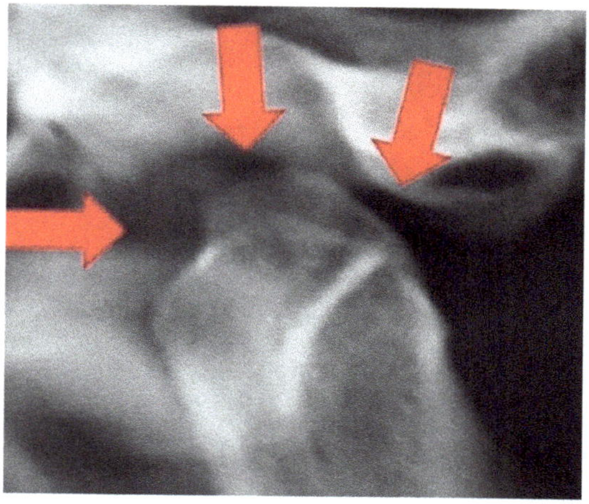

Fig. 35.6 Magnified view of TM joint showing presence of scooped out area of erosion in posterosuperior aspect of the head of condyle giving the appearance of a mouthpiece of flute [14]

Histopathology:
Histopathologically, laryngeal lesions and nodules carry similarities with rheumatoid nodules present elsewhere in the body. The nodule carries areas of fibrinoid necrosis surrounded by palisading epithelioid macrophages, vascular granulation tissue, lymphocytes, plasma cells, eosinophils, and occasional giant cells.

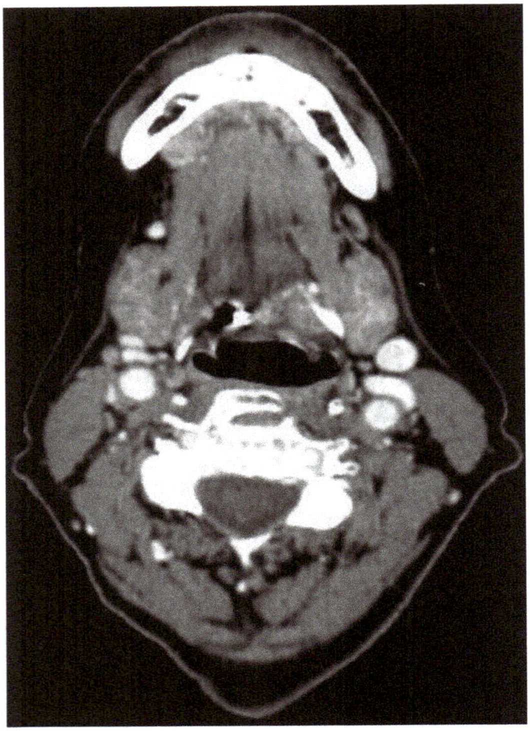

Fig. 35.7 Post-contrast axial CT. Post-contrast axial CT scan demonstrating a heterogeneous, well-circumscribed lesion (rheumatoid nodule) in the left pre-epiglottic space abutting the posterior surface of the hyoid bone at the junction of the body and the cornua [16]

Dense perivascular inflammatory infiltrates of T lymphocytes, plasma cells (often with eosinophilic cytoplasmic inclusions called Russell bodies), macrophages are evident (Fig. 35.8). The inflammation extends to subchondral bone [16].

Blood tests:

- Erythrocyte sedimentation rate (ESR) and C-reactive protein (CRP)—Elevated levels are not specific for RA but are useful tests for other inflammatory conditions or infections [13, 18].
- Anemia—Many people with RA also have coexistent anemia.[18].
- Rheumatoid factor—If an antibody known as a rheumatoid factor is present in the blood, it can indicate that RA is present. However, not everyone with RA is positive for this factor [19].

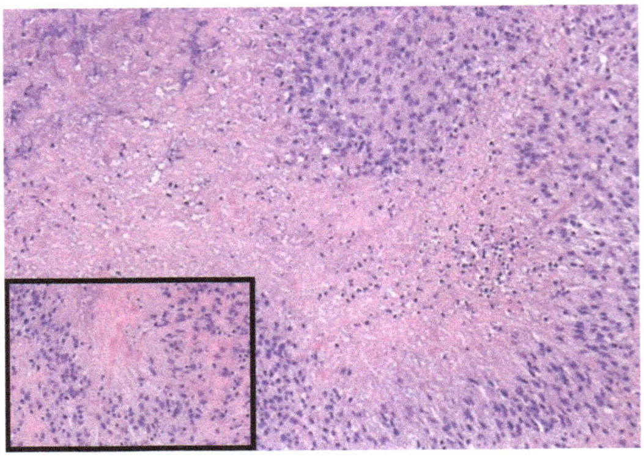

Fig. 35.8 The lesion composed of multiple irregular, fairly demarcated nodules with central eosinophilic necrosis (×20) lined by thick peripheral layer of palisading mononuclear cells (inset ×40) characteristic of rheumatoid nodules [16]

Serology:

- Serum Anti-citrullinated protein antibodies (ACPAs measured as anti-CCP antibodies)—It is positive in 75–85%, but a negative CCP antibody does not rule out RA, rather, the arthritis is called seronegative, which is in about 15–25% of people with RA [12, 19].
- 80% have IgM autoantibodies to Fc portion of IgG (rheumatoid factor), which is not sensitive or specific [12, 13, 18, 19].
- Other antibodies include antikeratin antibody (specific, not sensitive), antiperinuclear factor, anti-rheumatoid arthritis-associated nuclear antigen (RANA) [18, 19].

Molecular assay:

A validated real-time quantitative PCR (Q-PCR) Q-PCR is a flexible, sensitive, and extract-based method for measuring gene expression in the target tissue. The use of a cellular standard generated with activated PBMC cDNA significantly improves assay reliability by reducing variation and by simplifying assay development.

35.6 Treatment

Pharmaecotherapy, physiotherapy, occupational therapy, counseling, and surgery form the mainstay of treatment.

The medical treatment consists of administering steroids or nonsteroid anti-inflammatory drugs to avoid the formation of nodules and fibrosis. Steroids are given systemically or intraarticular in the joint [18, 20].

Disease-modifying antirheumatic drugs (DMARDs):
DMARDs can slow the progression of the RA and prevent permanent damage to the joints and other tissues by interfering with the overactive immune system. This is usually a life-long treatment. It is most effective if the patient uses it in the early stages, but it can take from 4 to 6 months to fully experience the benefits. Some people may have to try different types of DMARD before finding the most suitable one.

Examples include [20]:
- Leflunomide—100 mg once a day for 3 days is the loading dose, followed by a maintenance dose of 10–20 mg/day.
- Methotrexate—7.5–10 mg/week. May be increased to 20–25 mg/week as per the severity of the disease.
- Sulfasalazine—0.5–1 g/day to be increased weekly to a maintenance dose of 2–3 g/day.
- Minocycline—100 mg 12 hourly.
- Hydroxychloroquine—400–600 mg as a single dose followed by a maintenance dose of 200–400 mg/day.

Side effects can include hepato-toxicity and immune-related problems, such as bone marrow suppression, and a higher risk of severe lung infections. Other types of immunosuppressants include Cyclosporine, Azathioprine, and Cyclophosphamide [19, 20].

Tumor necrosis factor-alpha inhibitors (TNF-alpha inhibitors):
The human body produces tumor necrosis factor-alpha (TNF-alpha), an inflammatory substance. TNF-alpha inhibitors prevent inflammation. It can reduce pain, morning stiffness, and swollen or tender joints. People usually notice an improvement 2 weeks after starting treatment [13, 18–20]. Examples include Infliximab and Adalimumab.

Possible side effects include:
- a higher risk of infection
- blood disorders
- congestive heart failure
- demyelinating diseases, involving an erosion of the myelin sheath.
- lymphoma

Occupational therapy:
An occupational therapist can help the patients to learn new and effective ways of carrying out daily tasks. This can minimize stress to painful joints. For example, a person with painful fingers might learn to use a specially devised gripping and grabbing tool [20].

Surgical management: Surgery is indicated to repair damaged joints, to correct deformities or to reduce pain.

Surgical procedures:
- Arthroplasty
- Tendon repair: If tendons have loosened or ruptured around the joint, surgery may help restore them.
- Synovectomy: This procedure involves the removal of the synovium if it is inflamed and causing pain.
- Arthrodesis: The surgeon will fuse a bone or joint to decrease pain and realign or stabilize the joint.
- With respect to the Bamboo nodes, these lesions may be treated either surgically or conservatively. In cases of unilateral fixation, medialization using either injection laryngoplasty or laryngeal framework surgery is recommended. When both vocal folds are fixed in the midline, a tracheostomy, temporary or permanent, may be indicated to alleviate the obstructed airway [19].

RA reduces life expectancy by 3–7 years. Death is usually due to amyloidosis, vasculitis, GI bleeds from NSAIDs, infections from steroids.

35.7 Essential Features

- Rheumatoid arthritis (RA) is a chronic systemic inflammatory disorder affecting the synovial lining of joints, bursae, and tendon sheaths. May also affect the skin, blood vessels, heart, lungs, and muscles.
- Produces nonsuppurative proliferative synovitis, may progress to destruction of articular cartilage and joint ankylosis. In Head Neck region, particularly affects temporo-mandibular joint, cricoarytenoid joint; rarely cricothyroid joint, ossicular joints, and cervical spine.
- Triggered by exposure of the immunogenetically susceptible host to an arthritogenic microbial antigen
- Common symptoms are malaise, fatigue, musculoskeletal pain, then joint involvement; joints are warm, swollen, painful, stiff in the morning.
- Laryngeal involvement varies from cricoarytenoid joint fixation and neuropathy of the recurrent laryngeal nerve to myositis and presence of laryngeal nodules
- Diagnosis is aided by typical symptoms of morning stiffness, arthritis in more than one joint areas, arthritis in hand joints, rheumatoid nodules, positive rheumatoid factor, and typical radiographic changes (osteopenia, irregular erosions of articular surface, reduced joint space, and soft tissue swelling)
- HRCT is helpful in the diagnosis of RA of cricoarytenoid joint and ossicular joints.
- Histopathology of rheumatic nodule shows fibrinoid necrosis surrounded by palisading epithelioid macrophages. Rheumatic nodules in the larynx (vocal folds) give characteristic bamboo nodes appearance.
- Serum Anti-citrullinated protein antibodies (ACPAs measured as anti-CCP antibodies) are positive in 75–85% cases of RA.
- Nonsteroidal anti-inflammatory drugs (NSAIDs); Disease-modifying antirheumatic drugs (DMARDs)—Leflunomide, Methotrexate, Sulfasalazine, Minocycline, and Hydroxychloroquine are particularly helpful. Life-long treatment is required. Immunosuppressants and TNF-alpha inhibitors are given in severe cases.
- Microlaryngoscopic excision of bamboo nodes, thyroplasty for cricoarytenoid joint fixation, Ossiculoplasty in middle ear involvement. Arthroplasty, synovectomy, or arthrodesis may be necessary.
- Physiotherapy, occupational therapy, counseling also play important roles.

References

1. Landre-Beauvais AJ. La goutte asthénique primitive (doctoral thesis). Paris. Reproduced in Landré-Beauvais AJ (March 2001). "The first description of rheumatoid arthritis. Unabridged text of the doctoral dissertation presented in 1800". Joint Bone Spine. 1800;68(2):130–43.
2. Paget SA, et al. The hospital for special surgery rheumatoid arthritis handbook everything you need to know. New York: Wiley; 2002. p. 32. ISBN 9780471223344.
3. Alamanos Y, et al. Incidence and prevalence of rheumatoid arthritis, based on the 1987 American College of Rheumatology criteria: a systematic review. Semin Arthrit Rheumat. 2006;36(3):182–8.
4. Shah A. Harrison's principles of internal medicine. 18th ed. United States: McGraw Hill; 2012. p. 2738. ISBN 978-0-07174889-6.
5. Hua C, et al. Diagnosis, prognosis and classification of early arthritis: results of a systematic review informing the 2016 update of the EULAR recommendations for the management of early arthritis. RMD Open. 2017;3(1):e000406.
6. Boldt AB, et al. Relevance of the lectin pathway of complement in rheumatic diseases. Adv Clin Chem. 2012;56:105–53.
7. Mikkelson WM, et al. Unusual manifestation of rheumatoid nodules; report of three cases. J Michigan State Med Soc. 1955;54(3):292–7.
8. Grossman A, et al. Rheumatoid arthritis of the cricoarytenoid joint. Proc Canadian Otolaryngological Soc. 1960;140:40–54.
9. Takahashi Y, et al. Human parvovirus B19 as a causative agent for rheumatoid arthritis. Proc Natl Acad Sci U S A. 1998;95(14):8227–32.
10. Murano E, et al. Bamboo node: primary vocal fold lesion as evidence of autoimmune disease. J Voice. 2001;15(3):441–50.
11. Hamdan AL, Sarieddine D. Laryngeal manifestations of rheumatoid arthritis. Autoimmune Dis. 2013;2013:103081. https://doi.org/10.1155/2013/103081. Published online 2013 Jun 25.

12. Arnett FC, et al. The American Rheumatism Association 1987 revised criteria for the classification of rheumatoid arthritis. Arthrit Rheumat. 1988;31(3):315–24.
13. Kalugina Y, et al. Fine-needle aspiration of rheumatoid nodule: a case report with review of diagnostic features and difficulties. Diagn Cytopathol. 2003;28(6):322–4.
14. Ruparelia PB, et al. Bilateral TMJ involvement in rheumatoid arthritis. Case Rep Dent. 2014;2014:Article ID 262430, 5 pages. https://doi.org/10.1155/2014/262430.
15. Ozcan I, et al. Temporomandibular joint involvement in rheumatoid arthritis: correlation of clinical, laboratory and magnetic resonance imaging findings. B-ENT. 2008;4(1):19–24.
16. Gomez-Rivera F, et al. Rheumatoid arthritis mimicking metastatic squamous cell carcinoma. Head Neck Oncol. 2011;3:26. https://doi.org/10.1186/1758-3284-3-26. Published online 2011 May 14.
17. Upile T. Rheumatoid nodule of the thyrohyoid membrane: a case report. J Med Case Rep. 2007;1:123. https://doi.org/10.1186/1752-1947-1-123. Published online 2007 Oct 31.
18. Takase-Minegishi K, et al. Diagnostic test accuracy of ultrasound for synovitis in rheumatoid arthritis: systematic review and meta-analysis. Rheumatology. 2018;57(1):49–58.
19. Westwood OM, et al. Rheumatoid factors: what's new? Rheumatology. 2006;45(4):379–85.
20. Wasserman AM. Diagnosis and management of rheumatoid arthritis. Am Fam Physician. 2011;84(11):1245–52.

Lightning Source UK Ltd.
Milton Keynes UK
UKHW051032150922
408905UK00003B/28

9 789811 640490